CONTRIBUTORS

Richard Hector Bensimon, MD
Medical Director
Plastic Surgery
Bensimon Center,
Portland, OR, USA

Claudia Borelli, MD
Associate Professor of Dermatology
Director, Aesthetic Dermatology and Laser Unit
    Department of Dermatology Eberhard-Karls-
    University Tuebingen
President of German Aesthetic Dermatology and
    Cosmetology Working group ADK Past President
    International Peeling Society IPS
Tuebingen, Germany

**Desmer Destang, DDS, MSc (Ortho), MSc (Derm),
MSc (Aesth Med)**
Medical Director, Dermalogics Aesthetic Dermatology,
    St. Lucia
Lecturer in Cosmetic Medicine, University of South
    Wales, Cardiff, UK

Luc Dewandre, MD
Consultant, Internal Medical Service, Paris, France
Consultant in Aesthetic Medicine, Vitality Institute,
    Miami, FL, USA

Sabrina Fischer, MD
Associate Professor of Dermatology
Aesthetic Dermatology and Laser Unit Department of
    Dermatology Eberhard-Karls-University
    Tuebingen
Tuebingen, Germany

Marina Landau, MD
Senior Dermatologist
Dermatology
Wolfson Medical Center,
Holon, Israel

Joe Niamtu III, DMD
Private Practice
Cosmetic Facial Surgery
Richmond, VA, USA

Suzan Obagi, MD
Associate Professor of Dermatology,
Associate Professor of Plastic Surgery,
Director
UPMC Cosmetic Surgery & Skin Health Center,
Sewickley, PA, USA

Jeave Reserva, MD
Dermatology Resident
Division of Dermatology
Loyola University Medical Center,
Maywood, IL, USA

Barry Resnik, MD
Private Practice
Resnik Skin Institute Miami
Voluntary Clinical Professor
Dr Phillip Frost Department of Dermatology and
    Cutaneous Surgery
University of Miami Miller School of Medicine,
Miami, FL, USA

Peter Rullan, MD
Medical Director
Dermatology Institute
Volunteer Clinical Faculty
University of California San Diego,
San Diego, CA, USA

Jaishree Sharad, MBBS, DDV, MD
Cosmetic Dermatologist
Medical Director
Skinfiniti Aesthetic Skin and Laser Clinic,
Mumbai, India

David Surprenant, MD
Dermatology Resident
Division of Dermatology
Loyola University Medical Center,
Maywood, IL, USA

Alain Tenenbaum, MD, PhD, DSc
Swiss National Delegate
EAFPS,
Lübeck, Germany, President
SACDAM,
Engelberg, Switzerland, Vice President
IPSC,
Alpnach Dorf, Switzerland, Researcher
Research and Development
Styling Cosmetics AG,
Engelberg, Switzerland

Yardy Tse, MD
Assistant Clinical Professor,
Department of Medicine/Dermatology,
University of California, San Diego; SkinCare
Physicians and Surgeons Inc., Encinitas, CA, USA

Rebecca Tung, MD
Mohs and Dermatologic Surgeon
Florida Dermatology and Skin Cancer Centers,
Winter Haven, FL, USA

Carlos G. Wambier, MD, PhD
Assistant Professor of Dermatology, Clinician Educator
Department of Dermatology, The Warren Alpert Medical
    School of Brown University
Providence, RI, USA

Carolyn Willis, MD
Dermatology
University of Pittsburgh Medical Center,
Sewickley, PA, USA

SERIES PREFACE, FIRST EDITION

While dermatologists have been procedurally inclined since the beginning of the specialty, particularly rapid change has occurred in the past quarter century. The advent of frozen section technique and the golden age of Mohs skin cancer surgery has led to the formal incorporation of surgery within the dermatology curriculum. More recently, technological breakthroughs in minimally invasive procedural dermatology have offered an aging population new options for improving the appearance of damaged skin.

Procedures for rejuvenating the skin and adjacent regions are actively sought by our patients. Significantly, dermatologists have pioneered devices, technologies, and medications that have continued to evolve at a startling pace. Numerous major advances, including virtually all cutaneous lasers and light-source based procedures, botulinum exotoxin, soft tissue augmentation, dilute anesthesia liposuction, leg vein treatments, chemical peels, and hair transplants, have been invented or developed and enhanced by dermatologists. Dermatologists understand procedures, and we have special insight into the structure, function, and workings of skin. Cosmetic dermatologists have made rejuvenation accessible to risk-averse patients by emphasizing safety and reducing operative trauma. No specialty is better positioned than dermatology to lead the field of cutaneous surgery while meeting patient needs.

As dermatology grows as a specialty, an ever-increasing proportion of dermatologists will become proficient in the delivery of different procedures. Not all dermatologists will perform all procedures, and some will perform very few, but even the less procedurally directed among us must be well-versed in the details to be able to guide and educate our patients. Whether you are a skilled dermatologic surgeon interested in further expanding your surgical repertoire, a complete surgical novice wishing to learn a few simple procedures, or somewhere in between, this book and this series are for you.

The volume you are holding is one of a series entitled *Procedures in Cosmetic Dermatology*. The purpose of each book is to serve as a practical primer on a major topic area in procedural dermatology.

If you want to make sure you find the right book for your needs, you may wish to know what this book is and what it is not. It is not a comprehensive text grounded in theoretical underpinnings. It is not exhaustively referenced. It is not designed to be a completely unbiased review of the world's literature on the subject. At the same time, it is not an overview of cosmetic procedures that describes these in generalities without providing enough specific information to actually permit someone to perform the procedures. And importantly, it is not so heavy that it can serve as a doorstop or shelf filler.

What this book and this series offer is a step-by-step, practical guide to performing cutaneous surgical procedures. Each volume in the series has been edited by a known authority in that subfield. Each editor has recruited other equally practical-minded, technically skilled, hands-on clinicians to write the constituent chapters. Most chapters have two authors to ensure that different approaches and a broad range of opinions are incorporated. On the other hand, the two authors and the editors also collectively provide a consistency of tone. A uniform template has been used within each chapter so that the reader will be easily able to navigate all the books in the series. Within every chapter the authors succinctly tell it like they do it. The emphasis is on therapeutic technique; treatment methods are discussed with an eye to appropriate indications, adverse events, and unusual cases. Finally, this book is short and can be read in its entirety on a long plane ride. We believe that brevity paradoxically results in greater information transfer because cover-to-cover mastery is practicable.

Most of the books in the series are accompanied by videos that demonstrate the procedures discussed in that text. Some of you will turn immediately to the video and use the text as a backup to clarify complex points, whereas others will prefer to read first and then view the video to see the steps in action. Choose what suits you best.

We hope you enjoy this book and the rest of the books in the series and that you benefit from the many hours of clinical wisdom that have been distilled to produce it. Please keep it nearby where you can reach for it when you need it.

Jeffrey S. Dover, MD, FRCPC,
Murad Alam, MD, MSCI

SERIES PREFACE, THIRD EDITION

As this *Procedures in Cosmetic Dermatology* series undergoes another iteration, it is clear our mission that was initiated 15 years ago to provide succinct and current expert guidance regarding particular cosmetic procedures remains highly relevant. Our portable, travel-ready format continues to match the ever-shortening attention span of the overwhelmed physician. Indeed, similar series of slim volumes have emerged in this and other procedural specialties—versions of the sincerest form of flattery.

Even so, changes need to be made. As the evolution and exponential growth of cosmetic dermatology continues, new procedures are created, and multiple variants of existing drugs, devices, and techniques emerge. The volumes in the series have been updated to reflect these advances so that the books are now better but remain concise and highly practical.

We are also cognizant of the decline of paper publishing. To preserve the environment and provide content everywhere, all the time, and on all types of media, the series will be available in whole and chapter-by-chapter in various electronic formats and on several platforms. We have expanded the video offerings because they are worth many pages of text and are easier to follow.

As always, we are very grateful to our chapter book editors and authors. These practitioners are among the most prominent, bright, erudite, and skilled in the world. They have worked tirelessly to provide a uniform tone and structure. It is our hope that you find that these multiauthored books read like a single person wrote them, whose writing is a paragon of clarity.

Our thanks are also due to Elsevier, our publisher since the start. Elsevier has provided our rapid publishing window, which allows content to be put out and disseminated before it goes out of date.

Finally, thanks to you, the reader, for continuing to use these texts. We wish you the joy of learning something new and then delighting your patients with your freshly honed skills.

Jeffrey S. Dover, MD, FRCPC
Murad Alam, MD, MSCI

CHEMICAL PEELS, THIRD EDITION

It is with much excitement that I bring to you the third edition of *Chemical Peels*! This latest textbook on peels will take your knowledge to the next level, building on what was covered in previous editions. Chemical peels will be covered by experts recognized worldwide for their innovation, talent, and skills. This international group of thought leaders will cover the entire approach to the skin resurfacing patient from evaluation, to skin preparation, to performing peels ranging from light peels to the advanced deep peels, and finally to recognizing and managing complications. The new edition features many new chapters dedicated to an in-depth dive into a specific peel or skin condition. These new chapters include trichloroacetic acid (TCA) peels of the chest, neck, and upper extremities; peels as an adjuvant treatment of acne; chemical peels in male patients; several chapters on unique approaches to acne scars; a chapter on combining peels with surgical procedures; and several chapters that illustrate safely performing deeper, modified phenol peels with wonderful photographs to accompany the text. Videos of various procedures will allow easy incorporation of chemical peeling techniques into your practice.

Once again, chemical peels have shown themselves to be time-proven methods with unparalleled flexibility in their performance. Chemical peels have resurged in popularity as courses and didactic sessions are once again being offered to physicians. With a growing, ethnically diverse population, we need a tool such as chemical peels to allow us to treat every patient with any skin type that comes to us seeking cosmetic enhancement.

I am truly humbled and grateful to work with colleagues from all over the world on this edition, and I thank them for their hard work in bringing to you an exceptional textbook. I want to also recognize and give special thanks to Meghan Andress at Elsevier for the patience and guidance she offered all the authors. Furthermore, our series editors, Murad Alam, MD, and Jeffrey Dover, MD, deserve special recognition for their tireless efforts in creating a series of textbooks focused on cosmetic dermatology procedures and for their guidance when the content of this book was being developed.

Lastly, to my family, thank you, thank you, thank you! It was a busy year to say the least, but knowing I had your support made it all worthwhile! I survived many weekends and evenings of writing and editing but made sure to get to all the important family celebrations and school achievements. It was worth the effort!

I hope, as you read through this textbook, your interest in peels is kindled and your desire to hone your skills in this field is heightened. I am sure I speak on behalf of all my coauthors when I say, once a "peeler" always a "peeler." Hopefully you will join us as a fellow "peeler"!

Sincerely,

Suzan Obagi, MD

CONTENTS

LIST OF VIDEOS

1

The Chemistry of Peels: A Hypothesis of Mechanism of Action and Classification of Peels

Luc Dewandre, Alain Tenenbaum, Desmer Destang

A chemical peel is a treatment technique used to improve and smooth the facial and/or body skin's texture using a chemical solution that causes the dead skin to slough off and eventually peel off. The regenerated skin is usually smoother, healthier, and less wrinkled than the old skin.

It is advised to seek training with a specialist such as a dermatologist, plastic surgeon, otorhinolaryngologist (facial plastic surgeon), or oral-maxillofacial surgeon who is experienced in the specific types of peels you wish to perform.

INTRODUCTION

This chapter proposes a classification of chemical peels based on the mechanism of action of chemical peel solutions. The traditionally accepted mechanism has been based on the concept that the effect of a peeling solution on the skin is based purely on its acidity. By using elementary concepts in chemistry, three separate mechanisms of action for chemical peeling solutions are explained:

1. Acidity
2. Toxicity
3. Metabolic interactions

The literature devoted to chemical peels is full of information about the methodology, indications, contraindications, side effects, and results obtained. Without any proof, acidity has always been assumed to be the sole mechanism of action of peeling agents. All peeling agents were assumed to induce the three stages of tissue

replacement: destruction, elimination, and regeneration, all accompanied by a controlled stage of inflammation.

A brief study of the chemistry of the molecules and solutions used in chemical peels immediately questions the hypothesis that acidity is the only basis for the action of peeling solutions. In fact, with the exception of trichloroacetic acid (TCA) and nonneutralized glycolic acid solutions, the most commonly used peeling solutions are only weakly acidic, and phenol and resorcinol mixtures may not be acidic at all, having a pH greater than 7 in some formulations.

This chapter will discuss the elementary chemistry concepts that, along with a review of the chemistry of the skin, should help explain the possible interactions between different peeling solutions and the skin. Finally, two classifications of solutions for peelings will be proposed, one according to their mechanisms of action (classification of L. Dewandre) and the other according to chemical parameters (structure of the molecule, pK_a, etc; or classification of A. Tenenbaum).

USEFUL ELEMENTS OF BASIC CHEMISTRY

Understanding some of the basic concepts of chemistry is necessary to truly understand chemical peels. Mineral and organic chemistry are taught as biochemistry to medical students, but most practicing physicians do not remember these fundamental principles.

Also chemistry has been unfortunately neglected in cosmetic dermatology and aesthetic medicine courses, masters workshops, and congresses. A brief review of useful information should help update most practitioners.

Acids

An acid (from the Latin *acidus,* meaning "sour") is traditionally considered any chemical compound that, when dissolved in water, gives a solution with a hydrogen ion activity greater than in pure water, i.e., a pH less than 7.0. That approximates the modern definition of Johannes Nicolaus Brønsted and Martin Lowry, who independently defined an acid as a compound that donates a hydrogen ion (H^+) to another compound (called a *base*). Acid–base systems are different from redox reactions in that there is no change in oxidation state. Acids can occur in solid, liquid, or gaseous form, depending on the temperature. They can exist as pure substances or in solution. Chemicals or substances having the property of an acid are said to be acidic (adjective).

Arrhenius Acids

The Arrhenius concept is the easiest one retained by most peelers, because most peeling acids are ionic compounds, acting as a source of H_3O^+ when dissolved in water.

The Swedish chemist Svante Arrhenius attributed the properties of acidity to hydrogen in 1884. An Arrhenius acid is a substance that increases the concentration of the hydronium ion, H_3O^+, when dissolved in water. This definition stems from the equilibrium dissociation of water into hydronium and hydroxide (OH^-) ions:

$$H_2O(l) + H_2O(l) \rightleftharpoons H_3O^+(aq) + OH^-(aq)$$

In pure water most molecules exist as H_2O, but a small number of molecules are constantly dissociating and reassociating. Pure water is neutral with respect to acidity or basicity, because the concentration of hydroxide ions is always equal to the concentration of hydronium ions. An Arrhenius base is a molecule that increases the concentration of the hydroxide ion when dissolved in water. Note that chemists often write $H^+(aq)$ and refer to the hydrogen ion when describing acid–base reactions, but the free hydrogen nucleus, a proton, does not exist alone in water; it exists as the hydronium ion, H_3O^+.

Brønsted Acids

Although the Arrhenius concept is useful for describing many reactions, it is also quite limited in its scope. Brønsted acids act by donating a proton to water and,

differently than Arrhenius acids, can also be used to describe molecular compounds, whereas Arrhenius acids must be ionic compounds.

In 1923 chemists Johannes Nicolaus Brønsted and Thomas Martin Lowry independently recognized that acid–base reactions involve the transfer of a proton. A Brønsted–Lowry acid (or simply Brønsted acid) is a species that donates a proton to a Brønsted–Lowry base. Brønsted–Lowry acid-base theory has several advantages over Arrhenius theory. Consider the following reactions of acetic acid (CH_3COOH) (used as a chemical peel for the décolleté by some great peelers like L. Wiest), the organic acid that gives vinegar its characteristic taste:

Both theories easily describe the first reaction: CH_3COOH acts as an Arrhenius acid because it acts as a source of H_3O^+ when dissolved in water, and it acts as a Brønsted acid by donating a proton to water. In the second example CH_3COOH undergoes the same transformation, donating a proton to ammonia (NH_3), but it cannot be described using the Arrhenius definition of an acid because the reaction does not produce hydronium.

As with the acetic acid reactions, both definitions work for the first example, where water is the solvent and a hydronium ion is formed. The next reaction does not involve the formation of ions but can still be viewed as a proton transfer reaction.

Lewis Acids

The Brønsted–Lowry definition is the most widely used definition; unless otherwise specified, acid–base reactions are assumed to involve the transfer of a proton (H^+) from an acid to a base.

A third concept was proposed by Gilbert N. Lewis that includes reactions with acid–base characteristics that do not involve a proton transfer. A Lewis acid is a species that accepts a pair of electrons from another species; in other words, it is an electron pair acceptor. Brønsted acid–base reactions are proton transfer reactions, whereas Lewis acid–base reactions are electron pair transfers. All Brønsted acids are also Lewis acids, but not all Lewis acids are Brønsted acids. Contrast the following reactions, which could be described in terms of acid–base chemistry:

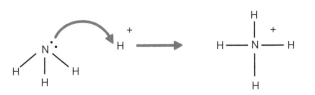

In the first reaction a fluoride ion, F^-, gives up an electron pair to boron trifluoride to form the product tetrafluoroborate. Fluoride "loses" a pair of valence electrons because the electrons shared in the B–F bond are located in the region of space between the two atomic nuclei and are therefore more distant from the fluoride nucleus than they are in the lone fluoride ion. BF3 is a Lewis acid because it accepts the electron pair from fluoride. This reaction cannot be described in terms of Brønsted theory, because there is no proton transfer. The second reaction can be described using either theory. A proton is transferred from an unspecified Brønsted acid to ammonia, a Brønsted base; alternatively, ammonia acts as a Lewis base and transfers a lone pair of electrons to form a bond with a hydrogen ion. The species that gains the electron pair is the Lewis acid; for example, the oxygen atom in H_3O^+ gains a pair of electrons when one of the H–O bonds is broken and the electrons shared in the bond become localized on oxygen. Depending on the context, Lewis acids may also be described as a reducing agent or an electrophile.

Dissociation and Equilibrium

Reactions of acids are often generalized in the form $HA \rightleftharpoons H^+ + A^-$, where HA represents the acid and A^- is the conjugate base. Acid–base conjugate pairs differ by one proton and can be interconverted by the addition or removal of a proton (protonation and deprotonation,

respectively). Note that the acid can be the charged species and the conjugate base can be neutral, in which case the generalized reaction scheme could be written as $HA \rightleftharpoons H^+ + A$. In solution there exists an equilibrium between the acid and its conjugate base. The equilibrium constant K is an expression of the equilibrium concentrations of the molecules or the ions in solution. Brackets indicate concentration, such that $[H_2O]$ means the concentration of H_2O. The acid dissociation constant K_a is generally used in the context of acid–base reactions. The numerical value of K_a is equal to the concentration of the products divided by the concentration of the reactants, where the reactant is the acid (HA) and the products are the conjugate base and H^+.

$$K_a = \frac{[H^+][A^-]}{[HA]}$$

The stronger of two acids will have a higher K_a than the weaker acid; the ratio of hydrogen ions to acid will be higher for the stronger acid because the stronger acid has a greater tendency to lose its proton. Because the range of possible values for K_a spans many orders of magnitude, a more manageable constant, pK_a, is more frequently used, where $pK_a = -\log_{10}K_a$. Stronger acids have a smaller pK_a than weaker acids. Experimentally determined pK_a at 25°C in aqueous solution are often quoted in textbooks and reference material.

Acid Strength

For peelers, the notion of acid strength is very important, because stronger acids have a higher K_a and a lower pK_a than weaker acids.

For our classification, two parameters have to be taken into consideration for peelers:
1. The pK_a, a synonym of the acid's strength.
2. The pH, a synonym of the penetration for the selected acid.

For chemists, the strength of an acid refers to its ability or tendency to lose a proton. A strong acid is one that completely dissociates in water; in other words, one mole of a strong acid, HA, dissolves in water, yielding one mole of H^+ and one mole of the conjugate base, A^-, and none of the protonated acid HA. In contrast a weak acid only partially dissociates, and at equilibrium both the acid and the conjugate base are in solution. In water each of these essentially ionizes 100%. The stronger an acid is, the more easily it loses a proton, H^+. Two key factors that contribute to the ease of deprotonation are the polarity of the H–A bond and the size of atom A, which determines the strength of the H–A bond. Acid strengths are also often discussed in terms of the stability of the conjugate base.

Caution is advised against simply classifying "cosmetic peels" for acids with $pK_a > 3$ and "medical peels" for acids with $pK_a < 3$, because some acids like phenol can be toxic substances even with a $pK_a > 3$.

Polarity and the Inductive Effect

The polarity of the H–A bond is the first factor contributing to acid strength.

As the electron density on hydrogen decreases, it becomes more acidic. Moving from left to right across a row on the periodic table, elements become more electronegative (excluding the noble gases).

In several compound classes, collectively called *carbon acids,* the C–H bond can be sufficiently acidic for proton removal. Inactivated C–H bonds are found in alkanes and are not adjacent to a heteroatom (O, N, Si, etc.). Such bonds usually only participate in radical substitution.

Polarity refers to the distribution of electrons in a bond, the region of space between two atomic nuclei where a pair of electrons is shared. When two atoms have roughly the same electronegativity (ability to attract electrons), the electrons are shared evenly and spend equal time on either end of the bond. When there is a significant difference in electronegativities of two bonded atoms, the electrons spend more time near the nucleus of the more electronegative element and an electrical dipole, or separation of charges, occurs, such that there is a partial negative charge localized on the electronegative element and a partial positive charge on the electropositive element. Hydrogen is an electropositive element and accumulates a slightly positive charge when it is bonded to an electronegative element such as oxygen or chlorine.

The electronegative element need not be directly bonded to the acidic hydrogen to increase its acidity. An electronegative atom can pull electron density out of an acidic bond through the inductive effect. The electron-withdrawing ability diminishes quickly as the electronegative atom moves away from the acidic bond.

Carboxylic acids are organic acids that contain an acidic hydroxyl group and a carbonyl (C–O bond).

Carboxylic acids can be reduced to the corresponding alcohol; the replacement of an electronegative oxygen atom with two electropositive hydrogens yields a product that is essentially nonacidic. The reduction of acetic acid to ethanol using $LiAlH_4$ (lithium aluminum hydride or LAH), and ether is an example of such a reaction.

The pK_a for ethanol is 16, compared with 4.76 for acetic acid.

Atomic Radius and Bond Strength

The size of the atom A or atomic radius is the second factor contributing to acid strength.

Moving down a column on the periodic table, atoms become less electronegative but also significantly larger, and the size of the atom tends to dominate its acidity when sharing a bond to hydrogen.

Hydrogen sulfide, H_2S, is a stronger acid than water, even though oxygen is more electronegative than sulfur. This is because sulfur is larger than oxygen and the H–S bond is more easily broken than the H–O bond.

Another factor that contributes to the ability of an acid to lose a proton is the strength of the bond between the acidic hydrogen and the atom that bears it. This, in turn, is dependent on the size of the atoms sharing the bond. For an acid HA, as the size of atom A increases, the strength of the bond decreases, meaning that it is more easily broken, and the strength of the acid increases.

Chemical Characteristics

It is important to keep in mind the difference between monoprotic acids (having one unique pK_a) and polyprotic acids (having two or more pK_a).

Monoprotic Acids

Monoprotic acids are those acids that are able to donate one proton per molecule during the process of dissociation (sometimes called *ionization*), as shown below (symbolized by HA):

$$HA(aq) + H_2O(1) \rightleftharpoons H_3O^+(aq) + A^-(aq)\ Ka$$

Common examples of monoprotic acids in organic acids indicate the presence of one carboxyl group, and mostly these acids are known as monocarboxylic acid. Examples in organic acids include acetic acid (CH_3COOH), glycolic acid, and lactic acid.

Lactic acid

Polyprotic Acids

Polyprotic acids are able to donate more than one proton per acid molecule, in contrast to monoprotic acids that only donate one proton per molecule. Specific types of polyprotic acids have more specific names, such as diprotic acid (two potential protons to donate) and triprotic acid (three potential protons to donate).

A diprotic acid (here symbolized by H_2A) can undergo one or two dissociations depending on the pH. Each dissociation has its own dissociation constant, K_{a1} and K_{a2}.

$$H_2A\,(aq) + H_2O\,(1) \rightleftharpoons H^3O^+(aq) + HA^-\,(aq)\ K_{a1}$$
$$HA^-\,(aq) + H^2O(1) \rightleftharpoons H_3O^+(aq) + A^{2-}(aq)\ K_{a2}$$

The first dissociation constant is typically greater than the second; i.e., $K_{a1} > K_{a2}$. For example, the weak unstable carbonic acid (H_2CO_3) can lose one proton to form bicarbonate anion (HCO_3^-) and lose a second to form carbonate anion (CO_3^{2-}). Both K_a values are small, but $K_{a1} > K_{a2}$.

Diprotic acids used for peelings are malic, tartaric, and azelaic acids.

Two dissociations mean that such acids can generate two peelings, depending on the pH, with the second one less acidic than the first one. In this case, we consider one peeling reaction per one dissociation.

A triprotic acid (H_3A) can undergo one, two, or three dissociations and has three dissociation constants, where $K_{a1} > K_{a2} > K_{a3}$.

$$H_3A\,(aq) + H_2O\,(1) \rightleftharpoons H_3O^+(aq) + H_2A^-\,(aq)\ K_{a1}$$

$$_2A\,(aq)\quad H_2O(1)\quad H_3O\,(aq)\quad HA\,(aq)\ K_{a2}$$

$$HA^{2-}(aq) + H_2O(1) \rightleftharpoons H_3O^+\,(aq) + A^{3-}(aq)\ K_{a3}$$

An organic example of a triprotic acid is citric acid, which can successively lose three protons to finally form the citrate ion. Even though the positions of the protons on the original molecule may be equivalent, the successive K_a values will differ, because it is energetically less favorable to lose a proton if the conjugate base is more negatively charged.

Weak Acid–Weak Base Equilibria

To lose a proton, it is necessary that the pH of the system rise above the pK_a of the protonated acid. The decreased concentration of H^+ in that basic solution shifts the equilibrium toward the conjugate base form (the deprotonated form of the acid). In lower-pH (more acidic) solutions, there is a high enough H^+ concentration in the solution to cause the acid to remain in its protonated form, or to protonate its conjugate base (the deprotonated form).

Solutions of weak acids and salts of their conjugate bases form buffer solutions.

Buffer Solution

A buffer solution is an aqueous solution consisting of a mixture of a weak acid and its conjugate base or a weak base and its conjugate acid. The property of buffer solutions is that the pH of the solution changes very little when a small amount of acid or base is added to it. Buffer solutions are used as a means of keeping pH at a nearly constant value in a wide variety of chemical applications. Many life forms thrive only in a relatively small pH range; an example of a buffer solution is blood.

Le Chatelier's Principle

In a solution there is an equilibrium between a weak acid, HA, and its conjugate base, A^-:

$$HA + H_2O \rightleftharpoons H_3O^+ + A^-$$

- When hydrogen ions (H^+) are added to the solution, equilibrium moves to the left, as there are hydrogen ions (H^+ or H_3O^+) on the right-hand side of the equilibrium expression.
- When hydroxide ions (OH^-) are added to the solution, equilibrium moves to the right, as hydrogen ions are removed in the reaction ($H^+ + OH^- \rightarrow H_2O$).

Thus, in both cases, some of the added reagent is consumed in shifting the equilibrium in accordance with Le Chatelier's principle, and the pH changes by less than it would if the solution were not buffered.

Henderson–Hasselbach Equation

The acid dissociation constant for a weak acid, HA, is defined as:

$$K_a = \frac{[H^+][A^-]}{[HA]}$$

Simple manipulation with logarithms gives the Henderson–Hasselbach equation, which describes pH in terms of pK_a:

$$pH = pK_a + \log_{10}\left(\frac{[A^-]}{[HA]}\right)$$

In this equation $[A^-]$ is the concentration of the conjugate base and $[HA]$ is the concentration of the acid. It follows that when the concentrations of acid and conjugate base are equal, often described as half-neutralization, pH = pK_a. In general, the pH of a buffer solution may be easily calculated, knowing the composition of the mixture, by means of an ICE table. An ICE (initial, change, equilibrium) table is a simple matrix formalism that used to simplify the calculations in reversible equilibrium reactions (e.g., weak acids and weak bases or complex ion formation).

One should remember that the *calculated* pH may be different from *measured* pH.

Buffer Capacity

Buffer capacity (Fig. 1.1) is a quantitative measure of the resistance of a buffer solution to pH change with the addition of hydroxide ions. It can be defined as follows:

$$Buffer\ capacity = \frac{dn}{d(pH)}$$

where dn is an infinitesimal amount of added base and d(pH) is the resulting infinitesimal change in pH. With this definition the buffer capacity can be expressed as:

$$\frac{dn}{d(pH)} = 2.303\left(\frac{K_W}{[H^+]} + [H^+] + \frac{C_A K_a [H^+]}{(K_a + [H^+])^2}\right)$$

where K_w is the self-ionization constant of water and CA is the analytical concentration of the acid, equal to $[HA] + [A^-]$. The term $K_w/[H^+]$ becomes significant at pH greater than about 11.5, and the second term becomes significant at pH less than about 2. Both these terms are properties of water and are independent of the weak acid. Considering the third term, it follows that:

1. Buffer capacity of a weak acid reaches its maximum value when pH = pK_a.
2. At pH = $pK_a \pm 1$ the buffer capacity falls to 33% of the maximum value. This is the approximate range within which buffering by a weak acid is effective. Note: at pH = $pK_a - 1$, the Henderson–Hasselbach equation shows that the ratio $[HA]:[A^-]$ is 10:1.
3. Buffer capacity is directly proportional to the analytical concentration of the acid.

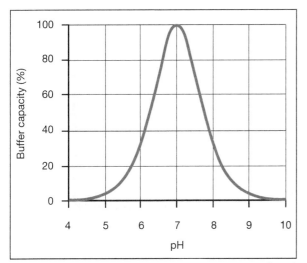

Fig. 1.1 Buffer capacity for pK_a = 7 as a percentage of maximum.

Current Applications of Buffer Solutions

Their resistance to changes in pH makes buffer solutions very useful for chemical manufacturing and essential for many biochemical processes. The ideal buffer for a particular pH has a pKa equal to that pH, since such a solution has maximum buffer capacity.

Buffer solutions are necessary to keep the correct physiological pH for enzymes in many organisms to work. A buffer of carbonic acid (H_2CO_3) and bicarbonate (HCO_3^-) is present in blood plasma, to maintain a pH between 7.35 and 7.45.

The majority of biological samples used in research are made in buffers, specifically phosphate-buffered saline (PBS) at pH 7.4.

Buffered TCA are more likely to create dyschromias.

Useful Buffer Mixtures

- Citric acid, sodium citrate, pH range 2.5 to 5.6.
- Acetic acid, sodium acetate, pH range 3.7 to 5.6.

Neutralization

There is among physicians a big confusion between a buffered peel (see above) and a neutralized peel. In chemistry, neutralization is a chemical reaction whereby an acid and a base react to form water and a salt.

In an aqueous solution, solvated hydrogen ions (hydronium ions, H_3O^+) react with hydroxide ions (OH^-) formed from the alkali to make two molecules of water. A salt is also formed. In nonaqueous reactions, water is not always formed; however, there is always a donation of protons (see Brønsted–Lowry acid–base theory).

Often, neutralization reactions are exothermic, giving out heat to the surroundings (the enthalpy of neutralization). On the other hand, an example of endothermic neutralization is the reaction between sodium bicarbonate (baking soda) and any weak acid—for example, acetic acid (vinegar).

Neutralization of the chemical peeling agent is an important step, the timing of which is determined by either the frost in the skin or how much contact time the peel has with the skin. Neutralization is achieved by a majority of peelers applying cold water or wet, cool towels to the face following the frost. According to physical chemistry, using water just after the frost provokes an exothermic reaction that can provoke a "cold" burn. Other neutralizing agents that can be used include bicarbonate spray or soapless cleansers. Peeling agents for which this neutralization step is less important include salicylic acid, Jessner's solution, TCA, and phenol.

In partially neutralized alpha-hydroxy acid (AHA) solutions, the acid and a lesser amount of base are combined in a reversible chemical reaction that yields unneutralized acid and a salt.

The resulting solution has less free acid and a higher pH than a solution that has not been neutralized. In partially neutralized formulations, the salt functions as a reservoir of acid that is available for second-phase penetration. This means that partially neutralized formulas can deliver as much, if not more, AHA than free acid formulas, but in a safer, "time-released" manner. Therefore the use of partially neutralized glycolic acid solutions seems prudent, because they have a better safety profile than low-pH solutions containing only free glycolic acid.

Clinical studies have shown that a partially neutralized lactic acid preparation improves the skin, both in appearance and histologically. Other studies using skin tissue cultures showed that partially neutralized glycolic acid stimulates fibroblast proliferation—an index of tissue regeneration. Looking at electrical conductance of the skin (an indicator of water content or moisturization), higher pH products (those that have been partially neutralized) are better moisturizers than lower pH preparations.

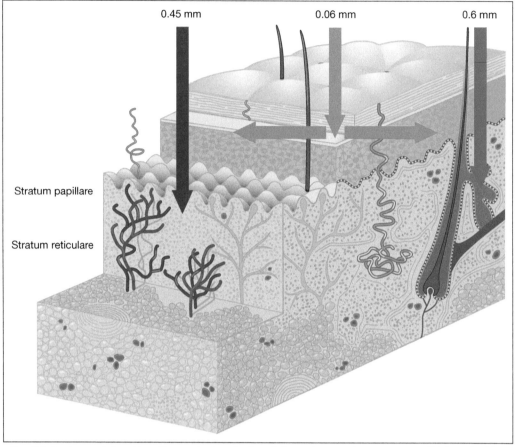

Fig. 1.2 Anatomy of the skin with penetration depths of the various peels: *green*, superficial peels; *blue*, medium-depth peels; and *red*, deep peels.

ANATOMY OF THE SKIN

Like the whole human organism, the skin can be considered an aqueous solution into which are dissolved a certain number of molecules (Fig. 1.2). These are molecules of proteins, lipids, and carbohydrates in variable quantities and proportions.

There is more water in the dermis than in the epidermis. This is due to the presence of blood, glycosaminoglycans (GAGs), and lymph in the dermis, all of which have a high water content, as well as the fact that the epidermis is in contact with a more or less dehydrated environment.

There are more proteins (keratin) in the epidermis than in the dermis, whereas more carbohydrates and lipids exist in the dermis, and there are even more in the subcutaneous layer than in the dermis.

The most important molecule in the epidermis is a fibrous and corneal protein, keratin, that protects and takes part, through its continuous production by the keratinocytes, in the complete replacement of the epidermis every 27 days.

The most important molecules of the dermis are collagen, elastin, GAGs, and the proteoglycans. Collagen and elastin are proteins, whereas GAGs (e.g., hyaluronic acid) and the proteoglycans are biological polymers formed mainly by sugars that retain water.

Collagen constitutes the skin's structural resource and is the most abundant protein in the human body. It is formed mainly by glycine, proline, and hydroxyproline. It is one of the most resistant natural proteins and helps give the skin structural support. Elastin is similar to collagen, but it is an extensible protein responsible for

In the figure:

0.45 mm   0.06 mm   0.6 mm

Stratum papillare

Stratum reticulare

elasticity; hence its name. It has two unique polypeptides, desmosine and isodesmosine.

The GAGs contain specific sugars such as glucosamine sulfate, *N*-acetylglucosamine, and glucosamine hydrochloride, all very capable of attracting water. They form long chains of molecules, such as hyaluronic acid, keratin sulfate, heparin, dermatin, and chondroitin, that retain up to 1000 times their weight in water.

The hypodermis or subcutaneous tissue consists mainly of fat, although this tissue accounts for a completely different chemical interaction with peeling solutions. Chemical peels are not meant to extend down into the subcutaneous layer, so this is not discussed.

The different molecular composition of the different levels of the skin may explain the variability of the interactions and the results obtained. These benefits are correlated to the penetration level achieved when using a given peeling agent.

It is likewise for the pH. Although the pH of the epidermis is a well-established number, the pH of the dermis is not an exact value and has been difficult to measure precisely.

The epidermal acid layer or mantle is the result of sebum secretion and sweat. It protects the skin and makes it less vulnerable from attacks by microorganisms such as bacteria and fungi. A healthy epidermis has a slightly acidic pH with a range between 4.2 and 5.6. It varies from one part of the skin to another and, in general, is more acidic in men than in women.

The pH of the epidermis also varies depending on its different layers. For a "skin" pH of around 5 we will find a pH near 5.6 in the corneal layer and one of 4.8 in the deep layers of the epidermis, which are rich in corneocytes and melanocytes. Finally, dry skin is more acidic than oily skin, which can reach pH 6.

Because the dermis contains a significant amount of fluid and blood, we can presume the pH to be 6 to 6.5, and it is slightly less acidic than the epidermis, with a pH of 6 for the papillary dermis and 7 for the vascular reticular dermis.

Skin Basic Chemistry

The approximate skin composition is seen in Box 1.1.

Acids and Cell Membranes

Cell membranes contain fatty acid esters such as phospholipids. Fatty acids and fatty acid derivatives

---

> ### BOX 1.1   Approximate Skin Composition
>
> Water 70%
>   Proteins 25.5%
>   Lipids 2.0%
>   Oligo mineral elements 0.5% (e.g., zinc, copper, selenium)
>   Carbon hydrates 2.0% (mucopolysaccharides)

---

are another group of carboxylic acids that play a significant role in biology. These contain long hydrocarbon chains and a carboxylic acid group on one end. The cell membrane of nearly all organisms is primarily made up of a phospholipid bilayer, a micelle of hydrophobic fatty acid esters with polar, hydrophilic phosphate "head" groups. Membranes contain additional components, some of which can participate in acid–base reactions. Cell membranes are generally impermeable to charged or large, polar molecules because of the lipophilic fatty acyl chains comprising their interior. Many biologically important molecules, including a number of pharmaceutical agents, are organic weak acids that can cross the membrane in their protonated, uncharged form but not in their charged form (i.e., as the conjugate base). The charged form, however, is often more soluble in blood and cytosol, both aqueous environments. When the extracellular environment is more acidic than the neutral pH within the cell, certain acids will exist in their neutral form and will be membrane soluble, allowing them to cross the phospholipid bilayer. Acids that lose a proton at the intracellular pH will exist in their soluble, charged form and are thus able to diffuse through the cytosol to their target.

BASIC CHEMISTRY OF THE MOST USED MOLECULES IN SOLUTIONS FOR CHEMICAL PEELINGS

It is interesting to consider the chemical nature of the molecules most commonly found in chemical peels. In the case of the alpha-hydroxy acids, the acid carboxyl group is on the first carbon (C1) and the hydroxyl is on the alpha carbon (C2). Salicylic acid is a beta-hydroxy acid with the hydroxyl group on C3.

How the Most Commonly Used Substances in Chemical Peel Solutions Work—A Hypothesis

Based on their different properties and the ways in which they work, L. Dewandre divides the substances most used for chemical peels into three categories: metabolic, caustic, and toxic (Table 1.1).

SUBSTANCES WITH MAINLY METABOLIC ACTIVITY

With the exception of glycolic and lactic acids, the metabolic substances described in the following sections are not used, properly speaking, in the solutions involved in chemical peels. Today, glycolic and lactic acids are nearly ubiquitous in medical cosmetology as a part of skin care regimens and in the office as chemical peel procedures.

Alpha Hydroxy Acids

The AHAs are a class of chemical compounds that consist of a carboxylic acid with a hydroxy group on the adjacent carbon. They may be either naturally occurring or synthetic. AHAs are well known for their use in the cosmetics industry. They are often found in products claiming to reduce wrinkles or the signs of aging and improve the overall look and feel of the skin. They are also used as chemical peels available in a dermatologist's office, beauty and health spas, and home kits, which usually contain a lower concentration. Although their effectiveness is documented, numerous cosmetic products have appeared on the market with unfounded claims of performance. Many well-known AHAs are useful building blocks in organic synthesis: the most common and simple are glycolic acid, lactic acid, citric acid, and mandelic acid.

AHA peels include aliphatic (lactic, glycolic, tartaric, and malic) and aromatic (mandelic) acids that are synthesized chemically for use in peels. Various concentrations can be purchased, with 10% to 70% concentration used for facial peels, most commonly 50% or 70%. AHAs are weak acids that induce their rejuvenation activity by either metabolic or caustic effect. At low concentration (<30%), they reduce sulfate and phosphate groups from the surface of corneocytes. By decreasing corneocyte cohesion, they induce exfoliation of the epidermis. At higher concentration, their effect is mainly destructive. Because of the low acidity of AHAs, they do not induce

enough coagulation of the skin proteins and therefore cannot neutralize themselves. They must be neutralized using a weak buffer.

Knowledge of the skin structure within the framework of cutaneous aging is helpful to understand the topical action of AHAs. Human skin has two principal components, the avascular epidermis and the underlying vascular dermis. Cutaneous aging, though it has epidermal involvement, seems to involve primarily the dermis and is caused by both intrinsic and extrinsic aging factors.

AHAs most commonly used in cosmetic applications are typically derived from fruit products including glycolic acid (sugar cane), lactic acid (sour milk), malic acid (apples), citric acid (citrus fruits) and tartaric acid (grapes and wine). For any topical compound, including AHA, it must penetrate into the skin, where it can act on living cells. Bioavailability (influenced primarily by small molecular size) is one characteristic that is important in determining the compound's ability to penetrate the top layer of the skin. Glycolic acid having the smallest molecular size is the AHA with greatest bioavailability and penetrates the skin most easily; this largely accounts for the popularity of this product in cosmetic applications.

- *Epidermal effects*: AHAs have a profound effect on keratinization, which is clinically detectable by the formation of a new stratum corneum. It appears that AHAs modulate this formation through diminished cellular cohesion between corneocytes at the lowest levels of the stratum corneum.
- *Dermal effects*: AHAs with greater bioavailability appear to have deeper dermal effects. Glycolic acid, lactic acid, and citric acid, on topical application to photodamaged skin, have been shown to produce increased amounts of mucopolysaccharides and collagen and increased skin thickness without detectable inflammation, as monitored by skin biopsies.

AHAs are generally safe when used on the skin as a cosmetic agent using the recommended dosage. The most common side effects are mild skin irritation, redness, and flaking. The severity usually depends on the pH and the concentration of the acid used.

The Food and Drug Administration (FDA) has also warned consumers that care should be taken when using AHAs after an industry-sponsored study found that they can increase photosensitivity to the sun.

TABLE 1.1	Classification of Chemical Peels (A. Tenenbaum)								
Acids Category	Acids Subcategory	pK_a >3 from Lower to Higher	pK_a = 3	pK_a <3	pK_{a1}	pK_{a2}	pK_{a3}	Classification of L. Dewandre	Number of Reactions
Alpha hydroxy	Aliphatic		Tartaric		3.04	4.37		Metabolic	Diprotic
		Citric			3.15	4.77	6.40	Metabolic	Triprotic
		Malic			3.40	5.13		Metabolic	Diprotic
		Glycolic			3.83			Metabolic	Monoprotic
		Lactic			3.86			Metabolic	Monoprotic
	Aromatic		Mandelic		3.37			Metabolic	Monoprotic
		TXA			4.3				Monoprotic
Alpha keto				Pyruvic	2.49			Not available	Monoprotic
Bicarboxylic		Azelaic			4.55	5.59		Metabolic	Diprotic
Beta Hydroxy			Salicylic		2.97			Toxic	Monoprotic
TCA				TCA	0.53			Caustic	Monoprotic
Phenol	Aromatic	Phenol			9.95			Toxic	Alcohol > acid

TCA, Trichloroacetic acid; TXA, tranexamic acid.

Comparison of the pH to the pK_a: The Interesting Cosmetic Actions of the Alpha-Hydroxy Acids

- *For a pH greater than the pK_a, the AHAs are essentially moisturizers.* The main differences between the moisturizing and caustic effects are related to the degree of neutralization of the AHA molecules. Neutralizing the AHA with sodium or ammonium creates a salt with more moisturizing and less caustic effect.
- *For a pH less than or equal to the pK_a, the AHAs are keratoregulators* that increase skin exfoliation and cell replacement. In such case, the acid form is preponderant, which is more absorbed and facilitates penetration.

Their antiaging action can be compared with retinoids, but their mechanism of action is different. They interfere with certain kinds of enzymes (sulfotransferases, phosphotransferases, kinases) whose function is to fix the sulfate and phosphate groups to the surface of the corneocytes. The reduction of these groups involves a decrease in electronegativity and corneocyte cohesion, which leads to a breaking away of the cells from each other, creating exfoliation and flaking. This activity can be characterized as a metabolic action. However, when used in strong concentrations of 30% to 70% free acid in aqueous solution for peeling, their effect is based on their acidity and results in destruction.

Aliphatic Alpha Hydroxy Acids (Glycolic, Lactic, Malic, Tartaric, Citric) With pK_a >3

Glycolic Acid (pK_a = 3.83) and Its Different Concentrations

Abbreviation: GA

Properties:
- Molecular formula: $C_2H_4O_3$
- Molar mass: 76.05 g/mol
- Appearance: white, powdery solid
- Density: 1.27 g/cm^3
- Solubility in water: 70% solution
- Solubility in other solvents: alcohols, acetone, acetic acid, and ethyl acetate
- Acidity (pK_a): 3.83

Glycolic acid (or hydroxyacetic acid) is the smallest AHA. This colorless, odorless, and hygroscopic crystalline solid is highly soluble in water. It is used in various skin care products.

Formulated from sugar cane, glycolic acid creates a mild exfoliating action. Glycolic acid peels work by loosening up the horny layer and exfoliating the superficial top layer. This peel also stimulates collagen growth.

Once applied, glycolic acid reacts with the upper layer of the epidermis, weakening the binding properties of the lipids that hold the dead skin cells together. This allows the outer skin to "dissolve," revealing the underlying skin.

In low concentrations, 5% to 10%, glycolic acid reduces cell adhesion in the top layer of the skin. This action promotes exfoliation of the outermost layer of the skin, accounting for smoother texture following regular use of topical glycolic acid. This relatively low concentration of glycolic acid lends itself to daily use as a monotherapy or a part of a broader skin care management for such conditions as acne, photo-damage, and wrinkling. Care needs to be taken to avoid irritation, as this may result in worsening of any pigmentary problems. Newer formulations combine glycolic acid with an amino acid such as arginine and form a time-release system that reduces the risk of irritation without affecting glycolic acid efficacy. The use of an anti-irritant like allantoin is also helpful. Because of its safety, glycolic acid at concentrations below 10% can be used daily by most people except those with very sensitive skin.

In medium concentrations, between 10% and 50%, its benefits are more pronounced but are limited to temporary skin smoothing without much long-lasting results. This is still a useful concentration to use because it can prepare the skin for more efficacious glycolic acid peels at higher concentrations (50%–70%) as well as to prime the skin for deeper chemical peels such as TCA peel.

At higher concentrations (called here *high concentrations*), 50% to 70% applied for 3 to 8 minutes (usually done by a physician), glycolic acid promotes disruption of the bonds between the keratinocytes and can be used to treat acne or photo damage (such as mottled dyspigmentation, or fine wrinkles). The benefits from such short contact application (chemical peels) depend on the pH of the solution (the more acidic the product, or lower pH, the more pronounced the results), the concentration of GA (higher concentrations produce more vigorous response), the length of application, and prior skin conditioning such as prior use of topical retinoids. Although single application of 50% to 70% GA will produce beneficial results, multiple treatments every 2 to 4 weeks are required for optimal results. It is important to understand that glycolic acid peels are chemical peels with similar risks and side effects as other peels.

Lactic Acid (pK_a = 3.86)

Lactic acid is derived from either sour milk or bilberries. This peel will remove dead skin cells and promote healthier, softer, and more radiant skin.

Properties:
- Molecular formula: $C_3H_6O_3$
- Molar mass: 90.08 g/mol
- Acidity (pK_a): 3.86 at 25°C

In our opinion, glycolic and lactic peel solutions must have a pH between 1.5 and 2.5 in order to combine a source of inflammation and stimulation, with their metabolic effects being, essentially, the turnover of epidermal cells.

Malic Acid (pK_{a1} = 3.4, pK_{a2} = 5.13)

This peel is the same type of mildly invasive peel derived from the extracts of apples. It can open up the pores, allow the pores to expel their sebum, and reduce acne.

Tartaric Acid (pK_{a1} = 3.04, pK_{a2} = 4.37)

This is derived from grape extract and is capable of delivering the same benefits as the above peels.

Citric Acid (pK_{a1} = 3.15, pK_{a2} = 4.77, pK_{a3} = 6.40)

Citric acid is usually derived from lemons, oranges, limes, and pineapples. These peels are simple and effective, though not incredibly invasive or capable of significant improvement with one treatment.

The citric acid is triprotic, having three pK_a values. It is quite interesting, because the first pK_a is lower than the pK_a of the monoprotic glycolic acid on one hand, and the three reactions are made of two peelings (pK_{a1} = 3.15, pK_{a2} = 4.77) that end with a buffer (third reaction) of a pK_{a3} = 6.40.

We can easily understand that citric acid used for peelings does not need any neutralization or a buffer.

Aromatic Alpha Hydroxy Acid with pK_a >3
Mandelic Acid: An Aromatic Alpha Hydroxy Acid (pK_a = 3.37)

Mandelic acid is an aromatic AHA with the molecular formula $C_8H_8O_3$. It is a white crystalline solid that is soluble in water and most common organic solvents.

Mandelic acid has a long history of use in the medical community as an antibacterial agent, particularly in the treatment of urinary tract infections. It has also been used as an oral antibiotic. Lately, mandelic acid has gained popularity as a topical skin care treatment for adult acne. It is also used as an alternative to glycolic acid in skin care products. Mandelic acid is a larger molecule than glycolic acid, which makes it better tolerated on the skin. Mandelic acid is also advantageous in that it possesses antibacterial properties, whereas glycolic acid does not.

Its use as a skin care modality was pioneered by James E. Fulton, who helped develop retinoic acid (tretinoin, Retin A) in 1969 with his mentor, Albert Kligman, at the University of Pennsylvania. On the basis of this research, dermatologists now suggest mandelic acid as an appropriate treatment for a wide variety of skin pathologies, from acne to wrinkles; it is especially good in the treatment of adult acne because it addresses both of these concerns. Mandelic acid is also recommended as a prelaser and postlaser resurfacing treatment, reducing the amount and length of irritation.

Mandelic acid peels are commercialized nowadays as gels with a specific viscosity, which make them user friendly for beginners.

Alpha Keto Acids With pK$_a$ <3
Pyruvic Acid: An Alpha Keto Acid (pK$_a$ = 2.49)

A solution of 40% to 50% pyruvic acid in ethanol is the most-used pyruvate in current practice.

Pyruvic acid is a ketone as well as the simplest alpha-keto acid. The carboxylate (COOH) ion (anion) of pyruvic acid, CH_3COCOO^-, is known as pyruvate and is a key intersection in several metabolic pathways.

It is often used to treat mild to moderate papulopustular acne with concentrations between 40% and 50% every 2 weeks for a total of 3 to 4 months. It reduces the sebum levels and does not affect the cutaneous hydration.

Bi Carboxylic Acid With pK$_a$ >3
Azelaic Acid (pK$_{a1}$ = 4.550, pK$_{a2}$ = 5.598)

Azelaic acid or 1,7-heptanedicarboxylic acid is a saturated dicarboxylic acid naturally found in wheat, barley, and rye. It is active in a concentration of 20% in topical products used in a number of skin conditions, mainly mild to moderate acne and papulopustular rosacea. It works in part by inhibiting the growth of skin bacteria that cause acne and by keeping skin pores clear.

It has some interesting properties:
- Antibacterial: It reduces the growth of bacteria in the follicle (*Propionibacterium acnes, Staphylococcus epidermis*)
- Keratolytic and comedolytic: It returns to normal the disordered growth of the skin cells, lining the follicle.
- Scavenger of free radicals and reduces inflammation
- Reduces pigmentation by acting as a weak tyrosinase inhibitor
- Nontoxic and is well tolerated by most patients

Azelaic acid does not result in bacterial resistance to antibiotics, reduction in sebum production, photosensitivity (easy sunburn), staining of skin or clothing, or bleaching of normal skin or clothing; however, 20% azelaic acid can be a skin irritant.

Azelaic acid is diprotic, having two pK$_a$ values. It is quite interesting, because its second pK$_a$ is almost equal to the pH of the skin (5.5).

We can easily understand that azelaic acid used for peelings may need to be neutralized but does not need any buffer.

In vitro, azelaic acid works as a scavenger (captor) of free radicals and inhibits a number of oxidoreductase enzymes, including 5-alpha reductase, the enzyme responsible of turning testosterone into dihydrotestosterone. It normalizes keratinization and leads to a reduction in the content of free oily acids in lipids on the skin surface.

Apart from that, azelaic acid has antiviral and antimitotic properties. Finally, it can also act as an antiproliferant and a cytotoxin via the blockage of mitochondrial respiration and DNA synthesis.

Beta Hydroxy Acid Peels With pK$_a$ Around 3

It is becoming common for beta hydroxy acid (BHA) peels to be used instead of the stronger AHA peels due to BHA's ability to get deeper into the pore than AHA. Studies show that BHA peels control oil and acne as well as remove dead skin cells to a certain extent better than AHAs because BHAs are more lipophilic than AHAs.

Salicylic acid (from the Latin Salix meaning: willow tree) is a biosynthesized, organic BHA that is often used. Sodium salicylate is converted by treating sodium phenolate (the sodium salt of phenol) with carbon dioxide at high pressure and temperature. Acidification of the product with sulfuric acid gives salicylic acid. Alternatively, it can be prepared by the hydrolysis of aspirin (acetylsalicylic acid) or oil of wintergreen (methyl salicylate) with a strong acid or base.

Salicylic Acid (pK$_a$ = 2.97)

The most commonly used peeling currently is 30% salicylic acid in ethanol.

Salicylic acid is lipid soluble (lipophilic); therefore it is a good peeling agent for comedonal acne. Salicylic acid is able to penetrate the comedones better than other acids. The antiinflammatory and anesthetic effects of the salicylate result in a decrease in the amount of erythema and discomfort that generally is associated with chemical peels.

Salicylic acid is a key ingredient in many skin care products for the treatment of acne, psoriasis, calluses, corns, keratosis pilaris, and warts. It works as both a keratolytic and comedolytic agent by causing the cells of the epidermis to shed more readily, opening clogged pores and killing bacteria within, preventing pores from clogging up again by constricting pore diameter, and stimulating new cell growth. Because of its effect on skin cells, salicylic acid is used in several shampoos to treat dandruff. Use of high concentrations of salicylic acid may cause hyperpigmentation in patients with unconditioned skin, those with darker skin types (Fitzpatrick phototypes IV, V, VI), and in patients who do not regularly use a broad-spectrum sunblock.

Also known as 2-hydroxybenzoic acid, it is a crystalline carboxylic acid and classified as a BHA. Salicylic acid is slightly soluble in water but very soluble in ethanol and ether (like phenol and resorcinol). It is made from sodium phenolate, and this explains its direct relationship with phenol, with which it shares certain toxic properties that become apparent when used in great quantity and on large surface areas.

Salicylic acid is found naturally in certain plants (*Spiraea ulmaria, Andromeda leschenaultii*), particularly fruits.

Jessner's Peel

Jessner's peel solution, formerly known as the Coombe's formula, was pioneered by Max Jessner, a dermatologist. Jessner combined 14% salicylic acid, 14% lactic acid, and 14% resorcinol in an ethanol base. Its main effect is to break intracellular bridges between keratinocytes, whereas the salicylic acid component also allows better penetration across sebum-rich skin. It is a stronger peel than 30% salicylic acid.

Retinoic Acid Peels

Retinoic acid or vitamin A acid is not soluble in water but is soluble in fat; therefore retinyl palmitate or vitamin A palmitate is the elected retinoic agent for chemical peels.

Retinyl palmitate, or vitamin A palmitate, is the ester of retinol and palmitic acid. Tretinoin is the acid form of vitamin A and so also known as all-*trans* retinoic acid (ATRA). It is a drug commonly used to treat acne vulgaris and keratosis pilaris. Tretinoin is the best-studied retinoid in the treatment of photoaging. It is used as a component of many commercial products that are advertised as being able to slow skin aging or improve wrinkles.

The terpene family, to which retinoic acid belongs, includes numerous compounds whose common feature is that they are formed by a chain of isoprene units $CH_2=C(CH_3)–CH=CH_2$. Terpenes have a raw formula type $(C_5H_x)_n$, x being dependent on the amount of unsaturation. Their names depend on n:
- $n = 2$ æ C10: monoterpenes
- $n = 3$ æ C15: sesquiterpenes
- $n = 4$ æ C20: diterpenes
- $n \approx 1000$: polyterpenes (rubber).

The main representative of the family of diterpenes is vitamin A or retinol. Retinol is present in food (beta carotene) and converts completely in the skin into retinaldehyde (retinal). Subsequently, 95% of this is converted into retinyl ester and 5% into all-trans and 9-cis retinoic acids.

Retinoids have multiple properties in embryogenesis, growth control and differentiation of adult tissues, reproduction, and sight. In dermatology their use is well established for psoriasis, hereditary disorders of keratinization, acne, and skin aging. The most commonly used retinoids are ATRA (tretinoin; used topically), 13-*cis* retinoic acid (isotretinoin; used both orally and topically), and retinaldehyde/retinal and retinol (both of which are used topically). In addition, there are the synthetic retinoids such as etretinate, acitretin, adapalene, and tazarotene.

Only the natural retinoids are of relevance in chemical peelings: retinol, ATRA, and retinoic acid, the last two of which are useful in strong concentrations as peeling agents used under medical supervision.

SUBSTANCE WITH MAINLY CAUSTIC ACTIVITY

Trichloroacetic Acid Peels

Trichloroacetic Acid (TCA) (pK_a = 0.54)

UN 1839 is required to transport it because of its corrosive activity.

TCA is also called trichloroethanoic acid. It is obtained through distillation of the product from nitric acid steam on chloral acid. It is found as anhydrous (very hygroscopic), white crystals.

TCA can be found directly in the environment because it is used as a herbicide (as sodium salt) and indirectly as a metabolite derived from chlorination reactions for water treatment. At the same time, it is a major metabolite of perchloroethylene (PCE), which is used mainly in the field of dry cleaning. Its general toxicity when taken in low dose is almost nonexistent. Its molecular structure is very close to glycolic acid. The carbon in the alpha position has a hydroxyl group and two hydrogens in the case of glycolic acid, as opposed to three chlorines in TCA. TCA is a much stronger acid than any other current acids used for peelings; its pKa is the lowest of any current acids used for chemical peels. Like glycolic acid, TCA does not have general toxicity, even when applied in concentrated form on the skin.

When applied to the skin, it is not transported into the blood circulation. TCA's destructive activity is a consequence of its acidity in aqueous solutions, but in peels the acid is rapidly "neutralized" as it progresses through the different skin layers, leading to a coagulation of skin proteins (Fig. 1.3). As the proteins become coagulated, the TCA is used up. To penetrate deeper, more TCA must be applied (volume) or a higher concentration of TCA needs to be used. TCA action is simple, reproducible, and proportional to the concentration and to the amount applied. Unique to TCA and phenol, visual signs (light speckling to white frost) in the skin following application indicate the degree of coagulation of protein molecules and the depth of penetration of the acid.

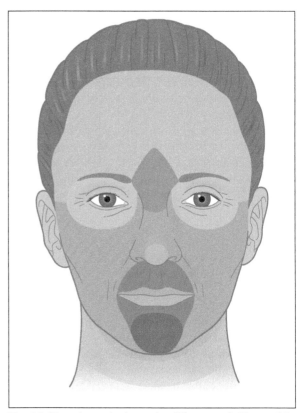

Fig. 1.3 The schematic shows the difference of skin reactivity to the coating with TCA. The darker the area, the higher the number of coats to be applied at the same concentration to achieve the same level of frosting.

TCA is used as an intermediate to deep peeling agent in concentrations ranging from 20% to 50%. Depth of penetration is increased as concentration increases, with 50% TCA penetrating into the reticular dermis.

The quality of manufacture of a particular TCA depends of 14 parameters linked to the raw material itself and one parameter linked to the manufacturer (material of protection if necessary like dust mask, eye shield, face shield, full face particle respirator, gloves, respirator cartridge, respirator filter):

1. The density of the vapor. Example: Relative vapor density (air = 1): 5.6.
2. The grade of purity.
3. The quality (analytical specification of the pH).
4. The index of refraction.
5. The temperature of ebullition per liter.
6. The density in g/ml at 25°C.
7. If present, the residual traces of anions and/or cations may cause tattooing due to increased penetration

depth correlative to pH. For this reason, we do not recommend using buffered TCA or neutralizing with plain water, which contains metallic ions. We prefer to use TCA prepared unbuffered, completed with bidistilled water and rose oil mosqueta.

8. Other residual chemical elements (such as SO_4): whether they should be considered as ignored.
9. The flash point (high flash point offers greater safety).
10. The impurities if they exist—for example, nonsoluble material.
11. The solubility in water in mole at 20°C, with the clearness or colorlessness (without any color) of the obtained solution.
12. The turbidity.
13. The pressure of the vapor (for low vapor pressure sealing and lubrication in high vacuum applications). Example: Vapor pressure, Pa at 51°C: 133.
14. Designed for use in electrophoresis, suitable as a fixing solution (designed for use in IEF and PAGE gels), ≥99%. Isoelectric focusing (IEF) separates proteins on the basis of their isoelectric point.

TCA peel solution must be stored separately from food and foodstuffs; it should be stored in a secure cool, dry area in a well-ventilated room. The packaging must be unbreakable; if it is breakable, it should be transferred to a closed unbreakable container. It is preferable to keep TCA peel solutions in opaque glass bottles.

In addition to this detailed chemistry data, clinical scenarios are helpful to highlight the action of TCA on the skin. TCA is the most aggressive acid (lowest pK_a of all acids used for peels), and the depth of penetration is correlated with its pH. The TCA application is linked to the pressure of application, the time, the number of coats, the total quantity used, and the neutralization.

We prefer special creams called "frosting stoppers" instead of water to neutralize the TCA, thus avoiding an exothermic reaction, which would provoke a "cold" burn. In our view, unbuffered TCA prepared with pure crystals and completed with bidistilled water with rose oil mosqueta is less likely to provoke pigmentary rebound or postinflammatory hyperpigmentation versus buffered TCA. It is recommended not to use water or primary or secondary alcohols before or after the application of an unbuffered TCA to prevent an exothermic reaction as a reversible reaction of esterification.

Some authors mix TCA and phenol for the comfort of the patient, arguing that phenol helps reduce the burning sensation of TCA. In fact, phenol has an anesthetic effect. Some combinations are TCA 35% w/w (weight/weight) and phenol without croton oil 15% to 25% w/w. However, the following must be kept in mind:

1. Both phenol and TCA are caustic, and adding both of them will not reduce the toxicity.
2. Phenol can be diluted into TCA or vice versa to reduce the concentration of the phenol and/or TCA. All calculations have to be made in w/w and never in v/v (volume/volume), because only mass are additive.

Why add another toxic substance to get a lower concentration of TCA or phenol for peels? It is safer to choose a lower concentration of TCA or phenol for the peel. Furthermore, the main caustic effect of phenol is due to croton oil and not the phenol itself.

SUBSTANCES WITH MAINLY TOXIC ACTIVITY

Phenol ((pK_aphoh$_2^+$/phoh) – 6.4 (pK_aphoh/pho$^-$) 9.95)

Phenol is also named phenic acid, or hydroxybenzene. It is a colorless, crystalline solid that melts at 41°C and boils at 182°C, is soluble in ethanol and ether, and is sometimes soluble in water.

Alcohols are organic compounds that have a functional hydroxyl group attached to a carbon atom of an alkyl chain. Benzene hydroxyl derivatives and aromatic hydrocarbons are called *phenols,* and the hydroxyl group is directly attached to a carbon atom in the benzene ring. In this case, phenol is an alcohol but not an alkyl alcohol: the group C_6H_5– is named *phenyl,* but the C_6H_5OH compound is called *phenol* and not *phenylic alcohol.*

Phenol is an aromatic alcohol with the properties of a weak acid (it has a labile H, which accounts for its acid character). Its three-dimensional structure tends to retain the H+ ion from the hydroxyl group through a so-called mesomeric effect. It is sometimes called *carbolic acid* when in water solution. It reacts with strong bases to form the salts called *phenolates.* Its pK_a is high, at 9.95. Phenol has antiseptic, antifungal, and anesthetic pharmacological properties.

Carbolic acid is more acidic than phenol, and there are three differences between phenol and carbolic acid:

1. The aromatic ring allows resonance stabilization of the phenoxide anion. In this way, the negative charge on oxygen is shared by the orthocarbon and

paracarbon atoms. That is why carbolic acid is used instead of phenol for endopeel techniques (which lead to medical liftings obtained by chemical myoplasty, myopexy, and myotension).

2. Increased acidity is the result of orbital overlap between the oxygen's lone pairs and the aromatic system.

3. The dominant effect is the induction from the sp^2 hybridized carbons; the comparatively more powerful inductive withdrawal of electron density that is provided by the sp^2 system compared with an sp^3 system allows for great stabilization of the oxyanion.

Resorcinol (pK_a = 11.27)

HO

Resorcinol is a phenol substituted by a hydroxyl in position meta. Hydroquinone is a phenol substituted by a hydroxyl in position para; pyrocatechol is a phenol substituted by a hydroxyl in position ortho.

Resorcinol is also named *resorcin, m*-dihydroxybenzene, 1,3-dihydroxybenzene, or benzenediol-1,3. It is a crystalline powder that melts at 111°C, boils at 281°C, and is soluble.

Like phenol, resorcinol is a protoplasmic poison that works through enzymatic inactivation and protein denaturation with production of insoluble proteins. Apart from that, both phenol and resorcinol act on the cellular membrane, modifying its selective permeability by changing its physical properties. This change in permeability then leads to cell death.

Phenol alone is a more powerful poison, with a secondary anesthetic effect due to inhibition of sensory nerve endings.

Phenol and (to a lesser extent) resorcinol are cardiac, renal, and hepatic toxins that are eliminated from the body at 80% concentration either unchanged or conjugated with glucuronic or sulfuric acid.

HOW THE MOST COMMONLY USED SUBSTANCES IN CHEMICAL PEELS WORK: A PROPOSAL FOR CLASSIFICATION

When making reference, even superficially, to the chemical and pharmacological properties of these diverse molecules, we realize that acidity is far from being the only mechanism of action that causes the previously documented peel-induced modifications of the skin. The pH alone is only destructive in the case of trichloroacetic acid. The other substances act mainly through toxic effects (phenol, resorcinol, less so- salicylic acid) or through metabolic effects in the case of AHAs and azelaic and retinoic acids and by interfering with cell structure and synthesis without destroying them, but merely modifying or stimulating them.

Thus we can propose to classify the substances used in the peels into three categories: caustic, metabolic, and toxic. Caustic effects are localized only to the areas that come into contact with the chemical, whereas toxic effects, although mainly localized in nature, can also affect cells distant from where the chemical has been applied.

Classification of Substances Used for Chemical Peels (L. Dewandre)

- Caustic: trichloroacetic acid
- Metabolic: AHAs, azelaic acid, retinoic acid
- Toxic: phenol, resorcinol, salicylic acid

When acidity is not the main mechanism of action, the pH seems to be the factor that allows certain other substances present in the solution (that have mainly metabolic effects) to penetrate the skin. The skin and its constituent molecules, and water, act as a kind of buffer for the solution that makes contact and penetrates until it reaches the depth necessary for its relative neutralization. It acts as a blotter of the solution applied, which is more or less avid depending on the pH and, most of all, on the pH gradient between this solution and the depth of the skin involved.

Toxins, particularly phenol, have little if any caustic action (unless solutions are used that contain croton oil); phenol solutions have a pH of 5 or 6.

We understand that there is an interest in using peeling mixtures of different substances to minimize complications and to take advantage of the various mechanisms of action (caustic, toxic, and metabolic effects). This explains the interest in Jessner's solution (a mixture of resorcinol, lactic acid, and salicylic acid); Monheit's formula (a version of a modified Jessner's solution with the resorcinol replaced with citric acid) followed by the application of a TCA peel; other "secret" modified phenol formulas; and others (Fintsi, Kakowicz, De Rossi Fattaccioli, etc.).

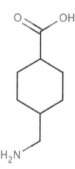

Fig. 1.4 The molecular structure of tranexamic acid.

The classification of A. Tenenbaum makes it easy to understand how even some acids with pKa >3 such as tartaric, mandelic, salicylic, and of course phenol may not be appropriate in the hands of novice peelers.

Therefore it is recommended that beginners start by using low concentrations of the nonaromatic diprotic or tripotic AHAs with pK_a >3.

Tranexamic Acid (pKa = 4.3) and Aromatic Carboxylic Acid

The Role of Tranexamic Acid in Chemical Peels

Proposed mechanisms of action. Tranexamic acid (trans-4-aminomethyl cyclohexane carboxylic acid; TXA) has a chemical composition as shown in Fig. 1.4. This agent was first introduced to the medical literature in 1962 by a Japanese husband-and-wife team and was first prescribed for heavy menstrual bleeding and dental extraction bleeding. It is a well-known plasmin inhibitor and is a synthetic derivative of the amino acid lysine. Its antifibrinolytic effects occur via the reversible blockade of lysine-binding sites on plasminogen molecules.

The figures show the molecular structure of TXA (see Fig. 1.4) and its inhibitory role in the plasminogen cascade (Fig. 1.5). Plasmin formation is inhibited by TXA, resulting in plasmin downregulation and inability to cleave the fibrin clot.

The effects of TXA on melanin production has been documented in the literature; however, the biochemical pathways and mechanisms of action are less well known. Studies on guinea pigs have demonstrated that TXA can reduce skin pigmentation. The mechanism of action is not by affecting the absolute numbers of melanocytes, but by decreasing the melanogenic activity of the melanocytes, resulting in a reduced synthesis of melanin.[1]

Plasminogen activity is also affected by TXA. Plasminogen exists in basal cell keratinocytes, and studies have confirmed that ultraviolet (UV) light stimulates plasminogen activation, and the resultant plasmin stimulates α-MSH (melanocyte-stimulating hormone), and therefore melanogenesis.[2] TXA has been found to act on UV-irradiated keratinocytes by reducing plasmin activity in these cells. As a result, factors promoting melanogenesis, such as prostaglandins, are downregulated and suppressed.[3,4]

Another proposed mode of activity is that TXA, having a similar molecular structure to tyrosine, functions as a competitive inhibitor to the enzyme tyrosinase, which is responsible for melanin production. This ultimately results in lowered melanin production.[5] A 2017 histological analysis of melasma patients treated with oral TXA revealed that not only was pigmentation decreased, but patients also experienced a decrease in associated facial erythema due to decreased vascularity and capillary numbers and a decrease in mast cell numbers.[6]

Based on current histochemical studies, TXA has been shown to have multiple effects on the skin and exhibits the following effects on cells within both the dermis and epidermis:

Dermis
- Fibroblasts irradiated by UVA demonstrate an increased expression of matrix metalloprotease 1 (MMP-1), an enzyme known to degrade collagen. MMP-1 activity is dependent upon plasmin activation. In tissue samples exposed to UVA radiation, TXA was found to decrease MMP-1 expression and as a result collagen degradation. It is proposed that TXA may confer antiaging benefits to UV-damaged skin via a decrease in collagen breakdown.[7]
- Capillary formation is suppressed by the action of TXA. Plasmin activates VEGF, an activator of neocapillary genesis. TXA has also been shown to suppress basic fibroblast growth factor (bFGF), which stimulates angiogenesis and repopulates the microvasculature. The antiplasmin effects of TXA therefore have shown clinical benefits by reducing the overall blood vessel count and reducing erythema.[6,8]

Epidermis
- TXA functions as a barrier membrane. In the epidermis, animal studies have demonstrated that TXA can improve xerosis, reduce transepidermal water loss (TEWL), and reduce inflammation by decreasing mast cell proliferation.[9]
- Another in vitro study supported the role of TXA in improving barrier function recovery because it showed an increase in upregulation of the protein occludin in cells treated with TXA.[5]

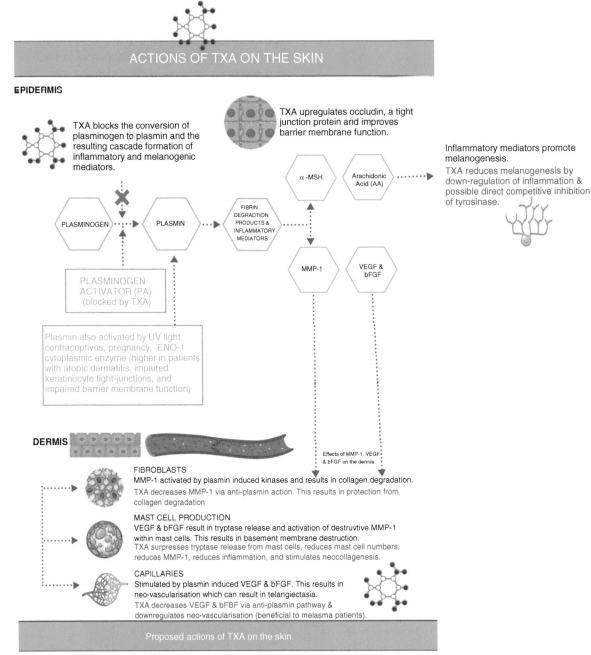

Fig. 1.5 Actions of tranexamic acid on the skin.

- TXA affects keratinocytes. Enolase-1 (ENO-1) is a ubiquitous cellular enzyme present both intracellularly and on the cell surface. It is a cell surface receptor for plasminogen. Patients with atopic dermatitis demonstrate increased levels of ENO-1 and plasminogen within the keratinocytes and basal layer. Upon treatment with TXA, it was found that in vitro tissue samples showed reversal of tight junction protein disruption. This implies that treatment with TXA improves the integrity of keratinocytes within the basement membrane.[10]

- TXA has been found to inhibit α-MSH production in melanocytes stimulated by ultraviolet B (UV B) radiation. In vitro studies propose that TXA can decrease α-MSH by decreasing the production of prohormone convertase 2 (PC2), an enzyme involved in the cleavage of POMC to α-MSH. PC2 is activated by plasmin and, via TXA's antiplasmin action, decreases melanogenesis.[4] Another pathway for TXA decreasing melanogenesis was found by investigating melanoma cells. This study determined that TXA enhanced the production of kinases (mitogen activated protein kinase [MAPK] and extracellular signal-regulated kinase [ERK]) involved in autophagy and downregulation of tyrosinase.[11]
- A histochemical study published in 2017 has confirmed that TXA can downregulate melanin synthesis via stimulation of the extracellular signal-regulated kinase (ERK) signaling pathway and the autophagy system. It means that production of melanogenesis-promoting proteins such as microphthalmia-associated transcription factor (MITF), tyrosinase, and tyrosinase-related protein 1 and 2 (TRP 1&2) can be reduced and downregulated by treatments with TXA. The research results suggest that TXA can result in a decrease in melanin synthesis by decreasing the production of tyrosinase and TRP 1&2, along with lowered MITF protein levels.[11]

It is known that melanocytes are immune cells highly responsive and communicative with cells of the dermis and epidermis. It is therefore reasonable to postulate that TXA having a positive regulatory effect on dermal and epidermal cells may create a favorable environment for pigmentation control via the multiple pathways on which it can act. TXA therefore has the ability to moderate cellular interactions, especially that between the keratinocytes and melanocytes.

Fig. 1.5 summarizes the proposed actions of TXA on the dermal and epidermal cells and melanogenesis.

Delivery of Tranexamic Acid to the Skin

As discussed, TXA has the ability to alter the physiological behavior of cutaneous tissue. TXA can be delivered to the skin via various modes: topical, intradermal, and oral delivery, with the topical and oral routes most widely studied. The ideal treatment route and delivery method for TXA is undetermined, and no consensus currently exists. Based on current publications, the following two regimens are often described.

Oral route: 500 mg daily (250 mg twice daily). Three recent clinical studies used this dose with reports that patients exhibited signs of skin lightening without adverse reactions. Lee et al have conducted the largest retrospective study to date on the efficacy of oral TXA. They concluded that 250 mg twice daily (BID) is an effective dose for the observance of skin lightening within 2 months. Studies confirming the efficacy and safety of this dosage were also reported by Del Rosario et al (2018), by Tan et al (2017), and by Wu et al (2012).[12-14]

Topical route. Topical serum 5% TXA in a suitable base for use BID.

Previous recent studies have shown effectiveness of topically applied TXA at 5% without adverse effects. Kanechorn et al used 5% in a liposomal gel base,[15] and Banihashemi et al[16] used 5% liposomal TXA and found it efficacious.

Tranexamic Acid and Its Usefulness With Chemical Peeling

Chemical peels are chemoexfoliants, with the underlying principle for their mechanism of action being to chemically alter the epidermis and/or the dermis in a controlled manner. As a consequence, peeling of the skin occurs, with the end result being a visible improvement in the aesthetic tone and texture of the skin. As previously described, TXA use can result in skin lightening, as well as improvement in skin barrier membrane function. Because of its positive effects on both the dermis and the epidermis, it stands to reason that TXA can be a useful adjunctive and supportive treatment to augment the resolution of postinflammatory hyperpigmentation (PIH) and cosmetic cutaneous dyschromias, while supporting the health of that ever-important barrier membrane. Barrier membrane function is often breached during chemical peels. TXA used by the clinician as both the prepeel treatment skin conditioning program and also postpeel use of the excellent agent is expected to produce enhanced results to the chemical peeling process.

CONCLUSION

If we look at the history and the evolution of chemical peels it is possible to distinguish two great developmental periods. The first period was from the 19th century to the end of the 1980s, during which great substances were discovered, classical formulas and mixtures were created, and their histological and clinical effects were studied. The second period includes the development and improved understanding of modified TCA, mainly influenced by Z. Obagi, and the development of AHAs. The rediscovery of AHAs, notably glycolic acid, by Van Scott et al popularized mild chemical peels for a large part of the population.

Despite this important progress, the science of chemical peels is still mainly empiric, and its applications are often intuitive. We believe that we might be entering a third period, characterized by a better understanding of the mechanism of action of peels, as discussed previously. Hopefully we will emerge from this period with the appearance of new, more scientific methods and products for use in chemical peeling.

Although some have predicted the disappearance of chemical peels in favor of physical peeling using lasers, quite the opposite has occurred, and we are witnessing a rekindled interest. This development in this field will be completely achieved when the application of chemical peels extends beyond the empiric and enters the scientific realm.

REFERENCES

1. Li D, Shi Y, Li M, Liu J, Feng X. Tranexamic acid can treat ultraviolet radiation-induced pigmentation in guinea pigs. *Eur J Dermatol*. 2010;20(3):289–292.
2. Handel AC, Miot LD, Miot HA. Melasma: a clinical and epidemiological review. *An Bras Dermatol*. 2014;89(5):771–782.
3. Maeda K, Naganuma M. Topical trans-4-aminomethyl-cyclohexanecarboxylic acid prevents ultraviolet radiation-induced pigmentation. *J Photochem Photobiol B*. 1998;47(2-3):136–141.
4. Hiramoto K, Yamate Y, Sugiyama D, Takahashi Y, Mafune E. Tranexamic acid suppresses ultraviolet B eye irradiation-induced melanocyte activation by decreasing the levels of prohormone convertase 2 and alpha-melanocyte-stimulating hormone. *Photodermatol Photoimmunol Photomed*. 2014;30(6):302–307.
5. Yuan C, Wang XM, Yang LJ, Wu PL. Tranexamic acid accelerates skin barrier recovery and upregulates occludin in damaged skin. *Int J Dermatol*. 2014;53(8):959–965.
6. Na JI, Choi SY, Yang SH, Choi HR, Kang HY, Park KC. Effect of tranexamic acid on melasma: a clinical trial with histological evaluation. *J Eur Acad Dermatol Venereol*. 2013;27(8):1035–1039.
7. Sonoki A, Okano Y, Yoshitake Y. Dermal fibroblasts can activate matrix metalloproteinase-1 independent of keratinocytes via plasmin in a 3D collagen model. *Exp Dermatol*. 2018;27(5):520–525.
8. Kim EH, Kim YC, Lee ES, Kang HY. The vascular characteristics of melasma. *J Dermatol Sci*. 2007;46(2):111–116.
9. Hiramoto K, Sugiyama D, Takahashi Y, Mafune E. The amelioration effect of tranexamic acid in wrinkles induced by skin dryness. *Biomed Pharmacother*. 2016;80:16–22.
10. Tohgasaki T, Ozawa N, Yoshino T, et al. Enolase-1 expression in the stratum corneum is elevated with parakeratosis of atopic dermatitis and disrupts the cellular tight junction barrier in keratinocytes. *Int J Cosmet Sci*. 2018;40(2):178–186.
11. Cho YH, Park JE, Lim DS, Lee JS. Tranexamic acid inhibits melanogenesis by activating the autophagy system in cultured melanoma cells. *J Dermatol Sci*. 2017;88(1):96–102.
12. Tan AWM, Sen P, Chua SH, Goh BK. Oral tranexamic acid lightens refractory melasma. *Australas J Dermatol*. 2017;58(3):e105–e108.
13. Del Rosario E, Florez-Pollack S, Zapata Jr L, et al. Randomized, placebo-controlled, double-blind study of oral tranexamic acid in the treatment of moderate-to-severe melasma. *J Am Acad Dermatol*. 2018;78(2):363–369.
14. Wu S, Shi H, Wu H, et al. Treatment of melasma with oral administration of tranexamic acid. *Aesthetic Plast Surg*. 2012;36(4):964–970.
15. Kanechorn Na Ayuthaya P, Niumphradit N, Manosroi A, Nakakes A. Topical 5% tranexamic acid for the treatment of melasma in Asians: a double-blind randomized controlled clinical trial. *J Cosmet Laser Ther*. 2012;14(3):150–154.
16. Banihashemi M, Zabolinejad N, Jaafari MR, Salehi M, Jabari A. Comparison of therapeutic effects of liposomal tranexamic acid and conventional hydroquinone on melasma. *J Cosmet Dermatol*. 2015;14(3):174–177.

FURTHER READING

Allinger NL, Cava MP, de Jongh DC, et al. *Chimie Organique [Organic Chemistry]*. Vols. 1–3. Montreal: McGraw-Hill; 1990.
Arnaud P. *Chimie Organique – Ouvrage D'initiation à la Chimie Organique. [Organic Chemistry – Introductory Work to Organic Chemistry]*. Paris: Dunod; 1992.
Brody HJ. *Chemical Peeling*. St Louis: Mosby; 1997.
Carlson BM. *Integumentary, Skeletal, and Muscular Systems. Human Embryology and Developmental Biology*. St Louis: Mosby; 1994:153–181.
Demas PN, Bridenstine JB, Braun TW. Pharmacology of agents used in the management of patients having skin resurfacing. *J Oral Maxillofac Surg*. 1997;55:1255–1258.

de Levie R. The Henderson–Hasselbach equation: its history and limitations. *J Chem Educ*. 2003;80:146.

de Levie R. The Henderson approximation and the mass action law of Guldberg and Waage. *Chem Educ*. 2002;7:132–135.

De Rossi Fattaccioli D. Histological comparison between deep chemical peeling (modified Litton's formulae) and ultra pulsed CO_2 laser resurfacing. *Dermatología Peruana*. 2005;15:1.

Ebbing DD, Gammon SD. *General Chemistry*. 8th ed. Boston: Houghton Mifflin; 2005.

Halaas YP. Medium depth peels. *Facial Plast Surg Clin North Am*. 2004;12:297–303.

Hasselbach KA. Die Berechnung der wasserstoffzahl des blutes aus der freien und gebundenen kohlensäure desselben, und die sauerstoffbindung des blutes als funktion der wasserstoffzahl. *Biochemische Zeitschrift*. 1917;78:112–144.

Henderson LJ. Concerning the relationship between the strength of acids and their capacity to preserve neutrality. *Am J Physiol*. 1908;21(4):173–179.

Hermitte R. Aged skin, retinoids and alpha hydroxyl acids. *Cosmetics Toiletries*. 1992;107:63–67.

Holbrook KA. Embryology of the human epidermis. In: Vincent C, ed. *Kelley's Practice of Pediatrics*. Hagerstown: MD: Harper and Row; 1980.

Holbrook KA. Structure and function of the developing human skin. In: Goldsmith LA, ed. *Physiology, Biochemistry, and Molecular Biology of the Skin*. New York: Oxford University Press; 1991.

Hornby M, Peach JM. *Foundations of Organic Chemistry*. Oxford: Oxford University Press; 1991.

Howard P, Meylan W, eds. *Handbook of Physical Properties of Organic Chemicals*. Boca Raton, FL: CRC/Lewis Publishers; 1997.

Kolbe H. *Liebig's Annals of Chemistry*. 1860;115:201.

Kortum G, Vogel W, Andrussow K. *Dissociation constants of organic acids in aqueous solution*. London: Butterworths; 1961[Reprint of Pure and Applied Chemistry, vol 1(2,3), 1961]

Lagowski J, ed. *Macmillan Encyclopedia of Chemistry*. New York: Macmillan; 1997.

Lee HC, Thng TG, Goh CL. Oral tranexamic acid (TA) in the treatment of melasma: a retrospective analysis. *J Am Acad Dermatol*. 2016;75(2):385–392.

Lespiau R. *La molécule Chimique [Chemical Molecule]*. Paris: Félix Alcan; 1920:285.

Methley AM, Campbell S, Chew-Graham C, McNally R, Cheraghi-Sohi S. PICO, PICOS and SPIDER: a comparison study of specificity and sensitivity in three search tools for qualitative systematic reviews. *BMC Health Serv Res*. 2014;14:579.

Montagna W, Parakkal PF. *The Structure and Function of Skin*. 3rd ed. New York: Academic Press; 1974.

Normant H, Normant J. *Chimie Organique [Organic Chemistry]*. Paris: Masson; 1968.

Pauwels. Les alpha-hydroxyacides en pratique dermatologique [The alpha-hydroxyacids in dermatological practice]. *BEDC*. 1994;2:437–453.

Pavia DL, Lampman GM, Kriz GS. *Organic Chemistry Volume 1: Organic Chemistry 351*. Mason, OH: Cenage Learning; 2004.

Perrin DD. *Dissociation constants of inorganic acids*. London: Butterworths; 1969 [Reprint of Pure and Applied Chemistry, vol. 20(2) 1969]

Po HN, Senozan NM. Henderson–Hasselbach equation: Its history and limitations. *J Chem Educ*. 2001;78:1499–1503.

Resnick SS, Resnik BL. Complications of chemical peeling. *Dermatol Clin*. 2005;13:309–312.

Rubin MG. *Manual of Chemical Peels: Superficial and Medium Depth*. Philadelphia: Lippincott Williams & Wilkins; 1995.

Schmitt R. [no title found]. *J Prakt Chem*. 1885;31:397.

Solomons TWG. *Organic Chemistry*. 3rd ed. New York: Wiley; 1984.

Streitwiezer A, Heathcock CH. *Introduction to Organic Chemistry*. 2nd ed. Macmillan; 1981.

Tenenbaum A. In: Laserpeel. Longo L, Hoffstetter AG, Pascu ML eds. Proceedings of the SPIE Laser Florence '99: a window on the laser medicine. 1999;4166:169–179.

Tenenbaum A. La tecnica Endopeel-Vol: la medicina estetica-A.Redaelli- 2009 Ed SEE Firenze; 2009:60–62, 71–73, 79, 227, 234.

Tenenbaum A, Tiziani M. The philosophy of synergy in rejuvenation's techniques-Tecniche Endopeel-Tecniche per il lifting non chirurgico del viso e del corpo- Ed Evolution MD.

Tenenbaum A. Medical facelifts by chemical myoplasty, myotension and myopexy (endopeel techniques or muscular SMAS repositioning). *Anaplastol*. 2013;2:116. https://doi.org/10.4172/2161-1173.1000116.

Van Scott EJ, Yu RJ. Control of keratinization with alpha-hydroxy acids and related compounds. *Arch Dermatol*. 1974;110:586–590.

Van Scott EJ, Yu RJ. Alpha-hydroxy-acids: procedures for use in clinical practice. *Cutis*. 1989;43:22–229.

Vollhardt KPC, Schore NE. *Traité de chimie organique [Organic Chemistry Handbook]*. Brussels: De Boeck-Wesmael; 1998:1350.

Zumdahl S, Zumdahl S. *Chemistry*. 8th ed. New York: Houghton Mifflin; 2009.

2

Choosing the Correct Peel for the Appropriate Patient

Yardy Tse, Suzan Obagi

INTRODUCTION

Chemical peels are a method of resurfacing the skin to address a variety of skin conditions. The benefits of understanding the peel–tissue interaction gives the physician the ability to selectively resurface various parts of the skin, thus allowing for control and artistry in the resurfacing process. By inducing a controlled wound to the skin, chemical peels can resurface part or all of the epidermis (very superficial and superficial peels), the papillary dermis (medium-depth peels), even down to the level of the upper or mid-reticular dermis (deep peels). By forcing turnover of skin cells, peels can improve photodamage, rhytides, pigmentation abnormalities, and scarring.

Chemical peels are divided into four categories depending upon the depth of the wound created by the peel (see Chapters 4 through 8). Very superficial peels only penetrate through the stratum corneum and the uppermost portions of the epidermis. Superficial chemical peels penetrate the epidermis but not more than the basal layer of the epidermis. Medium-depth peels penetrate the entire epidermis plus the papillary dermis. Deep chemical peels create a wound to the level of the upper and mid-reticular dermis.

Each category of peels addresses a different aspect of photodamage and pigmentary abnormality. Healing time and complications vary among the different categories of peels as well, with some peels being more appropriate for certain skin types. Therefore, to maximize the benefits of a peel for a patient and to minimize adverse effects, it is important to choose which, if any, peel is appropriate for each patient.

EVALUATION OF THE PATIENT

When evaluating a patient for a peel, an extensive history should be taken. The patient should be questioned regarding a history and frequency of herpes simplex virus (HSV) infection, human immunodeficiency virus (HIV) status (more so, viral load), keloid formation, previous x-ray therapy of the skin, nicotine use, oral isotretinoin use, and a history of a previous facelift or browlift.

Patients with a history of frequent HSV infections (more than 1 every 6 months) should be treated prophylactically to prevent an outbreak of herpes during the healing process. This is most important during medium-depth and deep peels. All patients having a medium-depth to deep peel should receive HSV prophylaxis with the dose adjusted so that it is higher in patients prone to more than one HSV breakthrough every 6 to 12 months. Typically patients having a medium-depth or deep peel are started on 500 mg valacyclovir twice a day for 7 to 14 days starting the day before the procedure. If they are at risk for HSV, the dose is increased to 1000 mg twice a day. If an HSV or varicella zoster virus (VZV) breakthrough is suspected during the healing process, the dose is increased to 1000 mg three times a day for 14 days.

Patients with detectable viral loads of HIV are poor candidates for a medium-depth or deep peel, because their immunocompromised state delays wound healing and increases the risk of wound infection and subsequent scarring. Transplant patients and patients on immunosuppressive medications for autoimmune diseases are similarly at risk for infection and poor wound healing.

The biggest controversy is the concern over timing of skin resurfacing in patients who have just completed isotretinoin treatment. The previous recommendation of waiting 6 to 12 months after isotretinoin use to have a chemical peel may have been overexaggerated. Isotretinoin does impair wound healing, but there is growing evidence that resurfacing patients with peels and lasers may be safe as early as 3 months after the medication is completed.

Although peels can be performed simultaneously with surgical procedures, the timing of skin resurfacing changes for patients who have had recent surgery in the same area. The safe window for resurfacing is either the same day as surgery or 6 to 12 months after a facelift or browlift procedure. The extensive undermining during facelifts and browlifts compromise the skin's lymphatic drainage, so it is best to wait 6 to 12 months to reduce the risk for prolonged postoperative edema.

Superficial x-ray therapy of the face (used many decades ago to treat acne) destroys the pilosebaceous units, which, in turn, leads to delayed reepithelialization, and nicotine use decreases the blood supply to the skin and delays wound healing. Both of these underlying factors can result in an increased risk of scarring.

The physician should also perform a physical examination and pay particular attention to the patient's skin type and degree of photodamage. Skin type can be classified using the Obagi Skin Classification System (Table 2.1). This skin classification system can be used to objectively assess the patient's skin and is an important tool for choosing the appropriate peel. This classification system incorporates more information than the traditional Fitzpatrick skin type or Glogau scales did. The five assessments are skin color, oiliness, thickness, laxity, and fragility (Figs. 2.1–2.5).

Color

Skin color involves a patient's variation within a particular ethnic or racial background. Patients who have very light Caucasian skin are less likely to experience hyperpigmentation than darker-skinned Caucasian patients. However, darker-skinned patients with Asian or African descent have more stable skin pigment and are at less risk of postinflammatory hyperpigmentation (PIH). Conversely, light-skinned patients with Asian or African descent and biracial fair-complexion patients are at increased risk for PIH. Patients at risk for PIH should receive a longer course of skin preconditioning (see Chapter 3). Risk of hypopigmentation also correlates with skin color (see Table 2.1).

Oiliness

The physician should also note the sebaceous quality of the skin, because oil is a significant hinderance to the penetration of the peeling solution. There is also an increased risk of postpeel acne flares if oiliness is not controlled. Patients with very sebaceous skin may require additional prepeel degreasing of the skin to achieve the same depth of penetration of the peeling agent as patients with very thin, nonsebaceous skin. Very oily-skinned patients may require several months of systemic isotretinoin before skin resurfacing if a medium-depth or deep peel is planned.

Skin Thickness

Thinner-skinned patients are at risk during deep skin resurfacing (peels or laser) due to a decrease in the amount of the adnexal structures that are required for reepithelialization. However, they benefit the most from skin resurfacing if performed properly. Thin skin is better treated with a series of medium-depth (papillary dermis level) peels to help build collagen and tighten skin. Thicker-skinned patients are safer for skin resurfacing with peels and lasers but will require more aggressive resurfacing to reach the desired depth of penetration.

Skin Laxity

Skin laxity must be differentiated from muscle laxity. Muscle laxity requires surgical intervention to help resuspend ptotic tissue. However, skin laxity improves with repeated papillary dermis level resurfacing because it increases the amount of anchoring fibrils at the dermal–epidermal junction (DEJ) and the papillary dermis–level collagen and elastin thickness, which in turn firms up skin.

Fragile Skin

Skin becomes more fragile as patients get older due to the flattening of the Rete ridges between the epidermis and dermis (DEJ) and the loss of anchoring fibrils at the DEJ. Patients usually present with easy bruising and delayed wound healing from minor wounds (mainly on the dorsal forearms). This is worsened with age, with long-term systemic prednisone use, and with taking blood-thinning medication. Repeated papillary dermis–level peels can help reduce the fragility of the skin.

TABLE 2.1   Obagi Skin Classification

Skin Variable	Skin Conditioning: Before and After Resurfacing	Suitable Procedures and Potential Complications

Color	Conditioning varies with skin color. More aggressive with darker Caucasian skin and with lighter skin in patients of Asian or African descent	Complications related to depth and skin color. Darker skin:
		• Hypopigmentation
		  • Superficial procedure: rare
		  • Medium-depth procedures: possible
		  • Deep procedures: more likely
		• Hyperpigmentation
		  • Common regardless of depth

Oiliness	Increased skin surface oil interferes with effectiveness of skin conditioning. It may contribute to postoperative acne flares. Topical or systemic therapy to control or reduce surface oiliness preoperatively[a]	Excessive oil hinders chemical peel acid penetration. Laser resurfacing is not affected by oiliness
Thickness	Thin skin needs papillary level procedures to thicken the papillary dermal collagen layer. Thick skin needs reticular dermis level procedures to effect a textural change	Thin skin: light to medium depth peels Medium-thick skin: good for peels, dermabrasion, fractionated lasers Thick skin: deeper chemical peels, dermabrasion, fractionated lasers
Laxity	Lax skin requires long-term collagen stimulation to prevent further laxity	Differentiate between skin and muscle laxity: Skin Laxity: Medium depth peel to the level of the papillary dermis Muscle laxity: Facelift alone or in combination with a medium depth peel (to correct any associated skin laxity)
Fragility	Goal is to maintain or possibly increase skin strength.	Fragility correlates with postsurgical scarring. Procedure depth should be limited to the papillary dermis in fragile skin

This classification looks at skin more critically using five categories: color, thickness, oiliness, laxity, and fragility. This helps guide depth of resurfacing to minimize complications while improving results.

[a]If systemic isotretinoin is used, it is prudent to delay medium or deep skin resurfacing at least 3 months (medium-depth resurfacing) to 6 months (deeper resurfacing).

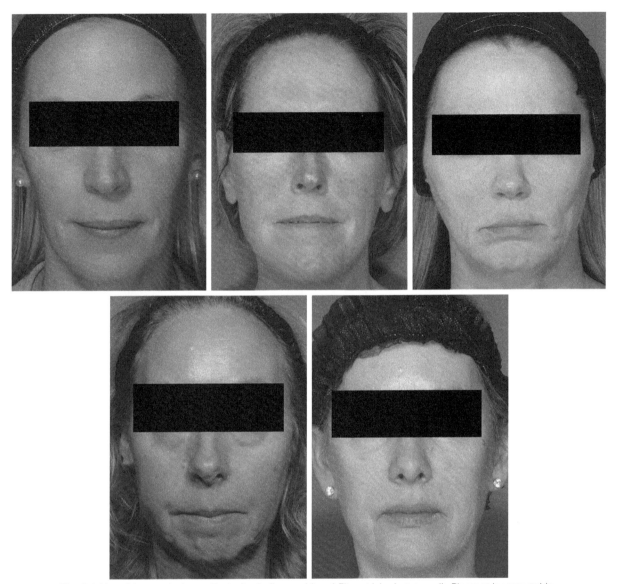

Fig. 2.1 Very fair complexion patients (typically considered Fitzpatrick phototype I). Pigment is very stable, postinflammatory hyperpigmentation is unlikely, fragility increases with age, and wrinkles are the predominant complaint. Rosacea is common.

Other Considerations

Perhaps the most important discussion that a physician must have with a patient preoperatively is one regarding realistic expectations. Without doubt, eliciting clearly a patient's chief complaint is of the utmost importance and can prevent any misunderstanding after the procedure. The physician should realistically describe the postoperative course, healing time, anticipated results, and potential risks of the procedure.

VERY SUPERFICIAL CHEMICAL PEELS

Although a single treatment of a very superficial peel can induce exfoliation, a series of these peels is necessary to achieve additional benefit. Improvement of skin texture, through the removal of the stratum corneum, induction of acanthosis, and an increase in thickness of the granular layer, as well as improvement of epidermal melasma and solar lentigines can be achieved through a

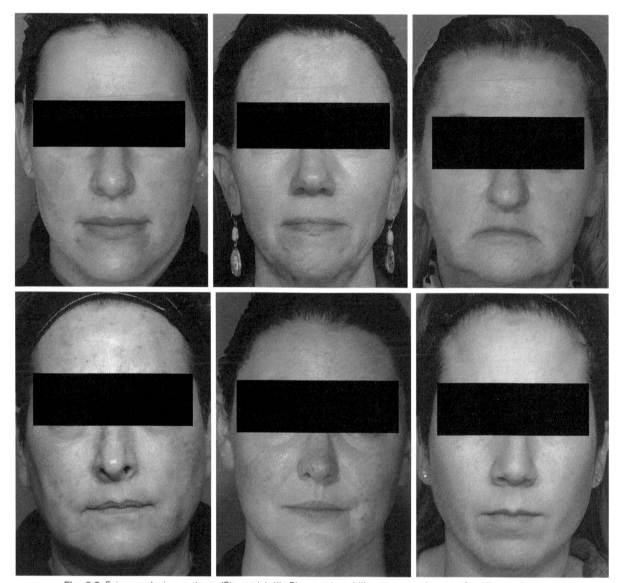

Fig. 2.2 Fair complexion patients (Fitzpatrick II). Pigment instability starts to show as freckling and uneven complexion, postinflammatory hyperpigmentation (PIH) is still unlikely, and wrinkles and rosacea are the predominant complaint. Patients with melasma are at increased risk for PIH. Skin thickness may begin to increase.

series of very superficial peels. PIH is not common with superficial peels, because they create minimal inflammation.

SUPERFICIAL CHEMICAL PEELS

Superficial chemical peels are more effective than the very superficial peels for the treatment of actinic keratoses, epidermal melasma, solar lentigines, and epidermal growths such as thin seborrheic keratoses.

Skin texture may also be improved. Erythema and scaling will occur postoperatively for 3 to 4 days; however, healing time is faster if patients are pretreated with the proper skin preconditioning (see Chapter 3).

Although all lighter peels can be used in virtually all skin types, caution must still be taken in patients at risk for PIH. A thorough knowledge of the subtleties of these chemical peels will allow the practitioner the ability to treat all skin types safely and effectively.

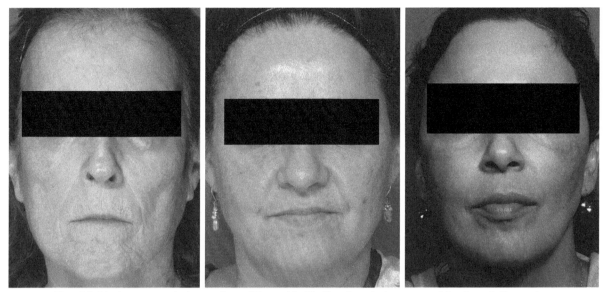

Fig. 2.3 Moderate complexion patients (Fitzpatrick III). Dyschromia increases, risk of postinflammatory hyperpigmentation increases, patients can present with a primary concern of wrinkles or dyschromia, or both. Oiliness, as well as skin thickness, may increase.

MEDIUM-DEPTH CHEMICAL PEELS

Medium-depth peels reach the papillary dermis level and thus take about 7 days to heal. With increased healing time comes an increased risk for complications such as scarring, hypopigmentation, and PIH. However, the benefit in skin firming, pore tightening, sun damage reduction, and pigmentation improvement make them very versatile peels.

DEEP CHEMICAL PEELS

Deep peels are comparable to traditional ablative CO_2 laser resurfacing and are most appropriate for patients with deep scars or deep wrinkles. However, due to the depth of penetration into the reticular dermis, textural change, permanent hypopigmentation, and scarring are real concerns. The recovery time associated with deep peels is on the order of 10 to 12 days.

SUMMARY

Chemical peels are a safe and versatile method of resurfacing the skin. However, it is critical for the physician to choose the appropriate peel for the appropriate patient to achieve the desired end point and to decrease the risk of complications. Superficial peels are safe in virtually all skin types. These peels can effectively treat melasma, acne vulgaris, and thin seborrheic keratoses and can lighten solar lentigines. They may also induce subtle changes in skin texture. Medium-depth peels are used to address deeper concerns such as dermal melasma, large pores, and fine wrinkles/laxity. The risk of PIH is greatly increased. Deep peels can dramatically improve deep facial rhytides, acne scarring, and photodamage. Newer phenol-croton oil combination peels have made these deeper peels safer to use in a wider range of patients.

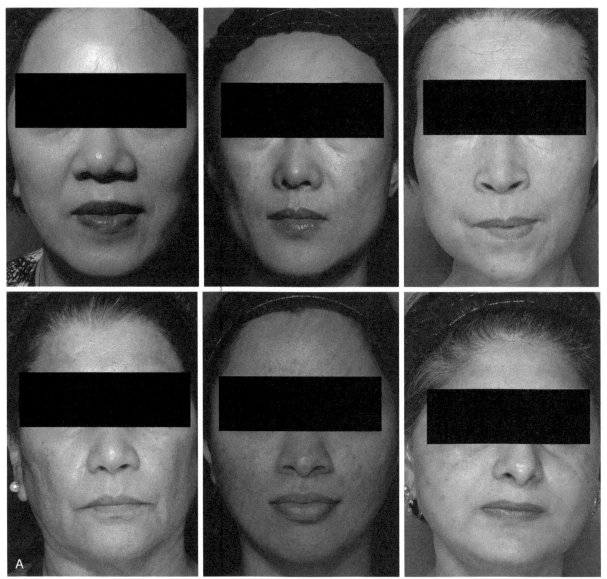

Fig. 2.4 These patients show the wide range of skin types in the Fitzpatrick IV group. Skin color alone does not help predict postinflammatory hyperpigmentation. Patients with melasma and freckling are more likely to develop PIH. Patients without dyschromia tend to have more stable pigment cells. Patients with freckling or melasma should be treated with longer skin-preconditioning regimens. Skin thickness and oiliness should be addressed before planning a resurfacing procedure.

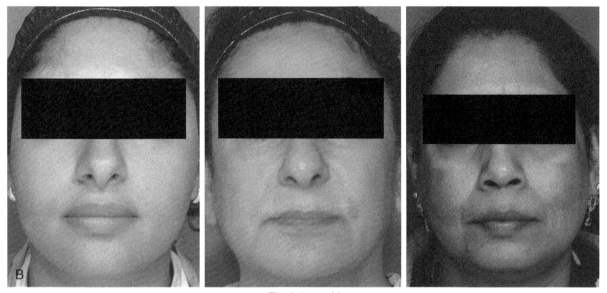

Fig. 2.4, cont'd

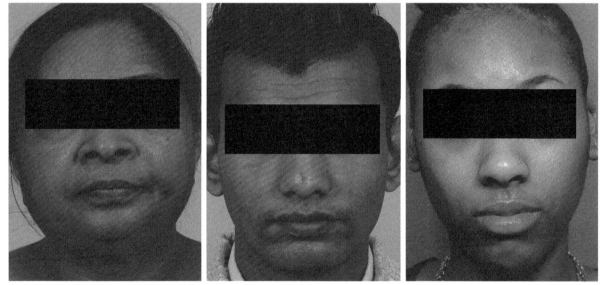

Fig. 2.5 More variability in the Fitzpatrick V group. Postinflammatory hyperpigmentation (PIH) is a significant concern with procedures; fragility is less of a concern. Patients with more even tone across their face are at less risk for PIH.

FURTHER READING

Ahn HH, Kim IH. Whitening effect of salicylic acid peels in Asian patients. *Dermatol Surg.* 2006;32:372–375.

Briden ME. Alpha-hydroxy acid chemical peeling agents: case studies and rationale for safe and effective use. *Cutis.* 2004;73(supply 2):18–24.

Brody HJ. *Chemical Peeling and Resurfacing.* 2nd ed. St Louis: Mosby-Year Book; 1997.

Buter PE, Gonzalez S, Randolph MA, et al. Quantitative and qualitative effects of chemical peeling on photo-aged skin: an experimental study. *Plast Reconstr Surg.* 2001;107(1):222–228.

El-Domati MB, Attia SK, Saleh FY, et al. Trichloroacetic acid peeling versus dermabrasion: a histometric, immunohistochemical, and ultrastructural comparison. *Dermatol Surg.* 2004;30:179–188.

Glogau RG, Matarasso SL. Chemical peels. Trichloroacetic acid and phenol. *Dermatol Surg.* 1995;13(2):263–276.

Fanous N, Côté V, Fanous A. The new genetico-racial skin classification: how to maximize the safety of any peel or laser treatment on any Asian, Caucasian or Black patient. *Can J Plast Surg.* 2011;19(1):9–16.

Halaas YP. Medium depth peels. *Facial Plast Surg Clin North Am.* 2004;12(3):297–303.

Hantash BM, Stewart DB, Cooper ZA, Rehmus WE. Facial resurfacing for nonmelanoma skin cancer prophylaxis. *Arch Dermatol.* 2006; 142:976–982.

Landau M. Cardiac complications in deep chemical peels. *Dermatol Surg.* 2007;33:190–193.

Monheit GD. Medium-depth chemical peels. *Dermatol Clin.* 2001;19(3):413–425.

Monhcit GD, Chastain MA. Chemical and mechanical skin resurfacing. In: Dermatology, Bolognia J, Jorizzo JL, Rapini RR, eds. St Louis: Mosby; 2003:2379–2396.

Obagi S, Obagi ZE, Bridenstine JB. Isotretinoin use during chemical skin resurfacing: a review of complications. *Am J Cosmet Surg.* 2002;19(1):9–13.

Obagi ZE, Obagi S, Alaiti S, Stevens MB. TCA-based blue peel: A standardized procedure with depth control. *Dermatol Surg.* 1999;25:773–780.

Resnik SS, Resnik BI. Complications of chemical peeling. *Dermatol Clin.* 13(2):309–312.

Stone PA, Lefer LG. Modified phenol chemical face peels. *Plast Reconstr Surg.* 2001;9(9):351–376.

Tse Y, Ostad A, Lee HS, et al. A clinical and histologic evaluation of two medium-depth peels: glycolic acid versus Jessner's trichloroacetic acid. *Dermatol Surg.* 1996;22(9):781–786.

3

The Role of Priming the Skin for Peels

Barry I. Resnik

INTRODUCTION

Foundation: That upon which anything is founded; that on which anything stands, and by which it is supported; the lowest and supporting layer of a superstructure; groundwork; basis
Webster's Revised Unabridged Dictionary 1998.

The art of chemical peeling has been a constant in dermatologic surgery for many years. From the use of phenol in the treatment of acne scars in the early 1950s through the delineation of trichloroacetic acid (TCA) as treatment for photodamage, through the use of high percentages of TCA in the treatment of acne scars and benign lesions to the advent of alpha-hydroxy acid (AHA) and beta-hydroxy acids and others, the chemical peel has been the "slow and steady" performer for a variety of conditions. Regardless of the indication, skin priming is a required first step to ensuring the best results. It may be the most valuable step in the peeling treatment of melasma, second only to aggressive sun protection. The various factors involved in skin priming are examined here.

The foundation of an effective chemical peel is skin preparation. This begins in the weeks leading up to the peel and also includes the actual preoperative steps before the peel. With adequate priming, the skin will frost rapidly and more uniformly than unprimed skin. TCA in particular is usually applied expeditiously to minimize discomfort; a more rapid and complete frost will enhance the patient's experience. Although relatively uncommon, adverse effects such as hypopigmentation or hyperpigmentation, delayed reepithelialization, and prolonged erythema may also be minimized, because skip areas are usually minimized as well. Finally, the postoperative phase can be shortened as a result of more rapid healing in primed skin.

Skin priming can be divided into two phases: (1) pretreatment and (2) preparation. These two phases are differentiated and determined by timing and the agents used. The pretreatment phase consists of topical agents applied in the days or weeks preceding the peel. The preparation phase encompasses those steps taken directly before the peel is performed. These include patient degreasing and cleansing just before and upon arrival at the office. The goal of both phases is to thin the epidermal barrier, enhance uniform active agent penetration, accelerate healing, and reduce postoperative side effects and complications, most importantly postinflammatory hyperpigmentation.

PRETREATMENT

Pretreatment refers to the period before the actual peel. A well-planned and executed regimen will enhance any chemical peel. The three major goals are thinning of the stratum corneum, reduction of postinflammatory hyperpigmentation, and faster wound healing. A valuable but less tangible goal is the ability to assess patient compliance and tolerance to the prepeel and postpeel peel regimens, including sunscreens, moisturizers, and other antiaging products. Agents commonly used during the pretreatment phase are hydroquinone, retinoids (tretinoin, retinol, adapalene, tazarotene), glycolic acid, and Kojic acid. Lactic acid, salicylic acid, and azelaic acid are rarely used. Aggressive sun protection may be the most important step in reducing the likelihood of postinflammatory pigment deposition and should accompany all agents.

Most practitioners will pretreat for 2 weeks to 3 months before the peel, with a longer pretreatment time for patients at risk for postinflammatory hyperpigmentation. This author has come to prefer a 1-month period of pretreatment. It is not mandatory, but it is more often than not beneficial to the outcome.

Retinoids, including tretinoin, or all-*trans* retinoic acid, retinol, adapalene, and tazarotene, are arguably the most popular pretreatment agents. Many studies have supported tretinoin's beneficial effects in wound healing. Pretreatment with 0.05% tretinoin cream for 2 weeks has been shown to significantly accelerate healing, regardless of body region. A more rapid and even frost in the pretreated areas has also been noted, regardless of location. Tretinoin pretreatment in dermabrasion cases has also been shown to enhance healing. In a study evaluating the effectiveness of hydroquinone and tretinoin as adjunctive therapy with TCA peels in the treatment of melasma in Indian skin, it was shown that although hydroquinone and tretinoin functioned equally well as adjunctive agents to TCA in the treatment of melasma, only hydroquinone showed a significant decrease in postinflammatory pigment deposition. However, in carbon dioxide (CO_2) resurfacing patients, no significant difference in the incidence of postprocedural hyperpigmentation was found in skin pretreated with 10% glycolic acid, 4% hydroquinone, or 0.025% tretinoin. Tazarotene is not commonly used as an adjunctive priming agent but does have utility in preparing the skin. Retinol (available over the counter in countless preparations) and adapalene, a popular acne therapy, are less irritating and are preferred by some practitioners.

The AHAs, of which glycolic acid is the best known, have been used in all three phases: pretreatment, preparation, and as a superficial peeling agent. Its utility is dependent on the concentration used. At low percentages, keratinocyte adhesion is reduced, whereas at high percentages, superficial to deep peeling can occur. A 2- to 3-week pretreatment period is sufficient to thin the epidermis and prepare the skin for the peel. In patients with keratotic lesions like actinic keratoses, AHAs help thin the hyperkeratotic tissue, increasing the penetration of the peeling agent. Glycolic acid does not have much effect on the incidence of postinflammatory hyperpigmentation. This AHA can also be used in combination with retinoids and hydroquinone. There have been no studies on whether glycolic acid has the same effect on postprocedural healing as tretinoin, but anecdotal experience has shown it to be beneficial in the postprocedural period as well.

Hydroquinone is a tyrosinase inhibitor used to treat conditions of pigmentation, including melasma and postinflammatory pigmentation. It is available commercially in 2% and 4% forms and is compounded in higher percentages. This agent, when used as a priming ingredient in both TCA and glycolic acid peels for melasma, was more effective than retinoic acid 0.025% in reducing this difficult-to-treat condition. Kligman and Willis's original formula consisted of hydroquinone 5%, tretinoin 0.1%, and dexamethasone 0.1%. This original formulation and many modified ones have been used successfully in reducing hyperpigmentation secondary to injury and melasma. The combination of hydroquinone 8%, tretinoin 0.025%, and hydrocortisone 1% (modified Kligman's formula) is one of the most common priming agents. Some physicians are concerned about aberrant pigmentation with higher percentages of hydroquinone. In the author's experience, aberrant pigmentation has not been noted with this formula. Some irritation can be seen in certain patients; expectations should be set appropriately.

Kojic acid is also a tyrosinase inhibitor that can be used in patients who cannot tolerate hydroquinone or have a sensitivity to it. It is most often used in combination with glycolic acid or a retinoid.

It should be noted that most priming regimens produce irritation. The regimen is generally discontinued at least one day before the actual peeling procedure. The degree of irritation noted may require an earlier cessation of the regimen.

Sun protection is important in the priming of skin for peeling. A broad-spectrum UVA/UVB sunscreen with a minimum SPF 30 and Heliocare dietary supplement should be used daily, along with appropriate sun protection measures.

The author's priming regimen of choice is as follows:
- Kligman's formula, modified (hydroquinone 8%, tretinoin 0.025%, and hydrocortisone 1%), applied nightly. This is custom-compounded by a local pharmacy for each patient.
- Glycolic acid foaming cleanser (Topix Pharmaceuticals, Amityville, NY) twice daily. Nondrying gentle cleanser (Topix Pharmaceuticals, Amityville, NY) is used postprocedure.

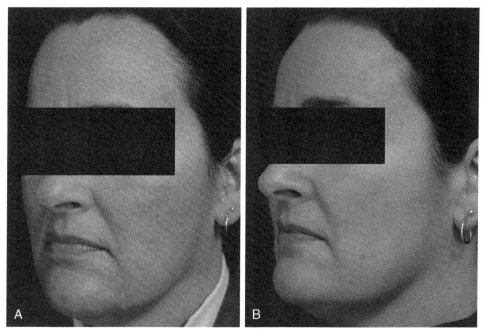

Fig. 3.1 Before (A) and after (B) using topical therapy. Photo courtesy of Suzan Obagi, MD.

- Extreme Moisture with hyaluronic acid moisturizing gel (Topix Pharmaceuticals, Amityville, NY) as needed.
- UltraSheer SPF 50+ sunscreen (Topix Pharmaceuticals, Amityville, NY) twice daily.
- Heliocare Dietary Supplement (Ferndale Laboratories, Ferndale, MI) daily.

This regimen begins 4 weeks before the peel, is stopped 1 day before the peel, and then is resumed at full healing for at least 4 weeks after the peel. Fig. 3.1 shows a patient with melasma treated for 6 weeks with tretinoin 0.05% nightly, 4% hydroquinone twice a day, 6% glycolic acid lotion every morning, and an SPF 50 mineral sunscreen.

PREPARATION

Preparation encompasses those steps that occur directly before, and sometimes those leading into, the peel itself. Uniformity of depth, as well as ease of application and enhanced healing, all figure into this phase of the peel. Degreasers; "depth-enhancing" agents such as Jessner's solution, glycolic acid, and solid CO_2; and applications of topical anesthetics all fall into this time period.

Most dermatologic surgeons will use alcohol, acetone, or a combination of both to degrease the skin before the peel. Chlorhexidine gluconate (Hibiclens), a popular antibacterial scrub, is also used in this manner. It should be noted that chlorhexidine gluconate can cause keratitis and therefore may not be the best choice for facial procedures. The amount of material used, as well as the force and time of application, will have an impact on the depth and uniformity of the peel. The use of different applicators will also have an impact on depth of peel. Cotton-tipped applicators, obstetrical swabs, and gauze squares have all been used to apply peeling agents. These will hold differing amounts of agent, release it at different rates, and allow for varying amounts of pressure during application. The search for the ideal degreasing agent prompted an examination of alcohol, acetone, chlorhexidine gluconate, and Freon Degreaser (trichlorotrifluoroethane) in 35% TCA peeling of the scalp. No differences between the various compounds were found, but the authors cautioned against the use of acetone in conjunction with possible igniters such as electrosurgical units.

Topical anesthetic preparations have been used as both preparatory and postprocedural agents. All contain combinations of "caine" anesthetics in differing vehicles.

They offer pain control as well as skin hydration. The initial formulations required occlusion, but there are multiple commercial and proprietary versions now available that are effective without occlusion. In the author's hands, a combination anesthetic gel obtained from a local compounding pharmacy (20% benzocaine, 6% lidocaine, 4% tetracaine) has proved to be very effective at pain control. The enhanced skin hydration usually combines with the other preparatory steps to deliver a more uniform peel. Differing results were reported with another proprietary formulation compounded in a methylcellulose base. Frosting occurred less rapidly, tended to be patchy, and went deeper than desired. Delayed stinging and discomfort occurred as well. These issues may have been due to the nature of the vehicle as well as to the topical anesthetic itself and do provide a cautionary note. This author has not encountered these issues when using the newer preparations and has determined that their use can be a valuable adjunct to the procedure.

Jessner's solution, consisting of lactic acid, salicylic acid, and resorcinol, is a mild peeling agent in its own right. It is a very safe peel, used primarily for acne treatment and to address light actinic damage. It produces a patchy blanching effect and has a mild postoperative course. Due to its ability to serve as cleanser, degreaser, and peel in one step, it is often combined with TCA in a combination peel, giving an excellent medium-depth peel. In this instance, the Jessner's solution is applied to the skin, and once it has penetrated, it is followed by the application of the TCA peel.

Glycolic acid in 70% strength was shown to promote even penetration of acid and facilitate uniformity of depth. In this instance, the glycolic acid solution is applied to the skin, and once it has penetrated and is neutralized, it is followed by the application of the TCA peel. Jessner's solution and solid CO_2 have also been used in this manner and have proven to be effective preparatory agents in combination with TCA 35% in both the aqueous and clay-chelated forms.

CONCLUSION

The palette approach to chemical peeling begins with a solid foundation. The first stratum is the pretreatment regimen. Epidermal effacement, reduction of potential hyperpigmentation, and enhanced healing are the goals. A more intangible asset of the pretreatment period is the ability to prepare the patient mentally for the procedure. Regular daily application of pretreatment medications enforces the habits necessary for safer and more effective healing postprocedure. Although a poorly executed regimen is not a contraindication to performing the peel, the dermatologic surgeon can better gauge the patient's commitment to treatment when assessing their adherence to the pretreatment regimen. The second stratum is the preparation period. The steps taken during this crucial time just before and during the peel itself are designed to ensure a more even application of agent, produce the desired depth of penetration, and reduce pain and discomfort. Combining a good foundation with excellent technique will help ensure an optimum result.

FURTHER READING

Ayres III S. Superficial chemosurgery in treating aging skin. *Arch Dermatol.* 1962;85:578.

Brody HJ, Hailey CW. Medium-depth chemical peeling of the skin: a variation of superficial chemosurgery. *J Dermatol Surg Oncol.* 1986;12(12):1268–1275.

Buchanan PJ, Gilman RH. Retinoids: literature review and suggested algorithm, for use prior to facial resurfacing procedures. *J Curan Aesthet Surg.* 2016;9:139–144.

Chiarello SE, Resnik BI, Resnik SS. The TCA Masque: a new cream formulation used alone and in combination with Jessner's solution. *Dermatol Surg.* 1996;8:687–690.

Chun EY, Lee JB, Lee KH. Focal trichloroacetic acid peel method for benign pigmented lesions in dark-skinned patients. *Dermatol Surg.* 2004;30(4):512–516; discussion 516.

Coleman III WP, Futrell JM. The glycolic acid trichloroacetic acid peel. *J Dermatol Surg Oncol.* 1994;20(1):76–80.

Garg VK, Sarkar R, Agarwal R. Comparative evaluation of beneficiary effects of priming agents (2% hydroquinone and 0.025% retinoic acid) in the treatment of melasma with glycolic acid peels. *Dermatol Surg.* 2008;34(8):1032–1040.

Hevia O, Nemeth AJ, Taylor JR. Tretinoin accelerates healing after trichloroacetic acid chemical peel. *Arch Dermatol.* 1991;127(5):678–682.

Hung VC, Yu-yun Lee J, Zitelli JA, et al. Topical tretinoin and epithelial wound healing. *Arch Dermatol.* 1989;125:65–69.

Kligman AM, Willis I. A new formula for depigmenting human skin. *Arch Dermatol.* 1975;111(1):40–48.

Koppel RA, Coleman KM, Coleman III WP. The efficacy of EMLA versus ELA-Max for pain relief in medium-depth chemical peeling: a clinical and histopathologic evaluation. *Dermatol Surg.* 2000;26(1):61–64.

Lee JB, Chung WG, Kwahck H, et al. Focal treatment of acne scars with trichloroacetic acid: chemical reconstruction of skin scars method. *Dermatol Surg.* 2002;28(11):1017–1021; discussion 1021.

MacKee GM, Karp FL. The treatment of post-acne scars with phenol. *Br J Dermatol.* 1952;64:456.

Mandy S. Tretinoin in the preoperative and postoperative management of dermabrasion. *J Am Acad Dermatol.* 1986;15(4):878–879, 888–889.

Matarasso SL, Glogau RG, Markey AC. Wood's lamp for superficial chemical peels. *J Am Acad Dermatol.* 1994;30(6):988–992.

Monheit GD. The Jessner's + TCA Peel: a medium depth chemical peel. *J Dermatol Surg Oncol.* 1989;15:924–930.

Moy LS, Howe K, Moy RL. Glycolic acid modulation of collagen production in human skin fibroblast cultures in vitro. *Dermatol Surg.* 1996;22(5):439–441.

Nanda S, Grover C, Reddy BSN. Efficacy of hydroquinone (2%) versus tretinoin (0.025%) as adjunct topical agents for chemical peeling in patients of melasma. *Dermatol Surg.* 2004;30(3):385–389.

Peikert JM, Krywonis NA, Rest EB, et al. The efficacy of various degreasing agents used in trichloroacetic acid peels. *J Dermatol Surg Oncol.* 1994;20(11):724–728.

Resnik SS, Lewis L. The cosmetic uses of trichloroacetic acid peeling in dermatology. *Southern Med J.* 1973;66(2):225–227.

Rubin MG. The efficacy of a topical lidocaine/prilocaine anesthetic gel in 35% trichloroacetic acid peels. *Dermatol Surg.* 1995;21(3):223–225.

Sarkar R, Arsiwala S, Dubey N, et al. Chemical peels in melasma: a review with consensus recommendations by Indian pigmentary expert group. *Indian J Dermatol.* 2017;62:578–584.

Van Scott EJ, Yu RJ. Alpha hydroxy acids: procedures for use in clinical practice. *Cutis.* 1989;43(3):222–228.

West TB, Alster TS. Effect of pretreatment on the incidence of hyperpigmentation following cutaneous CO2 laser resurfacing. *Dermatol Surg.* 1999;25(1):15–17.

4

Light Chemical Peels

Claudia Borelli, Sabrina Fischer

INTRODUCTION

Chemical peels are classified by their level of injury to the skin as very light/very superficial, light/superficial, medium-depth, or deep peels. They can also be classified by their mechanism of action as caustic, metabolic, or toxic peels. They induce a controlled destruction of parts or the whole epidermis with or without the dermis, producing exfoliation with ablation of superficial lesions. The ablation is followed by regeneration of new epidermal and dermal tissue.

Very light or very superficial peels (Table 4.1) are those that lead to a necrosis of the epidermis at the level of the stratum corneum. In contrast, light peels or superficial peels are those that penetrate through the epidermis and lead to necrosis of the entire epidermis down to the level of the stratum granulosum or the basal lamina. Light peels cause reduced corneocyte adhesion and increase the collagen formation in the dermis. In this way they improve the skin's radiance and luminosity.

Light peels are used to treat pigmentary disturbances like solar lentigines, melasma and hyperpigmentation, papulopustular rosacea, superficial acne scars and photoaged or light-damaged skin, as well as to improve skin tone.

The type of chemical peel and depth of the peel is selected according to the severity of the wrinkling, laxity, and the patient's downtime expectations. To enhance cosmetic improvement, topical skin-rejuvenating creams and dermal fillers can be used. Light peels should be repeated to achieve the best possible cosmetic improvement and to obviate recurrence of the skin lesions being addressed.

Schürer and Wiest divide the penetration depths more exactly into five levels (Fig. 4.1): very superficial peels only reach the stratum corneum (level A), and superficial/light peels reach the middle epidermal layers (level B) (Table 4.2). A deeper light peel to a medium-depth peel reaches just below the stratum basale (level C) and in this way causes epidermolysis.[1-5]

Very superficial peels can be repeated every 1 to 2 weeks, and light peels can be repeated every 2 to 4 weeks. Peeling too frequently can result in an increased risk for complications, in particular persistent erythema, postinflammatory hyperpigmentation, infections, and scarring. Because of the simplicity, low morbidity, cost effectiveness and simple availability of solutions, chemical peels still play an important role in treating photoaging and pigmentary disturbances, even though there are more modern techniques available such as lasers.[4,6,7]

PEELING AGENTS: CHEMISTRY AND CHEMICAL FORMULATIONS

Alpha-Hydroxy Acids

Alpha-hydroxy acids (AHAs) are a group of organic acids. They are often referred to as fruit acids, including glycolic acid from cane sugar, citric acid from citrus fruits, and malic acid from apples. The AHAs used for a chemical peeling are produced in chemical laboratories. Additional AHAs also include lactic and mandelic acid. Lactic acid decreases corneocyte cohesion, leading to a thinner stratum corneum. It moisturizes and brightens the skin and improves superficial acne scarring by improving the skin texture and appearance

TABLE 4.1 Agents for Very Light Peels

Peeling Agent	Concentration	Procedure
Trichloroacetic acid (TCA)	10%	Applied in 1 coat
Glycolic acid (GA)	20%–50%	Applied briefly for 1–4 minutes
Salicylic acid	10%–30%	4–6 minutes
Resorcinol	20%–30%	Applied briefly for 5–10 minutes
Jessner's solution	Salicylic acid 14 g, lactic acid (85%) 14 g, resorcinol 14 g with ethanol to make 100 mL	Applied in 1–3 coats
Retinoic acid	1%–5%	Washed off after 4–5 hours

Data from Drake LA, Dinehart SM, Goltz RW et al 1995 Guidelines of care for chemical peeling. Guidelines/Outcomes Committee: American Academy of Dermatology. *Journal of the American Academy of Dermatology* 33:497–503; Khunger N 2008 Standard guidelines of care for chemical peels. *Indian Journal of Dermatology, Venereology and Leprology* 74 Suppl:S5-12; Clark E, Scerri L 2008 Superficial and medium-depth chemical peels. *Clinical Dermatology* 26:209–218; and Committee for Guidelines of Care for Chemical Peeling. Guidelines for chemical peeling in Japan (3rd edition). *Journal of Dermatology.* 2012;39(4):321–325.

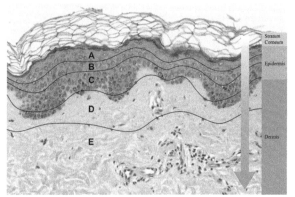

Fig. 4.1 Classification of the depth of peeling in five levels according to Schürer and Wiest. A. very superficial, B. superficial/light, C. medium-depth peel, D. and E. deeper peels (From Rubin MGS, Nanna Y, Wiest LG, Gout U 2014 *Illustrated Guide to Chemical Peels: Basics, Practice, Uses (Aesthetic Methods for Skin Rejuvenation)*. London, Quintessence)

of the scars.[8,9] Mandelic acid has slow skin penetration due to its large molecule size. Therefore, it is considered a safe, light peeling agent. In concentrations of 20% to 50% it has a skin-rejuvenation and lightening effect.[9]

AHAs are considered keratolytic agents because they cause a superficial exfoliation by breaking bonds between keratinocytes in the different layers of the stratum corneum and stratum granulosum. AHAs help to correct an abnormally thickened stratum corneum of the epidermis. This effect lasts for up to 14 days after the end of the therapy. The daily use of topical AHA lotion leads to an increased epidermal thickness.[8] In addition, AHAs lead to an increased dermal thickness by stimulating an increased deposition of collagen and glycosaminoglycans.[8] AHAs are particularly suitable for treating patients with very sensitive skin, a ruddy complexion, telangiectasias, or moderate sun damage.[8-11]

Beta-Hydroxy Acid

Both salicylic acid (SA) and beta-lipohydroxy acid (LHA), which is a derivative of SA, have antibacterial, antiinflammatory, antifungal, and anticomedogenic properties. Due to the additional fatty chain, LHA is more lipophilic than SA and has a more targeted mechanisms of action and a greater keratolytic and comedolytic effect. LHA penetrates well into the sebaceous follicle and through the epidermis, but less deeply into the skin compared with glycolic acids and SA. It is particularly effective in the superficial layers of the stratum corneum, specifically the stratum compactum/disjunctum interface, and focuses its effects on the follicle and epidermis. Neutralization is neither necessary nor possible when peeling with LHAs.[3,4,8]

Retinoic Acid

Retinoic acids (RAs) (all-*trans* retinal and retinoic acid) are usually used alone or in combination with AHAs or other ingredients. RAs lead to a thinner and more compact stratum corneum and a thicker epidermis. They can help to improve dyschromias by creating a more consistent distribution of melanin throughout the epidermis. Furthermore, RAs reverse the number of atypical keratinocytes, thus leading to an improvement or eradication of actinic keratosis.[8] By increasing production of collagen and capillary branching in the dermis, RAs improve skin texture and superficial dyschromias and lead to a pinker, rosier complexion.[8] The side effects of RAs include increased photosensitivity.[8] Exposure to sunlight during treatment should therefore be strictly avoided.[8]

AHAs act mainly on the stratum granulosum, compared with RAs, which mainly act on the stratum corneum.[8] Both AHAs and RAs lead to an increased and accelerated skin turnover from the normal 28 days to 10 to 12 days.

TABLE 4.2	**Agents for Light Peels**	
Peeling Agent	**Concentration**	**Procedure**
Trichloroacetic acid (TCA)	10%–30%	Applied in 1 coat
Glycolic acid (GA)	20%–70%	Applied for a variable time (2–20 minutes)
Salicylic acid	10%–30%	Applied in 1 coat and left on for 5–6 minutes
Mandelic acid	20%–25%	—
Pyruvic acid	40%–60%	Application until erythema occurs, 2–4 minutes
Jessner's solution	Salicylic acid 14 g, lactic acid (85%) 14 g, resorcinol 14 g with ethanol to make 100 mL	Applied in 4–10 coats
Resorcinol	40%–50%	Applied for 30–60 minutes

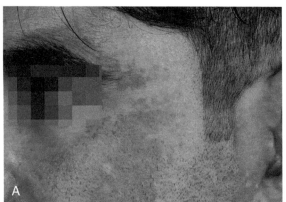
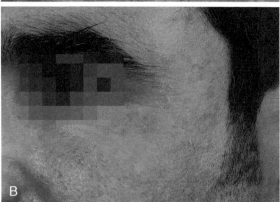

Fig. 4.2 A, Male patient with hyperpigmentation (darker skin type) who received five very superficial chemical peels with glycolic and salicylic acid (20%) every 2 weeks in combination with a 2.5% hydroquinone formulation: before treatment. B, Two weeks after treatment.

RAs and glycolic acids facilitate the distribution of melanin throughout the epidermis. This skin-lightening effect can be used for the treatment or reduction in the incidence of postinflammatory hyperpigmentation (Fig. 4.2).

In addition to the peels, topical products with a lightening effect such as hydroquinone, Kojic acid, or tyrosinase inhibitors can be used. They inhibit tyrosinase, thus blocking the conversion of tyrosine into L-dopa. This may reduce the melanin production of the skin and result in a lower risk of hyperpigmentation. Supplementary treatment with skin-lightening products should be started 2 to 4 weeks before the chemical peel, be continued during the peel, and not be finished until 2 to 3 months after cessation of the peels. The more pronounced the hyperpigmentation and the darker the pigment, the earlier the preconditioning should be started (see Chapter 3).[8]

Salicylic-Mandelic Combination Acid Peels

Salicylic-mandelic combination acid peels, in concentrations of 20% SA and 10% mandelic acid, are effective in treating acne vulgaris and acne scars. One study by Sarkar et al. showed that salicylic-mandelic combination acid peels are better tolerated and therefore more suitable in treating Indian patients with melasma compared with glycolic acid peels (35%).[9-12]

Pyruvic Acid

Pyruvic acid belongs to the α-ketoacids. Pyruvic acid is also effective in treating acne scars because of its keratolytic, antimicrobial, and sebostatic qualities and collagen-building ability. It is used in concentrations of 40% to 70% and causes desquamation during the treatment. It may cause a transient, intense stinging and burning sensation.[11,13]

INDICATIONS

The indications for a superficial peeling include the following:
- Coarse skin, large pores (Fig. 4.3)
- Acne comedonica, papulopustular acne (Fig. 4.4), acne excoriée
- Papulopustular rosacea

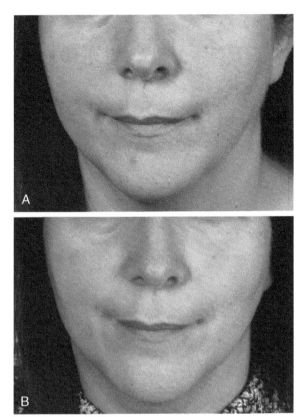

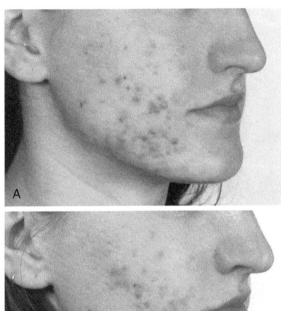

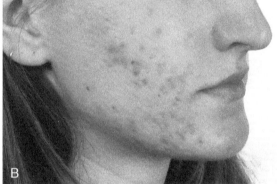

Fig. 4.3 A, Patient who received four superficial chemical peels with glycolic and salicylic acid (20%) every 2 weeks in combination for skin texture. B, Two weeks after treatment.

Fig. 4.4 A, Patient with papulopustular acne. B, After four very superficial chemical peels with glycolic and salicylic acid (20%) every 2 weeks.

- Keratosis pilaris (Fig. 4.5), including ulerythema ophryogenes
- Photodamaged and photoaged skin
- Actinic keratosis
- Dyschromias of the skin including ephelides, lentigines simplex, senile lentigines, flat seborrheic keratoses, melasma (Fig. 4.6), and postinflammatory hyperpigmentation
- Improvement of the skin appearance[1-5,9,10,15]

PATIENT PREPARATION

Priming or preprocedural treatment of the skin before the peel is recommended at least 2 to 4 weeks before the peel. The more pronounced the pigment and the darker the complexion, the longer the priming or preconditioning should be.

Adequate priming of the skin helps reduce wound healing time, facilitates uniform penetration of the peeling agent, reduces the risk of possible side effects, strengthens patient compliance, and helps detect intolerances at an early stage. In addition, a daily use of broad-spectrum sunscreen (SPF 50+) and sun avoidance are crucial for the treatment.

Patients should be instructed not to perform any bleaching, scrubbing, waxing therapies or depilatories, or massage in the treatment area throughout the time that chemical peels are being performed.

Prophylactic antiviral therapy is recommended for patients prone to herpes simplex infections, for example with acyclovir 200 mg four times per day (400 mg two times) or valacyclovir 500 mg one-two times per day, starting 1 day before the peel and for 5 to 14 days, until reepithelialization is completed.[1-4,8,9,11-13] Antiviral therapy is continued for a longer duration for deeper peels than for lighter peels.

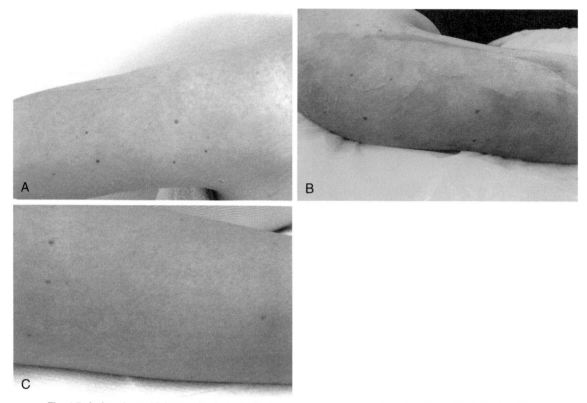

Fig. 4.5 A, A patient with keratosis pilaris. B, Scaling some days after peeling. C, After epithelialization. (Courtesy Dr. Luitgard Wiest.)

PEELING TECHNIQUE

Salicylic Acid Peel and General Instructions

Before starting the chemical peel, it is very important to ensure that the patient performed the skin priming and strict daily sun protection/sun avoidance reliably. There should be precise documentation of the dosage, duration, and condition of the treated skin after each peel, as well as a chemical peel consent form.

After exclusion of active viral, mycotic, or bacterial infections, the patient's face is cleaned with a mild soap and water. The hair is held back by a band or cap.

The patient should be positioned lying on the back with the head elevated at 45 degrees or less and is asked to keep the eyes closed throughout the whole procedure.

Because of the thinner stratum corneum, xerosis, and an increased sensitivity of certain areas, the acid can be absorbed more quickly in areas like the nasolabial fold, the lateral canthus of the eye, the oral commissures, and the chin. These sensitive areas should be protected with petroleum jelly before the application of the peel. Additionally, the eyes should be covered with 2-inch by 2-inch moist gauze pieces. The skin is then cleaned with alcohol-soaked 2-inch by 2-inch cotton gauze pieces and degreased with acetone.

The required peeling agent is poured into a glass beaker or cup. The neutralization solution or cream should be placed in a glass cup and a syringe filled with saline or water, to flush the eyes in case of accidental exposure of the eyes to the peel solution.

It is important to check the label of the bottle to make sure the correct acid is being used before applying the peel. The neutralization solution should also be ready, and this should be checked before starting the procedure. To avoid dripping of the peel solution into the eyes, the opened bottle or soaked applicator should never be passed over the patient's face/eyes.

The peeling agent is applied evenly and quickly to the face using a brush, cotton-tipped applicator, or gauze. The application starts from the forehead, then

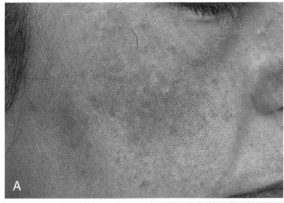

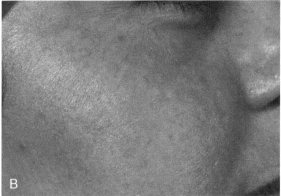

Fig. 4.6 A, Patient with melasma (darker skin type) who received four very superficial chemical peels with glycolic and salicylic acid (20%) every 2 weeks in combination with a 2.5% hydroquinone formulation: before treatment. B, Eight weeks after last chemical peeling (ongoing home care regimen with depigmenting formulation and alpha-hydroxy acids).

proceeds to the right temple and cheek, nose, left temple and cheek, to the chin. If a treatment of the upper or lower eyelids or perioral region is required, these areas are treated last. To avoid demarcation lines and to blend with the surrounding untreated skin, feathering strokes are applied on the edges.

The application of SA peels leads to crystallization, which leads to the formation of a "pseudofrost." In SA peels, one to three layers are usually applied to achieve an even pseudofrost. After 3 to 5 minutes, the peel is washed off with water once the burning has subsided. The patient is asked to continue washing the face with cold water until the burning sensation ceases. The face is then dabbed dry with gauze. Rubbing the skin should be avoided.

Tretinoin peels are yellow peels. They are left on for an exposure time of 4 to 5 hours and are then washed off.

Very superficial peels can be repeated every 1 to 2 weeks, superficial peels every 2 to 4 weeks.[2,4,8]

Glycolic Acid Peels

Glycolic acid is the most commonly used AHA as a peeling agent. AHA peels are nontoxic, systemically safe, and well tolerated by patients and are associated with a low incidence of manageable complications. In low concentrations (5% to 15%), glycolic acid can be used for daily skin care. Concentrations of 20% to 70% are used to perform chemical peels. The higher the concentration of the solution and the longer the exposure time, the deeper the penetration depth of the peel.

When using a glycolic acid peel, the peeling agent has to be neutralized after a certain, predetermined time, usually 3 to 5 minutes. Once the desired penetration depth has been reached or the predetermined application time is reached, AHA peels must be neutralized to terminate their effect.

If erythema or epidermolysis occurs, which often appears as a greyish white discoloration of the epidermis or small blisters (so-called "frost"), the peeling agent must be neutralized immediately regardless of the time. For neutralization, 10% to 15% sodium bicarbonate solution or neutralization lotion is used, which is then washed off with water, which causes a fizzing on the face. The acid can also be neutralized by washing the face with water. Care must be taken to make sure that the complete acid is neutralized.

Glycolic acid solutions with a low pH value cause erythema, irritation, stinging, and burning pain and are less tolerated by patients. They also do not penetrate the skin evenly. Therefore it is recommended to use solutions with a higher pH value.

According to the penetration depth of a superficial peeling, the skin first turns pink, then red, signifying intraepidermal wounding. The occurrence of frost signifies dermal injury. A bland emollient is suitable for posttreatment. Glycolic acid peels can be repeated at 2 to 4 week intervals until the desired result is achieved. These peels are particularly suitable for the treatment of mottled hyperpigmentation, fine wrinkles, and sun-damaged skin (Fig. 4.7). They can also be applied on other sun-damaged areas like the dorsum of the hands, the neck, and the chest, but the peel needs to be superficial outside the face to avoid scarring.[8] Dark pigmentation and moderate wrinkling are mostly resistant to the treatment with glycolic acid.

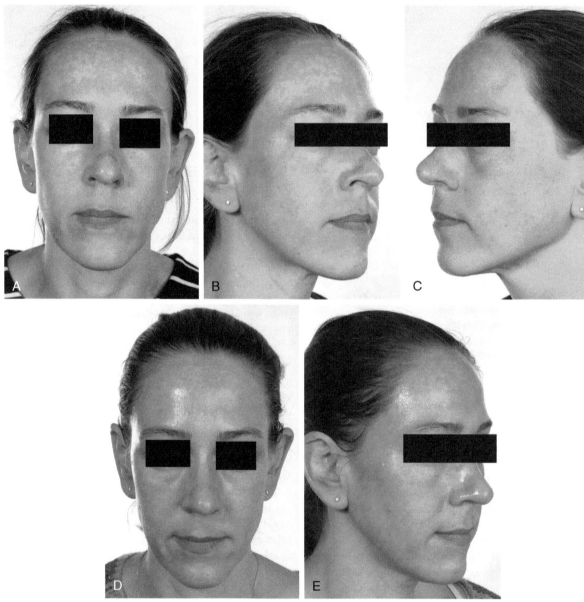

Fig. 4.7 A–C, Patient with mottled skin and melasma before treatment, baseline. D, Directly after chemical peeling (third time) with glycolic and salicylic acid (20%) every 2 weeks in combination with a 2.5% hydroquinone formulation. E–F, Immediately after the peel. G–I (see next page), After eight chemical peelings with glycolic and salicylic acid (20%) every 2 weeks in combination with a 2.5% hydroquinone formulation.

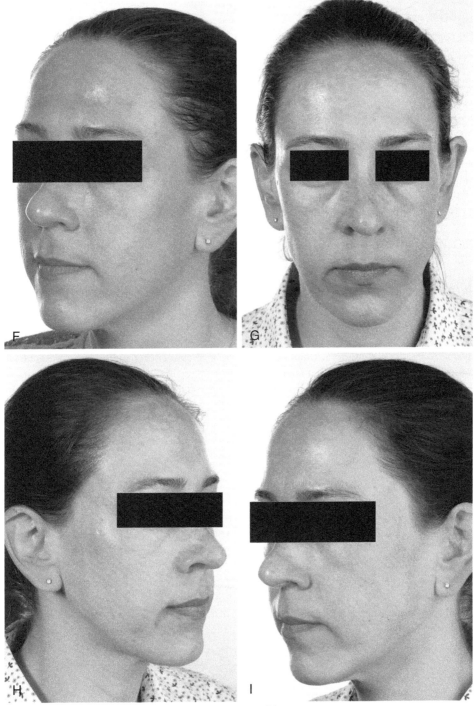

Fig. 4.7, cont'd

Jessner's Solution Peels

Jessner's solution consists of the following components: SA 14 g, lactic acid (85%) 14 g, and resorcinol 14 g with ethanol to make 100 mL.[8] It is used for light peels or as a priming agent before a TCA peel. The penetration depth of the peeling depends on the number of coats of solution applied.

For a very superficial peel (level A), one to three coats are applied. A slight erythema is formed, which can be associated with a slightly whitish-powdery appearance of the skin. This white precipitate is caused by the precipitation of SA on the skin and can easily be wiped off. There is no coagulation (frost). For 1 to 2 days a slight exfoliation of the skin may occur, or none at all.

For a superficial peel (level B) 4 to 10 coats are applied. An erythema is formed and pinpoints of white frost occur. For 15 to 30 minutes, mild to moderate burning and stinging occurs. The following 1 to 3 days, the skin turns slightly red-brown and feels very tight. For 2 to 4 days there is exfoliation with flaking, but rarely peeling of the skin.

If more layers of Jessner's solution are applied, a deeper penetration depth is achieved, which is accompanied by increasing formation of frost and subsequent exfoliation lasting 8 to 10 days.

The penetration depth depends not only on the number of coats of solution applied, but also on the preparation or priming of the skin, the thickness of the stratum corneum, and the sensitivity of the skin. It may therefore vary slightly from patient to patient. The solution should be left on the skin for 4 to 6 minutes to assess the full effect of the solution on the skin.

In the healing phase, a mild moisturizing treatment should be applied to offset the tight and mask-like feeling of the skin. In case of persistent stinging or persistent sensitivity, a mild topical steroid can be applied. Makeup may be used during the healing phase. Facial toners, peels, scrubs, masks, or RAs may only be used 48 hours after the peeling has healed.

The advantages of a Jessner's peel are its very superficial effect, that it goes rarely deeper than expected, and that it is safe and has few side effects. Because of the low amount of resorcinol and SA, toxicity only plays a role in the treatment of very large areas, such as the simultaneous treatment of face, chest, arms, and lower legs.[8]

Trichloroacetic Acid Peels

TCA peels with a concentration of 10% to 25% TCA are suitable for intraepidermal peels. With concentrations of 30% to 40%, a deeper peel reaching the papillary dermis can be achieved. TCA peels are often used as a medium-depth peel to treat pigmentation disorders and early facial rhytids.

The application of several coats or overlap of coats should be avoided to prevent deep wounding. It is recommended to treat the region of the eyebrows and also a little beyond the hairline and jawline. A very light peel results in some erythema, and irregular patches of light frosting (speckled frosting) may occur, which heals after 2 to 4 days of mild flaking. A light TCA peel that penetrates the entire epidermis results in erythema and an "almost" uniform white frost, which heals within 5 days (Figs. 4.8 and 4.9). The TCA peel is washed off with cold water and a gentle cleanser.[2,4,8]

POSTPEEL CARE

The goal of a good aftercare routine is to minimize the risk of side effects and complications and to achieve an early "restitutio ad integrum" regeneration of the skin. This is particularly important for darker skinned patients, who have an increased risk of postinflammatory hyperpigmentation. A careful postpeeling treatment is crucial for most patients to maximize the results of the peel.

After the chemical peel, erythema, mild edema, and desquamation occur. These last for 1 to 3 days in superficial peels. After 3 to 5 days, the epidermis is usually completely reepithelialized.

A mild soap or gentle nonsoap cleanser can be used. In case of crusting, a topical antibacterial therapy should be used to avoid bacterial superinfections. The patients must be given clear instructions for the postpeel period. To soothe the skin, cold compresses can be used. Patients should be instructed to the daily use of broad-spectrum sunscreen (SPF 50+) and sun avoidance and to use only light moisturizing lotions until the skin has completely healed. Patients are instructed to avoid manipulating, picking, or scratching the skin or treated areas. They must avoid all sports and sweating during the healing process. Usually analgesics are not necessary.

In addition, patients should be informed of early warning signs of complications such as severe and

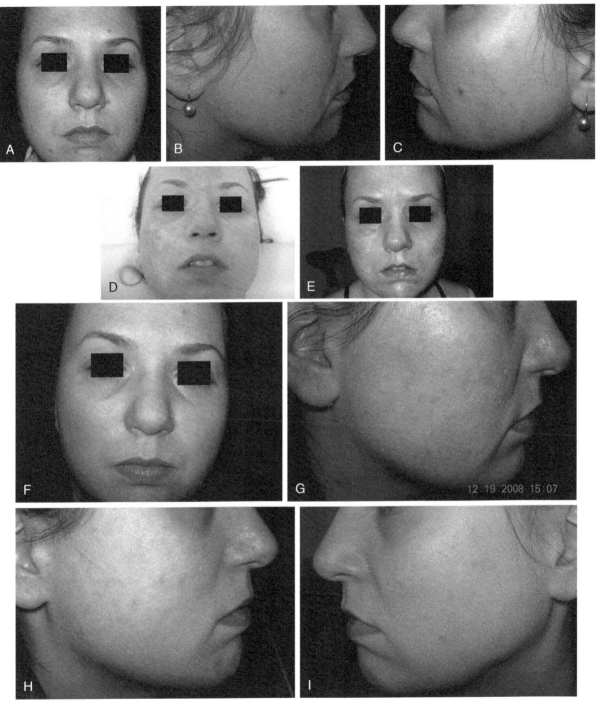

Fig. 4.8 A–C, Patient before treatment. D, Chemical peeling with trichloroacetic acid 20%, beginning of frost. E, Directly after, treatment with cream. F–G, After 1 month. H–I, After 2 months. (Courtesy Dr. Luitgard Wiest.)

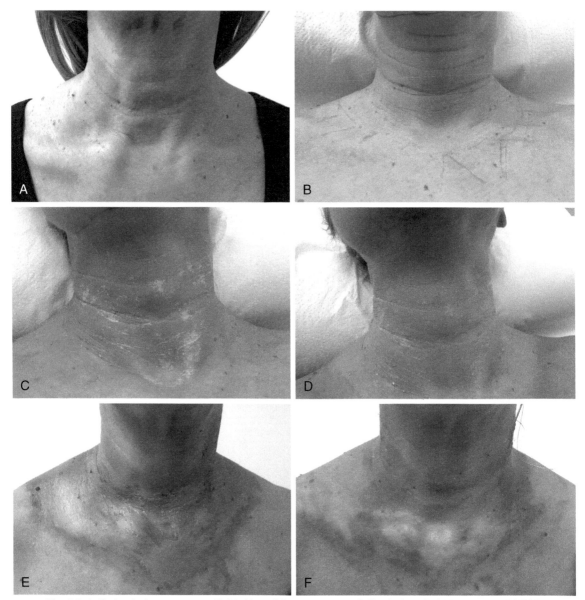

Fig. 4.9 A, Patient before treatment. B, Marking of the area to treat. C, Beginning of trichloroacetic acid (TCA) frost (15% TCA). D, TCA frost. E, Three days after chemical peeling. F, Seven days after chemical peeling. (Courtesy Dr. Luitgard Wiest.)

prolonged erythema, edema, burning sensation, crusting, hyperpigmentation, or formation of pustules or vesicles. In addition to close postpeel follow-up treatment, patients should be instructed to immediately report any early signs of complications to initiate a therapy at an early stage. Patients should be given a contact number for such emergencies.[1-4,8,9]

CONTRAINDICATIONS AND COMPLICATIONS

Contraindications

Absolute contraindications of superficial chemical peels include active bacterial, viral, or fungal infections; open wounds; pregnancy; and breastfeeding.

Additional relative contraindications include the use of photosensitizing drugs or the presence of inflammatory skin diseases. Patients with unrealistic expectations and noncompliant patients, for example patients who presumably do not adhere to strict sun protection and sun avoidance or do not perform the preconditioning or priming before and after treatment, should not be treated.[2,9]

Complications

Superficial peels are quite safe and have fewer side effects and complications than deeper peels (Table 4.3).[3]

TABLE 4.3	Complications
Tears	By tears running down the cheeks, the peeling agent in the area of the cheeks can be neutralized prematurely and may cause the tears to transfer the peel solution to areas such as the neck or the ears. It is very important to dab off all tears immediately and to wash and neutralize the fallen tears as quickly as possible with water.
Premature peeling	Premature peeling of the skin is associated with an increased risk of several side effects such as infection, persistent erythema, postinflammatory hyperpigmentation, and scarring. It may occur accidentally or by manipulation of peeled skin (e.g., picking at the treated skin). Early and aggressive therapy with oral antibiotic is recommended until complete reepithelialization.
Infections	The risk of infections increases with the depth of the peeling. • Bacterial infections (staphylococci, streptococci, pseudomonas, nitrobacteria) • Viral infections (herpes simplex, varicella) • Mycoses (Candida) An adequate, early, and aggressive therapy is indispensable to avoiding scarring.
Acneiform eruptions	Acneiform eruptions may present as multiple erythematous follicular papules and may occur during or shortly after the peel. They are treated with oral antibiotics, commonly used in the treatment of acne.
Postinflammatory hyperpigmentation (PIH)	Patients with dark skin type are particularly at higher risk for PIH. It may occur very soon or several months after the peel, is often associated with a too early sun exposure after the peeling, persists, and is very difficult to treat. The daily use of broad-spectrum sunscreen (SPF 50+) and sun avoidance is indispensable for the treatment. Epidermal PIH responds well to therapy with topical steroids, tretinoin, hydroquinone, Kojic acids, alpha-hydroxy acids, and light peels (e.g., with 10% trichloroacetic acid, Jessner's solution, or 50%–70% glycolic acid).
Persistent erythema	Erythema lasting longer than 3 weeks after the peeling may be a sign of an impending hypertrophic scarring. A therapy with highly potent topical corticosteroids (class 1) for about 2 weeks is recommended.
Scarring	Scarring is a rare side effect in light peels. The risk of scarring can be reduced with appropriate priming or prepeel treatment, the right choice of exfoliating agents, and appropriate follow-up treatment and care. Particularly at risk are patients with a history of poor wound healing, hypertrophic scars and keloids, a recent therapy with isotretinoin in the last 1–2 months, infection in the treatment area, deep peels, or too short of a time interval between peels, or a peel that is performed too soon after surgery in the treatment area.

Data from Drake LA, Dinehart SM, Goltz RW et al 1995 Guidelines of care for chemical peeling. Guidelines/Outcomes Committee: American Academy of Dermatology. *Journal of the American Academy of Dermatology* 33:497–503; Khunger N 2008 Standard guidelines of care for chemical peels. *Indian Journal of Dermatology, Venereology and Leprology* 74 Suppl:S5-12; Rendon MI, Berson DS, Cohen JL, et al 2010 Evidence and considerations in the application of chemical peels in skin disorders and aesthetic resurfacing. *Journal of Clinical Aesthetic Dermatology* 3:32–43; Clark E, Scerri L 2008 Superficial and medium-depth chemical peels. *Clinical Dermatology* 26:209–218; Kontochristopoulos G, Platsidaki E 2017 Chemical peels in active acne and acne scars. *Clinical Dermatology* 35:179–182; Garg VK, Sinha S, Sarkar R 2009 Glycolic acid peels versus salicylic-mandelic acid peels in active acne vulgaris and post-acne scarring and hyperpigmentation: a comparative study. *Dermatologic Surgery* 35:59–65; and Berardesca E, Cameli N, Primavera G, Carrera M 2006 Clinical and instrumental evaluation of skin improvement after treatment with a new 50% pyruvic acid peel. *Dermatologic Surgery* 32:526–531.

PRACTICAL TIPS AND CONCLUSION

The best way to avoid complications is to identify patients at risk and to use lighter peels or to avoid peels altogether. The deeper the chemical peel and the darker the skin type, the higher the risk of complications. Patients at risk are those with dark skin type, a history of hyperpigmentation, hypertrophic scarring or keloids, high exposure to sunlight, outdoor occupations (e.g., field workers), history of photosensitivity or patients taking photosensitizing drugs, patients who were treated with isotretinoin in the last 1 to 2 months, patients with very sensitive skin or atopic dermatitis or who do not tolerate topical sun protection or hydroquinone, those with dry skin and a reddish skin tone, patients with recurrent herpes infections, and uncooperative patients or patients with low compliance and unrealistic expectations.[2,3,8]

AHAs peels are particularly suited for priming patients with very sensitive skin, reddish complexion, or telangiectasias or patients with severe sun exposure. Glycolic acid peels are also suitable for other sun-damaged areas like the neck, dorsum of the hands, and the chest but are currently most popular in the treatment of melasma. They lead to an improvement of mottled hyperpigmentation and fine wrinkling. Glycolic acid peels are also used in the treatment of acne, postinflammatory hyperpigmentation, shallow acne scars, papulopustular rosacea, seborrheic and actinic keratoses, keratosis pilaris, and some verrucae that are resistant to conventional treatments. AHAs increase ultraviolet (UV) sensitivity, whereas LHA leads to an increased resistance of the skin to UV-induced damage.[3,8,16-18]

Beta-hydroxy acids peels, especially SA or LHA, are excellent for treating patients with acne because of their lipophilic and strong comedolytic effect. Kessler et al. showed in a split-face study that both glycolic acid and SA are similarly effective, but SA peels had better sustained efficiency 2 months after the treatment (blinded evaluator and number of acne lesions) and fewer side effects. SA peels are also effective in the treatment of dyschromias like melasma and postinflammatory hyperpigmentation, oily skin, rough skin texture, and mild photodamage, but less effective in patients with significant photodamage.

Salicylic-mandelic combination acid peels, in concentration of 20% SA and 10% mandelic acid, are proven effective in treating acne vulgaris and acne scars and seem to be well tolerated and therefore suitable in treating Indian patients with melasma, compared with glycolic acid peels (35%).[3,8,11,12,19-21]

RA peels are often used in combination with AHAs peels, particularly in patients with oily and thick skin. AHA peels act mainly on stratum granulosum, whereas RA peels mainly act on stratum corneum. LHA and RA improve the surface texture.[3,8]

Jessner's peels are ideal for patients with dyschromias because they create a fairly uniform peel with a distinctive amount of exfoliation. Jessner's solution peels are also used in the therapy of mild acne scarring, often as a combined peel with TCA. Disadvantages of Jessner's solution peels include erythema and discoloration, which are often not easy to cover up with makeup.[3,8]

RA peels are very suitable for treating patients with melasma and postinflammatory hyperpigmentation.

TCA peels are mostly used to treat pigmentation disorders and early facial rhytides with medium-depth peels.[3,8]

REFERENCES

1. Drake LA, Dinehart SM, Goltz RW, et al. Guidelines of care for chemical peeling. Guidelines/Outcomes Committee: American Academy of dermatology. *J Am Acad Dermatol.* 1995;33(3):497–503.
2. Khunger N. Standard guidelines of care for chemical peels. *Indian J Dermatol Venereol Leprol.* 2008;74(suppl):S5–S12.
3. Rendon MI, Berson DS, Cohen JL, Roberts WE, Starker I, Wang B. Evidence and considerations in the application of chemical peels in skin disorders and aesthetic resurfacing. *J Clin Aesthet Dermatol.* 2010;3(7):32–43.
4. Rubin MGS, Nanna Y. / Wiest, Luitgard G. / Gout, Uliana. *Illustrated Guide to Chemical Peels: Basics, Practice, Uses (Aesthetic Methods for Skin Rejuvenation).* 1st ed. London; Chicago: Quintessence Publishing/KVM; 2014:280.
5. Wiest LG, Habig J. [Chemical peel treatments in dermatology]. *Hautarzt.* 2015;66(10):744–747.
6. Baumann L. *Cosmetic Dermatology: Principles and Practice.* 2nd ed. United States: McGraw-Hill Education / Medical; 2009.
7. Rullan P, Karam AM. Chemical peels for darker skin types. *Facial Plast Surg Clin North Am.* 2010;18(1):111–131.
8. Clark E, Scerri L. Superficial and medium-depth chemical peels. *Clin Dermatol.* 2008;26(2):209–218.
9. Kontochristopoulos G, Platsidaki E. Chemical peels in active acne and acne scars. *Clin Dermatol.* 2017;35(2):179–182.

10. Bennett M L, Henderson R L. Introduction to cosmetic dermatology. *Curr Probl Dermatol.* 2003;15(2):43–83.
11. Sarkar R, Garg V, Bansal S, Sethi S, Gupta C. Comparative evaluation of efficacy and tolerability of glycolic acid, salicylic mandelic acid, and phytic acid combination peels in melasma. *Dermatol Surg.* 2016;42(3):384–391.
12. Garg VK, Sinha S, Sarkar R. Glycolic acid peels versus salicylic-mandelic acid peels in active acne vulgaris and post-acne scarring and hyperpigmentation: a comparative study. *Dermatol Surg.* 2009;35(1):59–65.
13. Berardesca E, Cameli N, Primavera G, Carrera M. Clinical and instrumental evaluation of skin improvement after treatment with a new 50% pyruvic acid peel. *Dermatol Surg.* 2006;32(4):526–531.
14. Guidelines for chemical peeling in Japan (3rd edition). *Jdermatol.* 2012;39(4):321–325.
15. Chen X, Wang S, Yang M, Li L. Chemical peels for acne vulgaris: a systematic review of randomised controlled trials. *BMJ Open.* 2018;8(4):e019607.
16. Erbil H, Sezer E, Tastan B, Arca E, Kurumlu Z. Efficacy and safety of serial glycolic acid peels and a topical regimen in the treatment of recalcitrant melasma. *J Dermatol.* 2007;34(1):25–30.
17. Rani S, Sharma P. Glycolic acid peel in disseminated facial verrucae. *J Cosmet Laser Ther.* 2017;19(8):475–478.
18. Sharad J. Glycolic acid peel therapy - a current review. *Clin Cosmet Investig Dermatol.* 2013;6:281–288.
19. Grimes PE. The safety and efficacy of salicylic acid chemical peels in darker racial-ethnic groups. *Dermatol Surg.* 1999;25(1):18–22.
20. Kessler E, Flanagan K, Chia C, Rogers C, Glaser DA. Comparison of alpha- and beta-hydroxy acid chemical peels in the treatment of mild to moderately severe facial acne vulgaris. *Dermatol Surg.* 2008;34(1):45–50; discussion 1.
21. Pierard GE, Rougier A. Nudging acne by topical beta-lipohydroxy acid (LHA), a new comedolytic agent. *Eur J Dermatol.* 2002;12(4):Xlvii–xlviii.

5

Medium-Depth Peels and Trichloroacetic Acid Blue Peel

Suzan Obagi

INTRODUCTION

Medium-depth chemical peels remain very important and highly versatile tools for skin resurfacing and rejuvenation. Although newer laser technology has added to the arsenal of tools for skin resurfacing, these lasers are either cost-prohibitive for certain patients, not advisable for certain skin types, or, most importantly, not as flexible for the physicians who like to tailor their skin-resurfacing approach for each patient. When performed correctly, chemical peels can play an important role in cosmetic surgery and can be tailored to address most skin issues. Advanced chemical peel techniques can be used in combination with laser resurfacing, nonablative lasers, and surgical procedures to enhance the overall outcome for patients.

INDICATIONS FOR MEDIUM-DEPTH CHEMICAL PEELS

Indications for light and deep peels will be covered in other chapters in this textbook. This chapter will focus on medium-depth peels. Knowledge of skin anatomy and where in the skin a particular skin pathology (wrinkles, lentigines, melasma, scars, actinic keratosis) exists is crucial to performing a safe and effective resurfacing procedure (Table 5.1). If one resurfaces too superficially, the patient's chief complaint may be missed. Conversely, resurfacing deeper than is required only increases the risk of complications and prolongs the recovery time.

AGING SKIN (INTRINSIC AND EXTRINSIC)

Many complex changes are occurring in the skin that reflect both intrinsic and extrinsic aging. Starting around the age of 18 years, there is a natural decline in fibroblast function resulting in decreased collagen and elastin production, which is referred to as "intrinsic aging." This reduction is on the order of approximately 1% per year starting at the age of 18 years. External factors such as ultraviolet radiation (UVR), high-energy visible light, and infrared light act on the skin to accelerate the aging process and is known as "extrinsic aging." At the epidermal level, the normal cycling of the keratinocytes slows with age, but with extrinsic aging, the epidermis begins to show roughness, dyschromia, and keratinocyte atypia.

PATIENT EVALUATION

Chapter 2 of this textbook covers patient evaluation in more depth. Some points worth reiterating are mentioned here. Of utmost importance is the proper selection of the resurfacing modality for the patient and the patient's concerns and the proper preparation of the patient's skin before and after skin resurfacing (see Chapter 3). Be sure to evaluate the patient for skin flaws and scars and to document skin imperfections at the time of consultation and to take high-quality before-and-after photographs for each procedure. Similarly, showing

TABLE 5.1   Clinical Indications for Skin Resurfacing

Anatomical Skin Level	Clinical Presentation	Treatment Options
Epidermis	Epidermal melasma Actinic keratosis Seborrheic keratosis[a] Solar lentigines (sunspots) Ephelides (freckles)	Topical products Superficial peels Pigment lasers[c]
Dermis	Dermal melasma Wrinkles: depth varies Scars: depth varies Telangiectasias[b] Sebaceous hyperplasias[a] Syringomas*	Medium-depth resurfacing to deep peels Vascular lasers
Epidermis and dermis	Mixed-type melasma	Medium-depth resurfacing

[a]Best treated with electrodessication (using an epilating needle for dermal lesions)
[b]Best treated with chromophore specific lasers
[c]Use cautiously in melasma patients

TABLE 5.2   Patient Social and Medical History

	Pertinent History	Relative Contraindications	Absolute Contraindications

Medical	Medications
	Systemic illnesses
	Psychiatric illnesses
	Depression
	  OCD
	  BDD
	MRSA history
	Radiation to the treated area
	HSV or VZV tendency
	Hormone contraceptives
	  including hormone IUDs
		Active inflammatory skin disease
		  such as acne, rosacea, CTD
		Vitiligo
		Bariatric surgery with nutritional
		  deficiency diabetes
		Isotretinoin current or recent
			Active infection at the treatment
			  site
			History of keloids at the treatment
			  site: avoid reticular dermis level
			  procedures
			Pregnancy

Social	Smoking history Chronic sun exposure	Smoking/vaping/nicotine use	Inability to follow instructions Unrealistic expectations

BDD, Body dysmorphic disorder; *CTD*, connective tissue disease; *HSV*, herpes simplex virus; *IUD*, intrauterine device; *MRSA*, methicillin-resistant *Staphylococcus aureus*; *OCD*, obsessive-compulsive disorder; *VZV*, varicella zoster virus.

patients high-quality before-and-after photographs is extremely useful and allows the patient to gauge whether this treatment is giving the amount of improvement they seek. Showing photographs also helps the physician to identify patients with unrealistic expectations.

Patient evaluation should include a thorough medical, social, and family history to identify any possible contraindication to skin resurfacing (Table 5.2). Patients should be examined with no makeup on in a well-lit room. Acne scar patients should be examined with indirect overhead light to allow shadows to be cast on the skin to better delineate scar morphology. Skin conditions that can Koebnerize to areas that are resurfaced should be identified as well (i.e., flat warts, vitiligo, psoriasis) (Fig. 5.1).

Patients being treated for melasma should be questioned about the use of hormone intrauterine devices (IUDs), hormone cervical rings, or oral contraceptives. The use of hormone contraceptives will continue to stimulate the melasma and may lead to treatment failure or worsening of the condition.

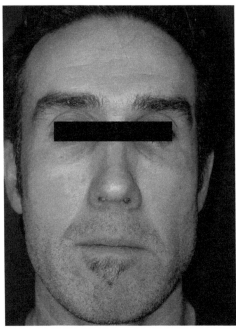

Fig. 5.1 A patient with vitiligo is at risk for Koebnerization.

CONSIDERATIONS IN MEDIUM-DEPTH SKIN RESURFACING

Chapter 2 offers a more detailed discussion on contraindications for skin resurfacing. The beauty of a properly performed chemical peel is that with the correct patient skin preparation and proper peel depth penetration, patients of most skin types can be treated. Furthermore, areas that are usually not amenable to laser resurfacing can be safely peeled with the proper chemical peel (Table 5.3), allowing for safe combination resurfacing in one sitting to give overall rejuvenation with no lines of demarcation. Similarly, with the proper skin preconditioning, patients of most ethnicities can be treated. Patients with darker complexions still remain at higher risk for temporary postinflammatory hyperpigmentation (PIH) with any peel and permanent hypopigmentation with peels that reach the reticular dermis. The risk of PIH in a darker-skinned patient can be reduced by extending the length of skin preconditioning to 3 months rather than the usual 6 weeks. Thus, although the risk of PIH is not a contraindication to resurfacing, it should be anticipated and addressed before resurfacing.

Medium-depth and deep peels require a healthy nutritional status and well-functioning immune system

TABLE 5.3 Anatomical Areas Safe for Light and Medium-Depth Peels

Peel Depth	Clinical Presentation	Anatomical Areas
Light peels to the basal layer of the epidermis	Epidermal melasma Actinic keratosis Solar lentigines (sunspots) Ephelides (freckles)	Hairline Eyebrows Eyelids Ears Lips Neck Décolletage of chest
Medium-depth peels to the papillary dermis level	Dermal melasma Lentigines Actinic cheilitis Wrinkles: depth varies Scars: depth varies	Hairline Eyebrows Eyelids Ears Lips Neck Décolletage of chest
Deep peels to the reticular or mid-reticular dermis[a]	Scars: ice-pick (CROSS[b] technique) Wrinkles: deep	Cheeks Perioral Periorbital[c]

[a]Proper patient selection is crucial.
[b]Chemical reconstruction of skin scars
[c]See chapters on phenol peels for various peel strengths to safely address these areas.

for uneventful wound healing. Patients who have undergone bariatric surgery often are deficient in vital nutrients, iron, and protein. Blood laboratory tests can help identify issues. Transplant patients or those on medications for autoimmune diseases are functionally immunologically impaired, putting them at risk for infection. These patients may require coverage with an oral antibiotic during the healing period (penicillin, cephalosporin, or trimethoprim/sulfamethoxazole).

Recent oral retinoid use was once considered an absolute contraindication for skin resurfacing due to concerns of increased hypertrophic scar formation in these patients. Many recent studies and case series have shown that this concern may not be valid. Patients having laser hair removal, laser skin resurfacing, or medium-depth peels in these studies did not demonstrate increased adverse outcomes. Although these studies may be small, they do show the complexities associated with keloid formation, and they challenge the conventional thinking that isotretinoin impairs wound healing. As described in Chapter 12, the author uses isotretinoin during the recovery phase if indicated to control oiliness and inflammation, but the same author does wait 6 months out from isotretinoin treatment before performing a deep peel. For medium-depth peels, it may be prudent to stop isotretinoin 3 to 4 months before the peel. If a patient has an inflammatory condition such as acne or rosacea, oral antiinflammatory antibiotics (doxycycline) can be used temporarily.

The timing of skin resurfacing with surgical procedures is important, because patients like the idea of maximizing their treatments and reducing the amount of time they have to take off from work or daily activities. Studies have shown the safety of skin resurfacing with browlifts, blepharoplasties, and rhytidectomies. Care has to be taken to minimize the depth of resurfacing over flaps (basal layer or papillary dermis level peel) and kept away from incisions, whereas the peel or laser resurfacing can be deeper over the central face (nonundermined skin).

As with any elective procedure, the absolute contraindications to resurfacing include pregnancy, active infection at the treatment site, significant tendency to develop keloids, and the inability to adhere to postoperative instructions.

MEDIUM-DEPTH SKIN RESURFACING

Mechanisms of Action

Peels are sometimes referred to as light or deep depending on the acid used and the concentration of the acid. However, by classifying peel depth solely by acid or concentration is misleading and dangerous, because there are many factors that affect peel depth. One should take into consideration the following variables that can affect peel depth: acid concentration, the volume of acid applied, skin thickness, percentage body surface area treated, skin preconditioning, and, in some cases, the duration of contact of the acid on the skin. Chapter 1 covers, in depth, the various types of chemical peel acids and their physical and chemical properties.

For medium-depth peeling, it is important to understand the main mechanism of action of the acid on the skin, especially when performing combination peels (Table 5.4). This is either a keratolytic effect or a protein denaturant effect. The keratolytics are mainly

TABLE 5.4	Chemical Peel Formulas
Acid Properties	**Commonly Used Concentrations & Formulations**
Keratolytics	Salicylic acid peels 15%–30%
	Glycolic acid 50%–70%
	Jessner's solution
	Phenol 25%–50%[a]
Protein denaturants	Trichloroacetic acid 15%–100%
	Phenol 60%–88%
	Baker-Gordon phenol peel: 50% phenol, 2.1% croton oil
	Hetter phenol peels: 50% phenol, 0.7% croton oil
	Hetter "all around": 35% phenol, 0.4% croton oil
	Hetter VL (neck and eyelid): 30% phenol, 0.1% croton oil
	Stone V-K: 62% phenol, 0.16% croton oil
	Stone 2: 60% phenol, 0.2% croton oil

[a]Phenol at concentrations below 50% has keratolytic properties.

used for superficial, exfoliative procedures, whereas the protein denaturants can be used for superficial or deeper peels.

Keratolytics

As the name implies, keratolytic agents disrupt the adhesion of the keratinocyte cells to one another. These agents can be used to break up the stratum corneum and various levels into the epidermis to allow for a light chemical exfoliation to occur. However, as will be discussed, keratolytic peels can also help enhance the depth of penetration of trichloroacetic acid (TCA) peels when used in combination. The two main acids used for combination peels are glycolic acid and Jessner's solution. Jessner's solution is composed of 14% each of resorcinol, salicylic acid, and lactic acid mixed in ethanol.

Jessner's solution has an advantage over glycolic acid in that the salicylic acid in it is lipophilic. Therefore Jessner's solution can penetrate acne lesions or oily skin better than a hydrophilic agent such as glycolic acid. An additional advantage of Jessner's solution is that the physician does not have to monitor the skin contact time closely as one would with a glycolic acid solution.

Protein Denaturants

Phenol and TCA are the two protein denaturant peeling agents. TCA is one of the main peeling acids used for medium-depth peels with a long, proven safety record. Similarly, phenol is the main peeling acid used in various formulas for deep peels. TCA and phenol work by causing protein coagulation and denaturation as they penetrate the skin. TCA and phenol coagulate proteins that make up the cells of the epidermis and dermis as well as the blood vessels. Once a certain amount of the acids have been applied, they will continue to coagulate proteins until they are used up. They cannot be neutralized once they begin to be absorbed into the skin. After about 2 minutes, the depth of TCA penetration can be observed and a decision can be made if more acid is needed to drive the peel deeper. Phenol is a lot more rapid in its penetration, and the depth is apparent almost immediately. Subsequent application of acid will continue to drive the peel deeper until it is used up by coagulating proteins deeper in the skin. When used correctly, these acids can be used to achieve a variety of peel depths ranging from exfoliation to deep peels.

There are four methods by which TCA concentration can be calculated. The safest and most agreed-upon method is the weight-to-volume (W:V) calculation. Thus it is of outmost importance that the physician purchase TCA from a reliable source. The author personally only purchases TCA from Delasco (Council Bluffs, IA). Similarly, there are many variations on phenol/croton oil peel formulas requiring a reliable pharmacy to formulate these solutions.

TRICHLOROACETIC ACID PEELS

As mentioned previously, it is incorrect to refer to TCA peels as light, medium, or deep solely based on TCA concentration. Acid concentration is only one variable affecting peel depth. For example, 1 mL of 40% TCA applied to the face will result in penetration to the basal layer, whereas 6 mL of 40% TCA applied over the same body surface area will result in penetration to the mid-dermis or deeper. Higher volumes will drive the peel even deeper.

One can perform peels of various depth with the same aptitude that one uses to dial in laser settings for skin resurfacing. The variations in peel formulas have given the physician unprecedented control over the depth of skin resurfacing.

TCA, 10% to 50%, can be used as a sole peeling agent. It is hydrophilic by nature; thus it may have patchy absorption through the lipid-containing and thickened stratum corneum. For this reason, higher doses of TCA are harder to work with. It is tough to reapply TCA at high concentrations in areas that need it without risking too deep of a peel. To facilitate even TCA penetration, the skin should be prepared in advance with a skincare regimen geared at making the stratum corneum more even and compact. Oily skin needs to have adequate oil control before performing the peel. This can be achieved with a short course of isotretinoin for a few months, ending about 3 to 6 months before the peel. On the day of the peel, the skin needs to be properly degreased with 70% alcohol and, in some instances, acetone.

To reduce the risks associated with high-concentration TCA peels, combination peels have been developed. These peels help to facilitate the penetration of the TCA solution, allowing for a lower concentration of TCA to be used while still allowing a medium-depth peel to be achieved.

The three most commonly used modified TCA peels are the Jessner's solution–TCA peel, glycolic acid–TCA peel, and the Blue Peel (Table 5.5). These peels are designed to peel to a depth of the papillary dermis and at most to the most superficial aspect of the reticular dermis. The main indications for TCA and modified TCA peels are for epidermal and upper dermal pathology: photodamage, actinic keratoses, lentigines, ephelides, fine rhytides, and very superficial, nonfibrotic (stretchable) scars. These peels are not suited for fibrotic scars, deep nonstretchable rhytides, or extensive laxity. If a rhytid or scar improves with stretching the skin, a medium-depth peel can help improve it. However, if the scar or rhytid is etched into the skin or is fibrotic, the tightening effect of the peel may not be enough to give adequate clinical improvement.

It is easiest to think of the combination TCA peels as being "accelerated" or "decelerated." Accelerated peels use a keratolytic agent such as Jessner's solution or glycolic acid to speed the penetration and depth of the TCA peel. The Jessner's–TCA peel uses Jessner's solution (keratolytic), applied before the application of TCA.

TABLE 5.5 Modified Trichloroacetic Acid Peel Formulas		
Modified Trichloroacetic Acid Peels	**Solutions**	**Technique**
Glycolic acid–TCA peel	70% glycolic acid 35% TCA	70% glycolic acid applied Neutralized after 2 minutes Light application of 35% TCA
Jessner's solution–TCA peel	Jessner's solution 35% TCA	Jessner's solution applied Rinsed with water after 6 minutes Light application of 35% TCA
TCA Blue Peel	Blue Peel base 30% TCA	2 mL (1 tube) Blue Peel base mixed with: 2 mL 30% TCA = 15% TCA Blue Peel 4 mL 30% TCA = 20% TCA Blue Peel 6 mL 30% TCA = 22.5% TCA Blue Peel 8 mL 30% TCA = 24% TCA Blue Peel

TCA, Trichloroacetic acid.

Application of the Jessner's solution allows for faster and deeper penetration of the subsequently applied 35% TCA. A similar mechanism is used with the glycolic acid–TCA peel, which uses 70% glycolic acid (keratolytic) before application of 35% TCA. The amount of 35% TCA required to peel into the papillary dermis is minimized by performing the preceding keratolytic peel.

A decelerated peel, such as the Blue Peel (Obagi Cosmeceuticals, Long Beach, CA), allows the entire peeling process to be slowed down so that one has greater control over the depth of penetration of the peel. The Blue Peel incorporates a nonionic blue dye, glycerin, and a saponin with a specific volume of 30% TCA to yield a 15%, 20%, 22.5%, or 24% TCA–Blue Peel solution (see Table 5.5). The blue coloring, which stains the stratum corneum, allows the physician to see where the solution has been applied while still allowing the signs of depth penetration, such as frosting and erythema, to be visualized. On the flipside, a regular TCA peel is a colorless solution that requires close attention to avoid reapplication over previously treated areas. Because TCA is hydrophilic, the use of a saponin as an emulsifying agent creates a homogenous TCA-oil-water emulsion that penetrates the skin in a slower and more even fashion.

Phenol Peels

Phenol peels are covered in several subsequent chapters in relation to the treatment of deeper skin pathologies such as deep/rigid rhytides, certain acne scars, or as a means to tighten and lift certain areas such as the eyelids or lips.

In a manner similar to TCA, phenol exerts its actions by protein denaturation and coagulation. The rapid speed by which phenol penetrates the skin requires careful application and constant vigilance by the physician. Additionally, when treating a large area such as the face, serum phenol levels can quickly become elevated, resulting in systemic toxicity and cardiac arrhythmias. Once absorbed, phenol is partially detoxified in the liver and excreted by the kidneys. Therefore all patients must be cleared from a cardiac, renal, and hepatic standpoint preoperatively. Intraoperative cardiac monitoring and high-volume intravenous fluid hydration are imperative to avoid cardiac issues. However, using lower-concentration formulas such as the Hetter VL and limiting the phenol peel to one cosmetic unit (perioral or periorbital), one can usually peel the patient without cardiac monitoring or IV hydration if the patient is healthy.

The systemic absorption of phenol is related to body surface area treated more so than the concentration used. To minimize toxicity, phenol peels are usually performed in small anatomical sections of the face with a 15-minute break before the application of the acid to the next anatomical unit. This allows the body to metabolize the phenol that is absorbed before the reapplication of the solution. The face is usually treated in sections such as the forehead, right cheek, left cheek, nose and perioral, and periorbital region.

Techniques
Trichloroacetic Acid Peels

TCA is usually used to peel to a medium-depth peel. The goal is to reach the papillary dermis with the peel solution.

BOX 5.1   Peel Tips

Ways to enhance peel depth	Degrease the skin with acetone
	Apply firmer pressure when applying the peel solution
	Apply more peel solution volume
	Apply a higher acid concentration
	Perform a light peel or microdermabrasion before applying the deeper peel solution[a]
Ways to enhance comfort	Cooling air units or strong fans
	Oral analgesics: ibuprofen, meperidine, hydrocodone
	Music or relaxing atmosphere
	Intravenous sedation
	Nerve blocks[b]

[a]Caution is recommended with more aggressive techniques.
[b]May not give complete analgesia

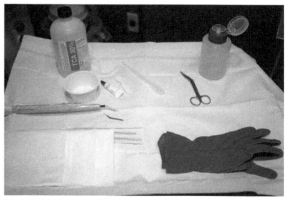

Fig. 5.2 Peel setup: Epilating needle, electrodessication needle, 70% alcohol, 30% trichloroacetic acid, one tube Blue Peel base, sponge, tissue, and cotton-tipped applicators.

Once applied to the skin, the TCA solution generates a stinging and burning sensation that builds up and peaks then subsides. Until the desired depth of penetration is achieved, more coats of TCA solution are applied, resulting in the cycle of burning/stinging then resolution. However, once the patient finishes the peel, there should only be little to no discomfort left. To make this peel easier to tolerate, a combination of oral meperidine (50–100 mg), hydroxyzine (50 mg), diazepam (5 mg), and ibuprofen (400–600 mg) is given (Box 5.1). Some physicians perform the peel under IV sedation or general anesthesia (usually in combination with a surgical procedure for which the patient is sedated). The author does not use topical anesthetics for fear of altering the TCA penetration by altering skin hydration. Additionally, topical anesthesia does not offer enough pain relief once the peel exceeds the depth of the epidermis. The use of a refrigerated air cooling unit (Zimmer Aesthetic Division, Germany) in combination with oral sedation can improve patient tolerance of the peel.

Chemical peel resurfacing is all about "reading" the skin depth signs. Regardless of the type of TCA peel performed, the evolving clinical depth signs remain the same. The only difference between the various peels is the speed by which these signs appear if one is using an accelerated or decelerated formula.

Until a physician has gained enough experience performing medium-depth peels, he or she should start with lighter peels and then proceed to deeper peels. In the same vain, it is best to start with relatively slower peeling techniques before proceeding to faster peels. As

mentioned, skin thickness can vary patient to patient and anatomically on the face: the cheeks, perioral region, and nose having thicker skin, the eyes having the thinnest skin, and the forehead being variable.

The peel setup is fairly simple with the TCA, 70% alcohol and/or acetone, the electrodessication tip, tissue (to blot tears or acid run off), cotton-tipped applicators (for the eyelids and nose), and the sponge to apply the acid (Fig. 5.2). Nearby there should be water or saline to flush the eyes if needed.

The patient is instructed to come to their appointment with clean skin and without any lotions or moisturizers. Residual oil or thick scale may lead to a patchy peel; therefore it is essential to cleanse and degrease the face well with 70% alcohol and possibly acetone before proceeding. While a peel is being performed, the physician should not leave the room, as one may miss some of the peel depth signs (Box 5.2) that are very transient.

The penetration of TCA in the skin starts to coagulate epidermal proteins first, resulting in a light, nonorganized frost (level 1 frost) (Fig. 5.3A). Further application of the peel solution will result in a solid frost with a reactive pink background (level 2 frost) (Fig. 5.3B). The pink background of the frost is referred to as the "pink sign" and will be apparent as long as the blood vessels of the papillary dermis are still intact with normal blood flow (Figs. 5.3A–C). The level 2 frost is the endpoint for the standard, papillary dermis–level peel. There may be noticeable edema in the skin upon pinching it. Yet further TCA application will penetrate to or into the upper

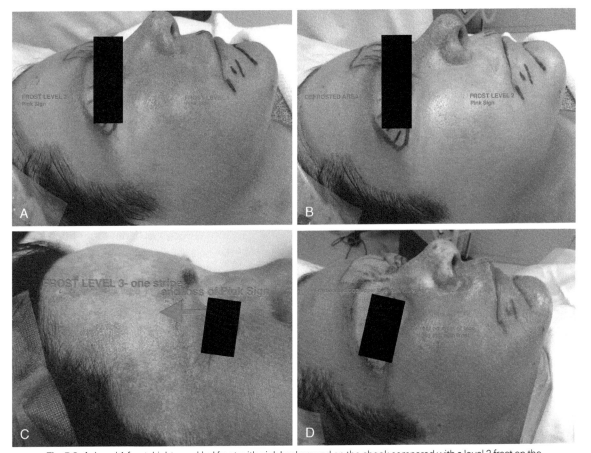

Fig. 5.3 A, Level 1 frost. Light speckled frost with pink background on the cheek compared with a level 2 frost on the forehead. B, Level 2 frost. Solid white frost with pink background on the cheek; pay attention to the area on the forehead that has already defrosted. C, Level 3 frost. Seen as a solid white frost with loss of the pink background suggesting that the superficial vascular plexus has been obliterated. D, Defrosting of skin occurs in the order in which the peel was performed. It is crucial to pay attention to this to avoid repeeling an area that has already been done.

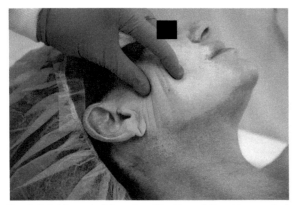

Fig. 5.4 Epidermal sliding sign. Pinching of the skin results in exaggerated skin wrinkling, suggesting the anchoring fibrils between the epidermis and dermis have been disrupted.

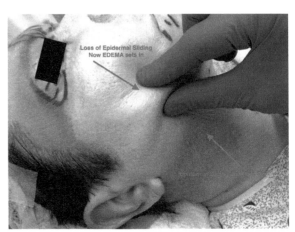

Fig. 5.5 Edema. Once the peel continues, the epidermal sliding sign is lost, and firm edema sets in as the epidermis and dermis are now fused together.

reticular dermis, resulting in a solid frost with a loss of the pink background (level 3 frost) (Fig. 5.3C). The level 3 frost implies that the whole papillary dermis is involved with the peel and the upper reticular dermis has been reached. This is the maximum recommended level for a TCA peel. Continued TCA application will drive the peel into the mid-reticular dermis, resulting in a "gray" appearance to the skin. Penetrating to this level correlates with an increased risk of scarring and permanent hypopigmentation.

On darker skin patient, the "pink sign" may be difficult to visualize. For this reason, on darker-skinned patients, one may have to rely on the "epidermal sliding" sign to gauge peel depth. The "epidermal sliding" sign is a transient sign that demonstrates exaggerated wrinkling of the skin that occurs before complete precipitation and coagulation of papillary dermis proteins (Fig. 5.4). Papillary dermal edema and disruption of anchoring fibrils allows the epidermis to be more freely movable, resulting in exaggerated wrinkling when the skin is pinched. This sign disappears when the papillary dermis proteins become coagulated and adherent to the epidermal coagulated proteins, thus indicating that the peel depth has reached the superficial reticular dermis. Once this is achieved, the pink background goes away and edema sets in (Fig. 5.5). In thicker skin, "epidermal sliding" may not be very obvious, and monitoring the "pink sign" alone has to be used to indicate the peel depth.

Glycolic Acid–Trichloroacetic Acid Peel

The skin is degreased by cleansing it with soap and water. Quickly and evenly, unbuffered 70% glycolic acid is applied. After 2 minutes of contact time, it is neutralized with a copious amount of water.

A small amount of 35% TCA is applied in even strokes to the skin using gauze or a large cotton swab. A 2 to 3 minute waiting time is given to allow the TCA to penetrate and to assess whether further application is indicated. To avoid lines of demarcation, the TCA should be feathered down along the jawline and should extend to the hairline.

Jessner's Solution–Trichloroacetic Acid Peel

The skin is adequately cleansed with soap (preferably a foaming cleanser) and water. The face is then further degreased by acetone.

A 2-inch by 2-inch gauze or cotton-tipped applicators are used to apply the Jessner's solution evenly, just enough to cause a very light frost. After 6 minutes, this is followed by the application of a small amount of 35% TCA in even strokes using either gauze or cotton-tipped applicators. A 2- to 3-minute waiting time is given to allow the TCA to penetrate and to assess whether further application is indicated. To avoid lines of demarcation, the TCA should be feathered down along the jawline and should extend to the hairline.

Trichloroacetic Acid–Blue Peel

The skin surface is gently cleansed with alcohol only or acetone for very oily skin. The Blue Peel base is mixed with 30% TCA immediately before use (see Table 5.5). Novice peelers should begin with lower concentrations and work themselves up. Similarly, the number of coats (volume) applied to the skin has to be adjusted to the skin thickness. Thinner skin requires fewer coats, whereas thicker skin may require additional coats. The solution is applied evenly to the face and feathered into the hairline, the earlobes, and along the jawline. The Blue Peel solution will only temporarily stain hair blue.

Each application or coat is allowed to penetrate for 2 to 3 minutes before further application so that the peel depth can be properly assessed. A level 2 frost is the usual endpoint of this peel. If more TCA is applied, there will be a loss of the pink background, indicating penetration beyond the papillary dermis and into the superficial reticular dermis (level 3 frost). A level 3 frost in certain areas is the maximum recommended depth of a facial TCA–Blue Peel. Fig. 5.6 shows the stages of frosting, epidermal sliding, pink background, and edema as they occur over time.

Peeling nonfacial skin can be rewarding and challenging at the same time, because nonfacial skin has fewer adnexal structures to repair the skin after the peel. For this reason, caution is necessary when peeling these areas. When feathering from the face to the neck, the deeper peel should be up closer to the jawline and should get progressively lighter as it nears the clavicles (Fig. 5.7A). This helps create a blending effect between the skin on the face and the neck.

Phenol Peels
Hetter VL Peel

Lighter phenol peels (less phenol and less croton oil) have made it easier to achieve a reticular dermis level peel with fewer complications than the traditional Baker-Gordon peels. The modified, lighter phenol peels, like the Hetter VL solution, can be used to treat a "single" cosmetic unit without the need for cardiac monitoring or IV hydration. Treating more than one area will require cardiac clearance, assessing hepatic and renal function, and appropriate IV hydration and cardiac monitoring.

Clean skin is further degreased by using 70% alcohol or acetone. The bottle is shaken gently to mix the various components, and some of the solution is pulled into another bowl using a pipette. While performing the peel and in between applications, the phenol mixture must be swirled, because the oil and water components of the solution have a tendency to separate (Fig. 5.8A–B). The solution is applied to the skin with a cotton-tipped applicator (Fig. 5.8C). Care must be taken not to let the

solution drip or run down the face. The frost appears very quickly following the application of the peel solution (Fig. 5.8D). The endpoint for deep wrinkles or redundant skin is an even white frost. The frost dissipates quickly, so one must pay close attention to make sure that one does not apply more solution and peel the skin too deeply.

Combination Procedures

In the day and age of fractionated laser resurfacing, one may feel that there is no role for chemical peels. However, this couldn't be further from the truth. Peels allow an unparalleled flexibility to treat areas on the face, neck, and chest that lasers cannot while also allowing a wider range of skin types to be resurfaced safely. In fact, peels can be safely combined with laser resurfacing, nonablative lasers, and surgical procedures.

The best method to plan out a combination procedure at the consultation noting which areas need a vascular laser, which need electrodessication of adnexal structures (syringomas, sebaceous hyperplasia, cherry angiomas, seborrheic keratosis), and which need medium-depth resurfacing and which need deep resurfacing. The order of the procedures is critical as well (Fig. 5.9). Peel solutions should be kept out of contact with open wounds created by surgery or laser resurfacing. Preoperative markings should be made to help demarcate the areas that will be treated more deeply from those to be treated more lightly.

During a facelift or eyelift procedure, a light- to medium-depth peel can be performed safely to improve skin appearance without compromising the flap. Undermined skin is peeled to a lighter level (not more than papillary dermis) than the skin that will not be undermined. The solution is kept away from the incisions. Alternatively, the resurfacing can be performed first, the skin cleansed, and then the surgery performed (Fig. 5.10).

Neck and chest rejuvenation is more challenging than facial skin rejuvenation, because the neck has fewer adnexal structures, which are crucial to wound healing. A series of papillary dermis–level peels may be more beneficial and less risky than one deeper peel on these areas. Some physicians will address more pronounced neck rhytides with a modified phenol peel using the Hetter VL formulation.

In summary, the correct order of procedures is crucial for controlling the depth of resurfacing when performing

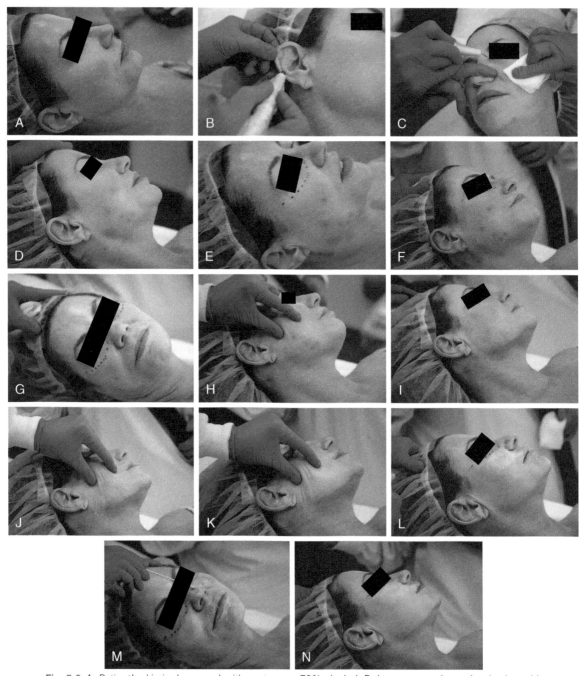

Fig. 5.6 A, Patient's skin is degreased with acetone or 70% alcohol. B, Low-energy electrodessication with a spatula tip for flat seborrheic keratosis, nevi, angiofibromas. C, Low-energy electrodessication with an epilating needle for dermal lesions such as syringomas, angiomas, and sebaceous hyperplasia. D, After electrodessication, some of the treated areas are now open wounds. E–N, The natural progression of the peel as each anatomical area is completed.

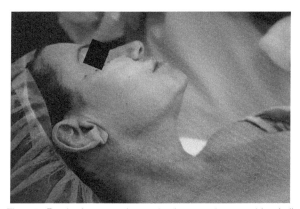

Fig. 5.7 Feathering onto the neck, chest, and ears to blend all the areas. It is important that the peel becomes less strong the more caudal one proceeds, to create a nice transition. Peels can be feathered onto the brows and into the hairline, and some can be applied to the mucosal lips.

combination procedures: (1) nonablative or minimally ablative lasers (vascular or pigment lasers) is performed first; (2) electrodessication next; (3) the medium-depth peel is performed next; (4) if a phenol peel is to be used in certain cosmetic units, this is then performed; (5) the skin is cleansed to remove all residual acids; and (6) the laser resurfacing of certain areas can then be performed (Fig. 5.11).

Postoperative Care

At the end of medium-depth and deep peels, the author prefers to cleanse the skin gently with soap and water. If a Blue Peel is performed, the blue dye is removed with a cleanser that comes in the kit or even with Dawn foaming dishwashing soap. The patient is told that some of the blue color will remain and will come off during the healing process. Any blue tinting of the hair will resolve with shampooing.

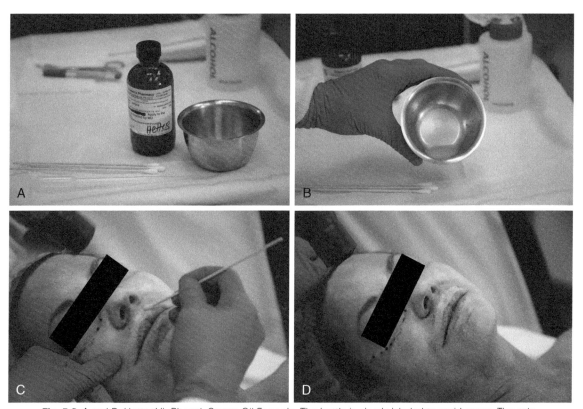

Fig. 5.8 A and B, Hetter VL Phenol–Croton Oil Formula. The bottle is clearly labeled to avoid errors. The solution separates, thus requiring constant mixing before application. C and D, The Hetter VL being applied to the cutaneous upper lip with a wet but not dripping cotton-tipped applicator. Firm, even strokes are applied until a solid white frost appears.

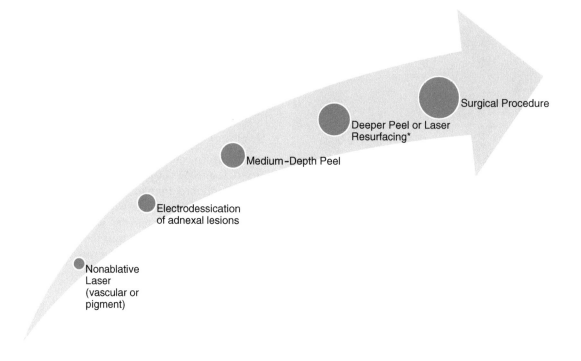

*Skin is cleansed with soap and water before laser resurfacing or surgery is performed.

Fig. 5.9 Algorithm for safely combining procedures. Procedures begin with the nonablative and minimally ablative procedures followed by the lighter of the peels, then the deepest peel, then, after the skin is cleansed, the laser resurfacing. Usually the last step is the surgical procedure. Alternatively, the surgical procedure can be performed first, but care must be taken to keep any acids away from the incisions.

Medium Depth Peels

Medium-depth peels usually take 6 to 7 days to heal fully. The first day patients are told to take it easy and apply frozen peas to the face 10 minutes per hour (no ice to nonfacial skin). Patients are asked to sleep at a 45-degree angle the first couple of days to reduce facial edema. Facial edema, especially with phenol peels, begins shortly after the procedure and peaks at 24 to 48 hours. By 72 hours, most of the swelling has resolved, but skin begins to look like a mask or a snake about to shed its skin. Patients will notice a progressive darkening and tightening of their skin into a mask-like appearance.

Areas that have been treated with phenol or laser resurfacing will have a fair amount of proteinaceous exudate that may look yellowish on appearance. These areas will look different during the entire healing process. This exudate may look like pus to the patient, so reassurance should be given that it is normal and will resolve.

There are variations among physicians in terms of postoperative regimens. The author has modified and simplified the postoperative care for patients based on 20 years of experience. Unless the patient is immuno-compromised or has had recent orthopedic surgery, prophylactic antibiotics are not given. To reduce the risk of postoperative staphylococcal infection, patients are instructed to start applying mupirocin ointment to the nostrils three times a day starting 1 week before resurfacing and continuing until the skin has fully healed. This simple step has reduced the number of postoperative infections tremendously.

The author does not routinely prescribe oral predni-sone for the swelling unless the patient has a history of very exaggerated swelling. Simple measures with sleeping at 45 degrees and applying frozen peas 10 minutes per hour the first day help reduce edema.

Patients should cleanse their skin twice a day using a gentle cleanser and avoiding the use of a washcloth. At

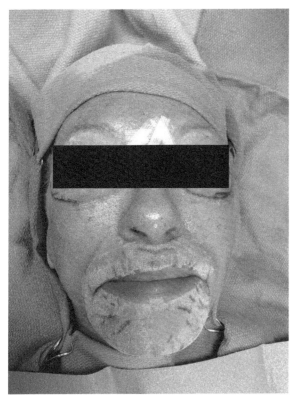

Fig. 5.10 Patient safely undergoing trichloroacetic acid Blue Peel followed by laser resurfacing, followed by an upper blepharoplasty.

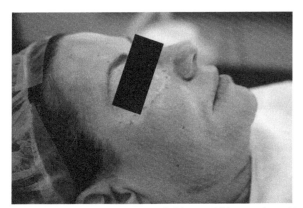

Fig. 5.11 Patient underwent a full-face trichloroacetic acid Blue Peel with feathering off of the face. The skin was then cleansed, eye protection was used, and periorbital resurfacing with a fractionated CO_2 laser was performed.

midday and late afternoon patients perform an astringent wash using gauze soaked in Domeboro Astringent Solution (Moberg Pharma, Cedar Knolls, NJ) for about 10 minutes. After each skin wash or soak, patients apply

an inert emollient onto the skin, such as Vaniply ointment (Pharmaceutical Specialties, Rochester, MN) or Aquaphor ointment (Beiersdorf, Hamburg, Germany).

All cleansing and ointment applications are performed using a "patting" technique. Patients are instructed to avoid rubbing their skin even when cleansing or applying ointments, because this can cause skin to come off prematurely.

Areas treated with phenol peels or laser resurfacing are treated with dilute vinegar soaks during the healing process. This is 1 teaspoon white vinegar in 2 cups of purified or distilled water. Patient will soak gauze in this solution, wring out the gauze, and lay it on the phenol or laser areas for 10 minutes per hour. This will soothe the skin, reduce the exudate buildup, and make for a much more comfortable recovery. After each skin wash or soak, patients apply an inert emollient onto the skin, such as Vaniply ointment or Aquaphor ointment.

The first day, the TCA areas should only feel slightly tight or warm. The phenol or laser resurfacing areas may feel like a light sunburn. After 24 hours, there should be no associated pain. In fact, pain is usually a hallmark of infection or an area that has been traumatized. This must be addressed promptly.

After 4 to 5 days, the skin will proceed to come off in thick sheets starting in areas of movement (perioral or periorbital) and last in areas of less movement (forehead). Papillary dermis peels should heal in 7 days, whereas peels reaching the superficial reticular dermis will take 10 days to heal. Any healing time that is faster or more prolonged is a sign that the peel was either too superficial or too deep, respectively. Compared with aggressive CO_2 laser skin resurfacing, chemical peeling is generally much easier for the patient, surgeon, and staff.

Patients are seen midweek at day 3 or 4 to make sure they are following instructions and to assess their level of compliance with the soaks and postoperative care. Any early signs of infection or contact dermatitis can usually be picked up early at this point. Patients are seen again at day 7 to make sure that all areas have healed and that any remaining exudate is soaked off in the office and the underlying skin is assessed. Furthermore, patients are seen to ensure they are using the mupirocin ointment and taking their valacyclovir as prescribed.

During the entire healing process, patients are to avoid exercise, heat exposure, bathtubs, swimming pools/Jacuzzis, and sun. They are to wash their hands after using the restroom or petting their animals. They are to keep their pets away from their faces and pillowcases.

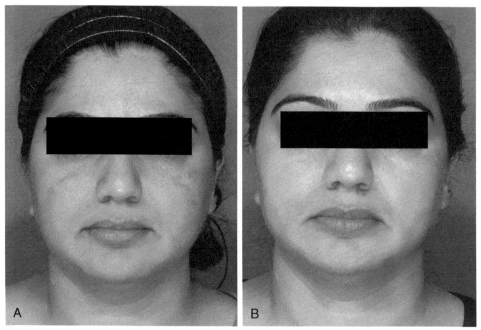

Fig. 5.12 A and B, Patient with melasma showing nice resolution of her dyschromia with a medium-depth trichloroacetic acid Blue Peel.

Patients should be encouraged to resume their skin-conditioning program upon complete reepithelialization of the skin. This is usually restarted 1 week after they have healed or even 2 weeks later to the laser or deeper peel areas. Absolute avoidance of sun exposure is recommended for the first 4 to 6 weeks postoperatively. Skin firming can become apparent in as little as a few weeks and continue for up to 3 months afterward.

CONCLUSION

All physicians performing skin rejuvenation procedures should be adept at chemical peel resurfacing to offer patients improved results either as stand-alone procedures or in combination with lasers and surgeries. Peels can be tailored to reach different depths, address areas that cannot be lasered, and be used on a wide variety of skin types. Peels have withstood the test of time despite the introduction into the market of a wide variety of laser and energy devices. In fact, many physicians who regularly perform chemical peels find them indispensable and would trade their lasers in before giving up their peels. Optimizing outcomes hinges on proper patient evaluation, procedure selection, depth selection, and proper technique (Figs. 5.12–5.15).

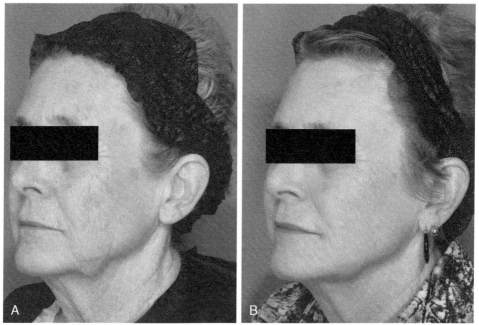

Fig. 5.13 A and B, Patient showing improvement of overall skin firmness, dyschromia, and wrinkles with electrodessication of adnexal structures and a full-face trichloroacetic acid Blue Peel, Hetter VL of the glabella, crow's feet, buccal region, and upper lip lines.

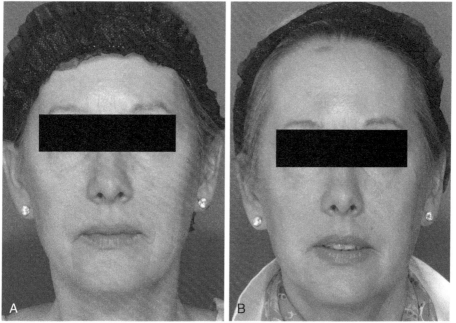

Fig. 5.14 A and B, Patient with improvement following a trichloroacetic acid Blue Peel of the face as well as a Hetter VL peel of the periorbital region and laser resurfacing of the perioral and glabellar region.

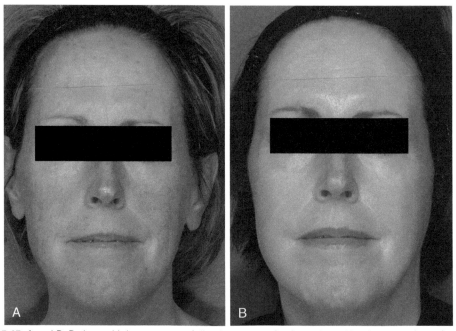

Fig. 5.15 A and B, Patient with improvement following a properly planned combination procedure of pulsed dye laser for telangiectasias; Q-Switch laser for lentigines; trichloroacetic acid Blue Peel of the face, neck, and chest; and a Hetter VL peel of the periorbital region and laser resurfacing of the perioral and glabellar region.

FURTHER READING

Abdel-Meguid Am, Taha EA, Ismail SA. Combined Jessner solution and trichloroacetic acid versus trichloroacetic acid alone in the treatment of melasma in dark-skinned patients. *Dermatol Surg.* 2017;0:1–6.

Agarwal N, Gupta LK, Khare AK, Kuldeep CM, Mittal A. Therapeutic response of 70% trichloroacetic acid CROSS in atrophic acne scars. *Dermatol Surg.* 2015;41:597–604.

Coleman WP, Futrell JM. The glycolic acid and trichloroacetic acid peel. *J Dermatol Surg Oncol.* 1994;20:76–80.

Dalpizzol M, Weber MB, Mattiazzi AP, Manzoni AP. Comparative study of the use of trichloroacetic acid and phenolic acid in the treatment of atrophic-type acne scars. *Dematol Surg.* 2016;42:377–383.

Hantash BM, Stewart DB, Cooper ZA, Rehmus WE, Koch RJ, Swetter SM. Facial resurfacing for nonmelanoma skin cancer prophylaxis. *Arch Dermatol.* 2006;142:976–982.

Hetter GP. An examination of the phenol-croton oil peel: part IV. Face peel results with different concentrations of phenol and croton oil. *Plast Reconstr Surg.* 2000;105(3):1061–1083; discussion 1084-1087.

Holzer G, Pinkowicz A, Radakovic S, Schmidt RB, Tanew A. Randomized controlled trial comparing 35% trichloroacetic acid peel and 5-aminolevulinic acid photodynamic therapy for the treatment of multiple actinic keratosis. *Br J Dermatol.* 2016.

Kumari R, Thappa DM. Comparative study of trichloroacetic acid versus glycolic acid chemical peels in the treatment of melasma. *Indian J Dermatol Venerol Leprol.* 2010;76:447.

Lee JB, Chung WG, Kwahck H, Lee KH. Focal treatment of acne scars with trichloroacetic acid: chemical reconstruction of skin scars method. *Dermatol Surg.* 2002;28:1017–1021.

Leheta T, El Tawdy A, Hay RA, Farid S. Percutaneous collagen induction versus full-concentration trichloroacetic acid in the treatment of atrophic acne scars. *Dermatol Surg.* 2011;37:207–216.

Li YT, Yang KC. Comparison of the frequency-doubled Q-switched Nd:YAG laser and 35% trichloroacetic acid for the treatment of face lentigines. *Dermatol Surg.* 1999;25:202–204.

Monheit GD. The Jessner's-trichloroacetic acid peel. An enhanced medium-depth chemical peel. *Dermatol Clin.* 1995;13(2):277–283.

Moubasher AE, Youssef EM, Abou-Taleb DA. Q-switched Nd:YAG laser versus trichloroacetic acid peeling in the treatment of melasma among Egyptian patients. *Dermatol Surg.* 2014;40:874–882.

Nofal E, Helmy A, Nofal A, Alakad R, Nasr M. Platelet-rich plasma versus CROSS technique with 100% trichloroacetic acid versus combined skin needling and platelet rich plasma in the treatment of atrophic acne scars: a comparative study. *Dermatol Surg.* 2014;40:864–873.

Obagi Z, Obagi S, Alaiti S, Stevens M. TCA-Based Blue peel: a standardized procedure with depth control. *Dermatol Surg.* 1999;25(10):773–780.

Puri N. Comparative study of 15% TCA peel versus 35% glycolic acid peel for the treatment of melasma. *Indian Dermatol Online J.* 2012;3(2):109–113.

Ramadan SA, El-Komy MH, Bassiouny DA, El-Tobshy SA. Subcision versus 100% trichloroacetic acid in the treatment of rolling scars. *Dermatol Surg.* 2011;37:626–633.

Raziee M, Balighi K, Shabanzadeh-Dehkordi H, Robati RM. Efficacy and safety of cryotherapy vs. trichloroacetic acid in the treatment of solar lentigo. *J Eur Acad Dermatol Venereol.* 2008;22(3):316–319.

Safoury OS, Saki NM, El Nabarawy EA, Farag EA. A study comparing chemical peeling using modified Jessner's solution and 15% trichloroacetic acid versus 15% trichloroacetic acid in the treatment of melasma. *Indian J Dermatol.* 2009;54(1):41–45.

Soliman MM, Ramadan AR, Bassiouny DA, Abdelmalek M. Combined trichloroacetic acid peel and topical ascorbic acid versus trichloroacetic acid peel alone in the treatment of melasma: a comparative study. *J Cosmetic Dermatol.* 2006;6:89–94.

Stone PA. The use of modified phenol for chemical face peeling. *Clin Plast Surg.* 1998;25(1):21–44. Review.

6

Trichloroacetic Acid Peels of the Neck, Chest, and Arms and Hands

Carolyn Willis

INTRODUCTION

The face is frequently the focus of antiaging and skin rejuvenation interventions. It is important to remember, however, that there are other areas that should be targeted for rejuvenation efforts to avoid a discordant appearance between the face and other visible areas. As we age, both intrinsic and extrinsic factors affect the appearance of the dorsal hands, neck, and décolletage and can "give away" a person's true age if care is not taken to treat them along with the face.

Typical signs of aging and sun damage include solar lentigines and other dyschromias. External factors, like ultraviolet light, smoking, and secondhand smoking, contribute to extrinsic aging of the skin. Extrinsic aging leads to skin changes that many patients find cosmetically unappealing and prompt them to seek evaluation and treatment.[1,2] These include actinic keratoses, seborrheic keratoses, and tactile and visible roughness. Intrinsic aging that results from internal factors, such as dermal and fat atrophy, contribute to wrinkles, prominent tendon and vein visibility, and bony prominence.[1,2] Procedures that target these common signs of aging will enhance a patient's overall rejuvenation results. The most cosmetically pleasing results often come from a combination of modalities focused on addressing the internal and external factors that are contributing to the appearance of the aged hand, neck, and chest (Figs. 6.1 and 6.2). Trichloroacetic acid (TCA) peels, when used appropriately, can be an important step in an overall rejuvenation plan.

INDICATIONS AND EVALUATION FOR CHEMICAL PEELS OF THE HANDS, NECK, AND CHEST

Chemical peels can address the extrinsic signs of aging. Proper patient selection is paramount for a reproducibly good outcome. It is important in the preprocedure consultation to identify the role that chemical peeling may play in overall rejuvenation and to discuss realistic expectations for improvement and review that the procedure is likely just one part of a therapeutic plan.

Unrealistic expectations or an inability to follow through on pretreatment recommendations should be red flags. A thorough medical history is necessary for identifying those at risk for poor or delayed healing. Those with diabetes mellitus, immunodeficiency, chronic kidney or liver disease, or connective tissue disease, or those on chronic steroids or immunosuppressive or immunomodulatory medications, deserve special attention. A history of medications that can lead to pigment deposition in areas of trauma, like minocycline, should also be elicited. Any allergies or medication sensitivities should be recorded. A history of herpes simplex virus (HSV), varicella zoster virus (VZV), or methicillin-resistant *Staphylococcus aureus* (MRSA) would indicate the need for more stringent preoperative and postoperative prophylaxis and surveillance. Patients with skin disorders with risk of Koebnerization, like psoriasis and lichen planus, should also be counseled about potential increased risk

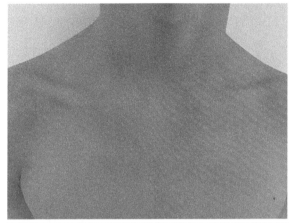

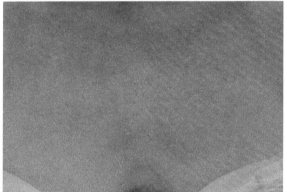

Fig. 6.1 Comparison of "youthful" chest (upper) with a "mature" chest (lower) showing changes due to aging, sun, and environmental factors.

from the procedure. It is important to solicit a social history as well. Smokers, including those who vape nicotine-containing solutions, due to reduced blood flow, are at increased risk for poor wound healing.[3] Occupation would also be relevant due to potential exposures that may affect healing. Those who work outdoors may be expected to have increased risk of ultraviolet (UV)-induced side effects like postinflammatory hyperpigmentation and dyschromia. Those who work in the healthcare setting may have increased risk for infection depending on their exposure level.

A patient's tendency to heal appropriately should be assessed and a history of poor healing, hypertrophic or keloidal scarring, or a tendency to postinflammatory hyperpigmentation should be elicited. Absolute contraindications to peels include pregnancy and active infection at the procedure site.

PREPROCEDURE SKIN PREPARATION

Proper preoperative skin conditioning is essential for an optimal outcome. The pretreatment regimen is preferably started a minimum of 6 to 8 weeks before the planned procedure to avoid the irritant dermatitis that may occur at the initiation of therapy and allow for the active ingredients to manifest their effectiveness (Table 6.1). It is used in combination with strict sun protection that includes sun avoidance, sun protective clothing, and a titanium dioxide or zinc oxide–containing sunblock. An antioxidant, usually

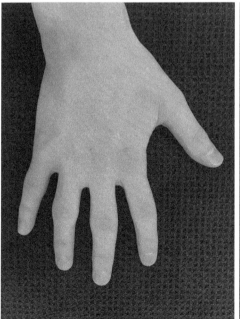

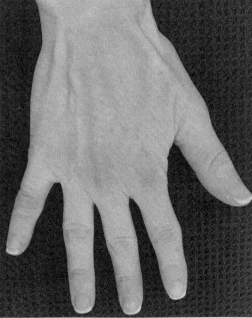

Fig. 6.2 Comparison of "youthful" hand on left with "mature" hand on right. Prominent veins, tendons, and tactile roughness characterize the aging hand.

TABLE 6.1	**Preoperative Skin Care Regimen**	
Product	**AM or PM Use**	**Reason for Use**
Sun protection	AM	Reduce further sun damage and protect the skin from the increased photosensitivity from topical retinoids
Vitamin C 10%	AM/PM, 6 drops	Antioxidant, epidermal barrier support; improves uneven skin tone
Hydroquinone 4%	AM/PM, 1 g	Bleaching cream; improves uneven skin tone, downregulates melanocyte activity
Retinoic acid/ tretinoin/ retinaldehyde	PM, 1 g	Promotes collagen production and cellular turnover, improves uneven skin tone

BOX 6.1   **Potential Complications**

- Infection
- Scarring
- Prolonged erythema
- Postinflammatory hypopigmentation
- Postinflammatory hyperpigmentation
- Unhappy patient

a vitamin C serum–containing stabilized L-ascorbic acid, is started as part of the regimen. Vitamin C has been shown in vitro to regulate keratinocyte viability and support epidermal barrier and basement membrane function.[4]

A topical retinoid is also initiated to promote dermal collagen production and to normalize keratinocyte turnover.[5] It has also been shown to speed healing after a TCA peel.[6] Tretinoin 0.05% cream is usually recommended for use two to three times per week on the neck and chest and 5 to 7 nights per week on the dorsal hands as tolerated. For those who cannot tolerate the tretinoin cream, a retinaldehyde 0.1% gel is recommended. The vitamin C and the retinoid also have a beneficial effect on melanocyte activity and appear to speed recovery and reduce the risk of postinflammatory hyperpigmentation.

Hydroquinone, a tyrosinase inhibitor, is also an important component of the preconditioning regimen, especially in the higher Fitzpatrick skin types. Suppression of melanogenesis has a beneficial effect on the preexisting pigmented lesions that patients complain about and is essential in reducing the risk of recurrence after the peel and the risk of postinflammatory hyperpigmentation. The treatment regimen has a synergistic effect, because the thinning of the stratum corneum induced by the retinoid allows for deeper and more uniform penetration of the chemical peel.

The preoperative period is also a good time to address any precancerous lesions on the areas to be treated. A course of topical 1% to 5% 5-fluorouracil or imiquimod 3.75% to 5% cream or ingenol mebutate will improve the health of the skin and improve the cosmetic appearance, because these lesions contribute to the tactile roughness and irregularity that is often part of the patient's complaint. Usually a full treatment course of one of these agents is prescribed and the area is allowed to fully heal before initiating the aforementioned preprocedure regimen.

TRICHLOROACETIC ACID PEEL COMPLICATIONS

With proper preprocedure preparation and diligent aftercare, the risk of complications from a properly performed TCA peel is low. It is important to recognize potential complications in the early stages, because prompt intervention can often improve the chance of a good outcome (Box 6.1). Infection is a risk because of the open wound that is created by the peel. It is important that the patient be aware of the risk and the importance of proper handwashing before wound care. Environmental risk factors include the patient's occupation and the presence of pets in the household. When the hands and forearms are treated, care must be taken with activities of daily living and household tasks like cooking and cleaning. One step we have taken to greatly reduce the risk of bacterial infections, especially staphylococcal infection, is to have all resurfacing patients swab the inside of their nostrils with mupirocin ointment three times a day starting 1 week before their procedure and continuing until postoperative day 7.

If an infection is suspected, the patient should be immediately evaluated in the office, and a skin swab should be sent for gram stains and proper cultures. Empiric antibiotics can be started if the suspicion for bacterial infection is high, keeping in mind the increasing rates of MRSA and the patient's occupation and exposures when choosing an antibiotic.

Herpes simplex and herpes zoster infections can also complicate the procedure and can lead to devastating scarring. The risk of viral infections occurring on non-facial skin is lower than when peeling the face. If a viral infection is suspected, a direct fluorescent antibody test can be taken, and the patient should be started immediately on antiviral therapy while awaiting results.

The postoperative use of occlusive ointments can sometimes lead to yeast infections. These can often be diagnosed clinically by the appearance of small, pruritic papules and pustules and confirmed by a KOH examination. Proper antiyeast medications can be initiated, and wound care can be adjusted.

The risk for scarring is higher on the hands, neck, and chest compared with the face because of the lower density of pilosebaceous units but should still be low in the setting of proper wound care. Risk of hypertrophic scarring should be reviewed and the treatment avoided in patients with increased susceptibility to such scarring or keloids. Prolonged erythema is often the first sign of impending scarring, and the patient should be counseled to call if the redness persists longer than expected. Early intervention with pulse dye laser (PDL) treatment and topical steroids can attenuate the risk of permanent scarring.[7]

Postinflammatory hyperpigmentation or hypopigmentation can also occur. These adverse effects can be mostly avoided by proper pretreatment and posttreatment preparation and vigilant sun protection. Initiation of bleaching agents once the skin has fully reepithelialized will play a role both prophylactically and therapeutically in management of hyperpigmentation. A series of light peels such as salicylic acid 30% or Jessner's solution can be used to hasten the resolution of the hyperpigmentation. Hypopigmentation is more common in higher Fitzpatrick skin types and is usually the result of inadvertently peeling too deeply. Mild hypopigmentation usually resolves without intervention (other than the regular aftercare regimen) over time. Marked hypopigmentation may be permanent.

TRICHLOROACETIC ACID PEEL PROTOCOL

Written informed consent should be obtained as the initial step in the peel protocol. Potential risks and adverse effects of the peel should be clearly reviewed with the patient, and the patient should be given an opportunity

---

BOX 6.2 Trichloroacetic Acid Blue Peel Protocol

- Verify patient name, date of birth, procedure, medications, and allergies.
- Determine whether any of the medications are new or there any new medical issues since preop.
- Ensure the patient has a driver.
- Ask whether the patient ate breakfast.
- Ask whether the patient feels well.
- Check blood pressure.
- Have the patient review and sign consent.
- Administer preoperative medications.
- Take photos.
- Review aftercare.
- Confirm 48-hour and 1-week postoperative appointments.
- Prepare for the procedure:
  - Prepare Blue Peel solution of the desired concentration.
  - Move the patient to the operating room.
  - Wipe the area to be treated well with alcohol.
  1) Electrodessicate adnexal lesions—sebaceous gland hyperplasia, milia, seborrheic keratoses—and/or treat lentigines with the appropriate wavelength laser.
  2) Apply the peel (while the assistant operates the dynamic cooler) with a slightly moistened sponge to one subunit at a time, making sure not to allow solution to pool in any one area, to achieve a uniform frost with a pink background.

Look for epidermal sliding or exaggerated wrinkling.
Have tissue ready for any drips.

  3) When all areas have been treated to the desired depth, apply EMLA cream, then gently cleanse the area with Dawn soap.
  4) Review aftercare.
  5) Call the patient the night of the procedure.

---

to ask questions and indicate understanding of the potential risks and benefits of the procedure. It is helpful to follow a consistent protocol to ensure reproducibly good outcomes (Box 6.2).

Preoperative photos should be taken to document the patient's baseline. Any scars or pigment or textural irregularities that are present before the peel should be pointed out to the patient.

TCA peels cause a mild to moderate amount of burning or "icy-hot" discomfort, and depending on the patient's pain threshold, dynamic cooling may be all that

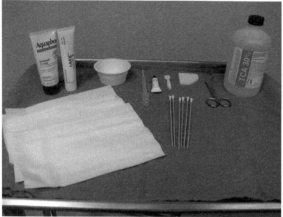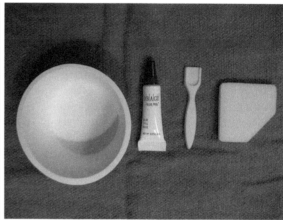

Fig. 6.3 Typical setup for an Obagi Blue Peel.

is needed for analgesia. Topical anesthetics should be avoided because they can affect the penetration of the peel solution. If analgesia is required, ibuprofen, meperidine, diazepam or hydroxyzine, or other agents depending on the provider's preference, can be used alone or in combination if the patient has no contraindications and there is a driver available to take the patient home.

The skin to be treated is degreased with one to two passes of either 70% alcohol or acetone to allow more even penetration of the TCA solution. TCA 10% to 25% is typically used for a superficial to superficial-medium depth peel of the neck, chest, dorsal hands, and forearms. These lower concentrations give the physician more control over peel depth. A deeper peel can be achieved by simply applying more layers of the peel solution. Higher concentrations should be reserved for patients with thicker skin and surgeons with more experience with cosmetic peels. The peel solution can be applied with either gauze or a sponge applicator. Care should be taken to apply the solution with the applicator saturated to the same degree and applied with the same pressure to all areas.

Conventional TCA peel solutions are colorless, making even application of the solution more difficult. An alternative solution would be to use a product with a color indicator. The Obagi Blue Peel (Obagi Cosmeceuticals, Long Beach, CA) incorporates a Blue Peel base containing glycerin, saponins, and a US Food and Drug Administration (FDA)–approved blue dye that can be combined with the TCA solution (Fig. 6.3). The homogeneous TCA-oil-water solution that is generated permits the surgeon to control the uniformity of application

TABLE 6.2	Blue Peel Solution Preparation	
Blue Peel Base	30% Trichloroacetic Acid	Final Trichloroacetic Acid Concentration
2 mL	2 mL	15%
2 mL	4 mL	20%
2 mL	6 mL	22.5%
2 mL	8 mL	24%

by using the intensity of the blue color as a guide.[8] An appropriate amount of 30% (W:V) TCA solution is added to the 2 mL Blue Peel base to generate the desired concentration of the peel solution (Table 6.2). The combination solution slows the penetration of the acid, allowing for even application and more precise control of the depth of the peel, because the clinical endpoints occur at a slower rate, making the different stages of the peel easier to identify. This reduces the risk of "overpeeling" the area as a result of too rapid absorption related to the excessive volume application of the colorless TCA solution. Regardless of the peel solution chosen, adequate time needs to be given between coats to allow for the penetration of the acid and frost development—typically 2 to 6 minutes between coats. Proceeding with caution, additional coats should be applied to achieve the desired level of frost. For the chest and neck, it is recommended to stop at a pink background with speckled or nonorganized frost (frost level 1) (Figs. 6.4 and 6.5). For the dorsal hands, the peel can be taken slightly deeper, to barely a uniform frost with a pink background. For the dorsal forearms, where there is a significant density of pilosebaceous units, the peel can be taken to a more uniform light, even frost with a pink background (frost level 2) (Figs. 6.6 and 6.7). It may be especially desirable to peel to a deeper level at this location in individuals with significant actinic damage and for patients prone

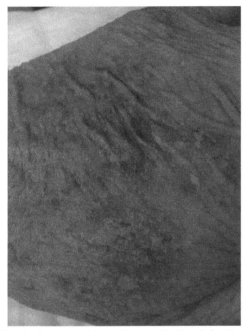

Fig. 6.4 Background pink erythema with "lacy" frosting indicating a level 1 peel.

to senile purpura. By repeatedly peeling to the papillary dermis on the forearms, it will significantly cut down on the density of precancerous lesions and will thicken the papillary dermis, thus helping to minimize easy bruising.

It is important to feather the peel solution lightly to the surrounding areas to avoid lines of demarcation between treated and untreated areas. When using the Blue Peel kit, the blue dye can be washed off at the conclusion of the peel with a gentle foaming cleanser. A bland ointment like Vaniply ointment (Pharmaceuticals Specialties, Inc., Rochester, MN), Aquaphor (Beiersdorf AG, Hamburg, Germany), or petroleum jelly should be applied postprocedure.

For optimal results, a series of TCA peels may be necessary, and it is reasonable to consider a repeat treatment at 3- to 6-month intervals until the desired endpoint is met (Fig. 6.8).

POSTPEEL WOUND AND SKIN CARE

Written postpeel wound care should be provided to the patient. In the immediate postoperative period, cool compresses and nonsteroidal antiinflammatory drugs are beneficial. The discomfort after a TCA peel is usually minimal, because the pain usually subsides shortly after the completion of the peel itself. Patients can be instructed to cleanse with a mild unscented foaming wash, making sure to only pat the area and not scrub or rub the area. Burow's soaks are also useful because

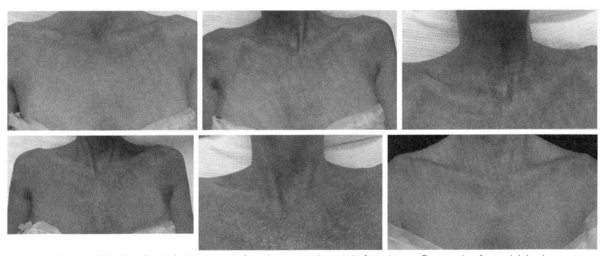

Fig. 6.5 TCA Blue Peel of the chest: before, intraoperative, and after photos. Progression from pink background with "lacy" frosting to the desired endpoint of a pink-red background with an almost uniform "see-through" frost is evident. The after photo shows improvement in texture and tone.

of their astringent and antiseptic properties. The area should be gently patted dry after cleansing and a bland ointment applied. The patient should be given strict instructions to avoid sun and any exercise that would induce sweating. Follow-up visits at postoperative days 2 or 3, day 7, and if needed, day 10 or 12, allow close monitoring and early identification of healing issues (Fig. 6.9). The patient should be reminded that they should not pick or try to peel of the desquamating skin prematurely, as this can lead to scarring. Reepithelialization typically takes 10 to 14 days, and the patient can switch to a regimen of mild foaming cleanser and bland emollients at that point. Daily sun protection should also be initiated. The preprocedure regimen of topical retinoids, vitamin C serum, and hydroquinone should be restarted approximately 2 weeks after the peel.

COMBINATION AND ADJUNCT PROCEDURES

Additional procedures can be performed along with the TCA peel to address other signs of aging. Epidermal growths, such as seborrheic or actinic keratoses, can be treated with electrodessication (ED) the same day of

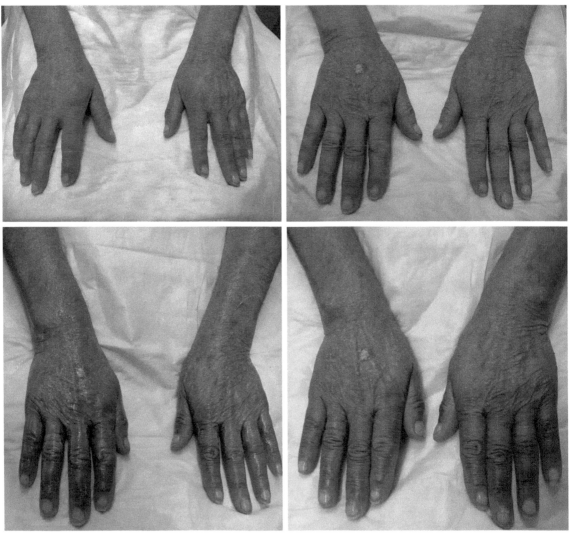

Fig. 6.6 Progression of Blue Peel on hands. Note that "thinner" skin will defrost more quickly, and close observation is necessary to identify safe peel endpoints.

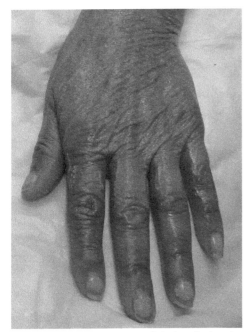

Fig. 6.7 Exaggerated wrinkling—a clinical endpoint—is apparent.

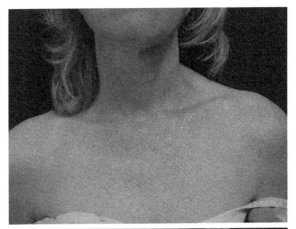

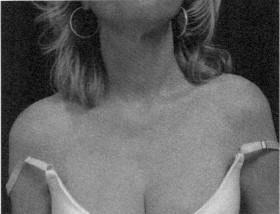

Fig. 6.8 Before (upper) and after (lower) trichloroacetic acid Blue Peel of the chest.

the peel, just before the application of the peel solution. Lentigines may also respond to light ED or alternatively to a laser of the appropriate wavelength (Fig. 6.10). Epidermal melanin has a broad absorption spectrum (250 to 1200 nm) and will respond to a variety of lasers; the proper choice of device is based on patient skin color and the nature of the pigmented lesion.[9] Q-switched lasers (ruby [694 nm], Alexandrite [755 nm], Neodymium-doped:yttrium aluminum garnet [Nd:YAG, 1064 nm] or frequency doubled Nd:YAG [532 nm]), or picosecond lasers are frequently used for this indication. For significant poikiloderma on the neck and chest, a series of PDL and pigmented lesion–specific laser treatments before the peel (on the same day) may yield a superior cosmetic outcome.

TCA peels may induce some tissue tightening, but for optimal results in patients with significant skin laxity of the décolletage it may be preferred to perform a tissue-tightening procedure several months before the peel. Ultherapy (Merz Aesthetics) and Thermage (Solta) both have an indication for tissue tightening in this area.

Volume loss contributes to formation of wrinkles on the chest and hands and is a main factor contributing to the appearance of prominent vessels and tendons on the dorsal hands. Volume restoration is an important step in an overall rejuvenation plan. There are a variety of fillers that are appropriate for these indications.

Poly-L-lactic acid (Sculptra, Galderma, Fort Worth, TX), which is a synthetic polymer of lactic acid, exerts its volumizing effect through the induction of neocollagenesis.[10] It has been used successfully to revolumize both the décolletage, neck, and the dorsal hands.[11,12] Poly-L-lactic acid is supplied as a sterile freeze-dried preparation that needs to be reconstituted with sterile water before use (Sculptra package insert). The advantage of a biostimulatory filler is that it yields a natural and longer-lasting result than synthetic fillers. The disadvantage is the risk of nodule formation. To reduce the risk, it is recommended to reconstitute the product a minimum of 72 hours in advance, to only inject a highly diluted preparation, and ensure that the patient understands

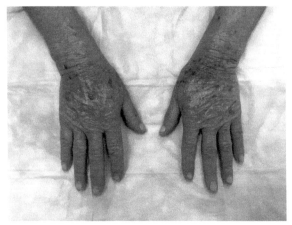

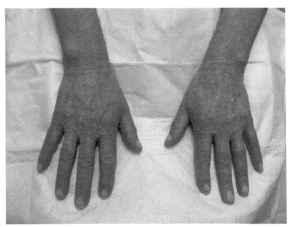

Fig. 6.10 Left hand after treatment with the Medlite (Cynosure, Westford, MA) q-switched 532 nm laser and right hand treated by electrodesiccation.

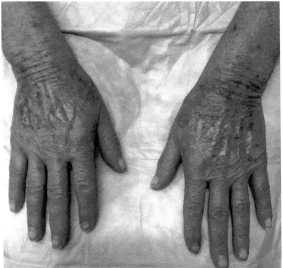

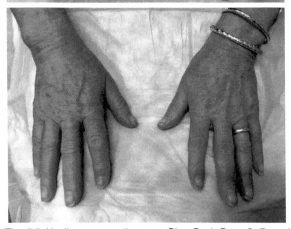

Fig. 6.9 Healing progression post–Blue Peel. Days 2, 7, and 14 are shown.

the importance of regular massage during the first 3 to 5 postprocedure days. The product is typically injected with 25- to 27-gauge, 1.5-inch needles into the subcutaneous plane. A 27-gauge cannula may also be used for the dorsal hands. Retrograde fanning or cross-hatching techniques can be used. It may helpful to mark the chest into quadrants to ensure an even distribution of product. Product placement should be followed immediately by vigorous massage, and the technique should be demonstrated to the patient. Caution should be used to not "overcorrect," because the neocollagenesis will lead to greater volumization than initially obtained.

Calcium hydroxylapatite (Radiesse, Merz Aesthetics, Raleigh, NC) is an FDA-approved filler for soft tissue augmentation of the dorsal hands. It is composed of calcium hydroxylapatite microspheres suspended in a sterile water/glycerin/sodium carboxymethylcellulose gel carrier (Radiesse package insert). The gel provides immediate correction, whereas the microspheres trigger fibroblast proliferation and collagen production, which contributes to prolonged volume correction.[13] The product can be mixed with 0.2 to 0.5 mL 2% lidocaine or 1% lidocaine with epinephrine solution before injection. It is typically administered in 0.5- mL boluses with a 25- to 27-gauge needle or cannula from a point at the dorsal wrist crease. The skin should be tented with the nondominant hand to avoid vessels and tendons and place the filler in the correct deep subcutaneous plane. Two depot injections are typically made, and the hand is then massaged to distribute the product. There can be a fair amount of swelling, and cool compresses and hand elevation postprocedure may be beneficial. As with poly-L-lactic acid, it is important to anticipate further volume correction through collagen induction and to not "overcorrect."

Hyaluronic acid fillers are another option for revolumization. Restylane Lyft (Galderma USA, Fort Worth, TX) is an FDA-approved hyaluronic acid filler for the treatment of the dorsal hands. There are multiple options for filler choice and injection techniques.[14-16] They can be used in both the décolletage and the dorsal hands. These fillers have the advantage of being reversible. One of their disadvantages is the lack of longevity of the result.

Autologous fat transfer is a good option for the dorsal hands and is an excellent "add-on" treatment when doing a facial revolumization procedure. Autologous fat is soft, natural appearing, and cost effective when comparing the per-milliliter cost of various fillers. The fat is harvested under local anesthetic, processed, and injected with a cannula via small incisions made at the dorsal hand crease. Because autologous fat is considered a graft and requires the development of its own blood supply, there are more posttreatment activity restrictions than would be the case with biostimulatory or synthetic fillers. As an added benefit, improvement has also been noted in overlying skin texture and appearance after fat transfer.[17] Platelet-rich plasma (PRP) may also play an increasing role in rejuvenation efforts, whether combined with fat transfer or as a stand-alone procedure.

All filler procedures come with potential complications. Discomfort with injection can be managed with topical and local anesthetic. Bruising or hematoma formation may occur from injection. Bromelain or arnica supplements and cool compresses can be of benefit. For hand injections, elevation of the extremity may hasten the clearance of swelling. The most feared complication is inadvertent blood vessel injection leading to the potential for skin necrosis and scarring. Slow, low-pressure injections and the use of cannulas can help to reduce this risk.

MAINTENANCE OF RESULTS

Once the patient has completed their therapeutic plan, they will need a maintenance regimen to preserve their results. Continued vigilance regarding sun protection is of central importance. Sunblock containing titanium dioxide or zinc oxide should be used on a daily basis—patients often need to be reminded to use them on their neck, chest, forearms, and hands because they may not realize how much unintended UV exposure they are receiving. Topical retinoid and antioxidant use should continue indefinitely. The hydroquinone can usually be discontinued 3 months postoperatively.

Nonablative fractional lasers, such as the Clear and Brilliant laser (1440/1927 nm) or the Fraxel DUAL (1550/1927 nm) (both by Solta Medical, Hayward, CA), are useful in maintaining and augmenting the results of chemical peel treatments. It is reasonable to suggest a follow-up maintenance treatment every 6 to 12 months to address the continued aging process.

The cosmetic surgeon can enhance the results of patient-specific antiaging regimens by paying attention to maintaining and improving the appearance of the neck, décolletage, and hands as part of an overall rejuvenation plan.

REFERENCES

1. Abrams HL, Lauber JS. Hand rejuvenation: the state of the art. *Dermatol Clin.* 1990;8(3):553–561.
2. Butterwick K, Sadick N. Hand rejuvenation using a combination approach. *Dermatol Surg.* (42):S108-S118.
3. Khunger N, Force IT. Standard guidelines of care for chemical peels. *Indian J Dermatol Venerol Leprol.* 2008;74(suppl):S5–S12.
4. Boyce ST, Supp AP, Swope VB, Warden GD. Vitamin C regulates keratinocyte viability, epidermal barrier, and basement membrane in vitro, and reduces wound contraction after grafting of culture skin substitutes. *J Invest Dermatol.* 2002;118(4):565–572.
5. Kircik LH Histologic improvement in photodamage after 12 months of treatment with tretinoin emollient cream. *J Drug Dermatol.* 2012;11:1036–1040.
6. Hevia O, Nemeth AJ, Taylor JR. Tretinoin accelerates healing after trichloroacetic acid chemical peel. *Arch Dermatol.* 1991;127:678–682.
7. Khatri KA, Mahoney DL, McCartney MJ. Laser scar revision: a review. *J Cosmet Laser Ther.* 2011;13(2):54–62.
8. Obagi ZE, Obagi S, Alaiti S, Stevens MB. Tca-based Blue peel: a standardized procedure with depth control. *Dermatol Surg.* 1999;25:773–780.
9. Patil UA, Dhami LD. Overview of Lasers. *Indian J Plast Surg.* 2008;41(suppl):S101–S113.
10. Stein P, Vitavska O, Kind P, Hoppe W, Wieczorek H, Schurer NY. The biological basis for poly-L-lactic-acid-induced augmentation. *J Dermatol Sci.* 2015;78(1):26–33.

11. Peterson JD, Goldman MP. Rejuvenation of the aging chest: a review and our experience. *Dermatol Surg.* 2011;37:555–571.

12. Palm MD, Woodhall KE, Buterwick KJ, Goldman MP. Cosmetic use of poly-l-lactic acid: a retrospective study of 130 patients. *Dermatol Surg.* 2010;36:161–170.

13. Berlin AL, Hussain, Goldberg DJ. Calcium hydroxylapatite filler for facial rejuvenation: a histologic and immunohistochemical analysis. *Dermatol Surg.* 2008;34(suppl 1):S64–S67.

14. Man J, Rao J, Goldman M. A double-blind, comparative study of nonanimal-stabilized hyaluronic acid versus human collagen for tissue augmentation of the dorsal hands. *Dermatol Surg.* 2008;34(8):1026–1031.

15. Fabi SG, Goldman MP. Hand rejuvenation: a review and our experience. *Dermatol Surg.* 2012;38:1112–1127.

16. Sadick NS, Anderson D, Werschler WP. Addressing volume loss in hand rejuvenation: a report of clinical experience. *J Cosmet Laser Ther.* 2008;10:237–241.

17. Coleman S. Structural fat grafting: more than a permanent filler. *Plast Reconstr Surg.* 2006;118(suppl 3):108S–120S.

7

Phenol-Croton Oil Peels

Richard H. Bensimon

INTRODUCTION

The history of phenol–croton oil peels dates back to the 1920s, when they were introduced into the United States by "lay peelers" coming from Europe. The formulas involved boiling crystals to obtain liquid phenol, to which were added drops of the caustic acid croton oil, among other ingredients. How these original formulas came to be is unknown, but what is clear is that the treatments were quite effective. Eventually these peels came to the attention of the medical community, and in 1961, plastic surgeon Thomas Baker from Miami published a formula that was straightforward and easily reproduced. The formula contained liquid phenol, three drops of croton oil, water, and the surgical soap Septisol, which acted as a surfactant to allow the aqueous and oily parts to mix. The belief at the time was that the phenol was the peeling agent and the purpose of the croton oil was unclear.

In 1962, Dr. Baker altered the volumes of the ingredients but left the three drops of croton oil unchanged. This simple change raised the concentration of the croton oil to 2.1% and became the standard formula, unchanged for decades. This peel was highly effective in treating deep wrinkles, but this was always at the cost of creating significant hypopigmentation and an unnatural alabaster look. Due to the need to constantly wear makeup, this peel was reserved for older, significantly wrinkled individuals with light eyes.

The peel was considered difficult to perform, and phenol had the reputation of having an "all-or-none" quality that was out of the practitioner's control. A weaker concentration of phenol was thought to be problematic, because it would peel deeper, and phenol also had the reputation of being cardiotoxic. These beliefs became ingrained in the fields of dermatology and plastic surgery and went unchallenged for decades. Despite the remarkable results, the risks were too intimidating, and "phenol peels" did not see widespread acceptance.

The next significant step in the evolution of the peels was brought about by plastic surgeon Gregory Hetter in Las Vegas. Hetter experimented with the ingredients of the Baker peel and convincingly proved that croton oil and not phenol was the peeling agent. Moreover, the Baker formula contained a high concentration of croton oil at 2.1%, responsible for the results and the feared complications. With this information, the croton oil concentration could be manipulated to be clinically effective while avoiding hypopigmentation. An important difference is that the peel could be performed superficial or deep, increasing the versatility.

The ability to alter the croton oil concentration has great utility and completely changes the nature of the peel. By using weaker croton oil concentrations the application technique becomes one of the important factors in determining the depth reached. The entire process is slowed down, and now the surgeon can observe the skin changes and have the opportunity to stop at whatever depth seems appropriate. The all-or-none phenomenon seen with the Baker peel was simply that the croton oil concentration was so high that it immediately resulted in a peel deep enough to cause hypopigmentation. The peel can now be customized, and by choosing the appropriate concentration and how the solution is applied, the practitioner is in precise control.

It is now feasible to peel to the desired clinical result without reaching a depth that causes hypopigmentation. A critical difference is that now the practitioner can choose different concentrations on different areas of the face depending on need and relative skin thickness. The Baker formula was all one high concentration, and many practitioners were reluctant to treat the eyelids because of fear of scarring. With the modern formulas, a weak concentration such as 0.1% can now safely and effectively treat the eyelid skin.

During my career as a plastic surgeon, the term "comprehensive facial rejuvenation" is frequently mentioned as an idealized goal. An excellent facelift that leaves prominent lip lines and an etched periorbital area is an aesthetic failure. Now at last there is an excellent tool available for facial resurfacing; the goal is to understand the process, simplify the delivery, and explore the potential.

PATIENT SELECTION

As a plastic surgeon, I have historically promoted surgery, but now that I have a viable option, I have learned that many patients place greater importance on the overall appearance of their skin and may be satisfied by a peel alone. Lighter peels that can be done on younger patients to target pigmentation and segmental peels, particularly around the eyes, are a useful adjunct to treatment plans. The main contraindication is a patient who is expected to be uncooperative in the postoperative care and may not refrain from picking. A relative contraindication is a patient whose skin is severely sun damaged and judged to be fragile. Staged lighter peels may be an option in these situations.

PREOPERATIVE PLANNING

Preparation of the skin before the peel is done to prevent hyperpigmentation and put the skin in a hyperproliferative state. The treatment begins 4 to 6 weeks before peeling, with tretinoin 0.05% or 0.1% and hydroquinone 4% twice daily (see Chapter 3). An exfoliating agent such as glycolic acid or phytic acid may be used to remove desquamated cells. The preparation is stopped 4 to 5 days before the peel to allow the epidermis to normalize. There is controversy whether this skin preparation is absolutely necessary, but my recommendation is to use it, especially in darker-skinned individuals.

Preparation of the Solution

The preparation of the acid solutions is a critical step that should be performed by the operator. The ingredients are the same as the Baker peel and consist of water, phenol, croton oil, and Septisol/Novisol.

Liquid phenol is 88% or 89%, and its corrosive effect allows passage into the dermis.

Croton oil is extracted from the seeds of *Croton Tiglium*, a tree indigenous to Asia. Full-strength croton oil is highly caustic and will result in a full-thickness burn if applied to the skin. However, when correctly diluted and appropriately applied, croton oil will yield remarkable aesthetic improvement.

Septisol is a surgical soap that has been historically used as a surfactant to allow miscibility of the aqueous and oil components. Septisol contains triclosan as a preservative, and this has become problematic as of late. Safety issues regarding triclosan have been raised resulting in a ban of Septisol in Europe and more recently by the Food and Drug Administration (FDA) in the United States. The triclosan is inconsequential to the peel, but the reality is that Septisol is no longer available.

Pure soaps may work, but recent work by Young Pharmaceuticals (Wethersfield, CT) has resulted in a viable alternative for Septisol and further understanding into the role of the surfactant. The necessity of replacing Septisol may have brought about an unexpected improvement.

Analysis of Septisol as a surfactant shows that it is an anionic detergent and results in a cruder, larger particle emulsion. The action of this emulsion is that the ingredients separate within seconds and a gradient forms. As the solution is applied, there may be different concentrations presented across the gauze leading to uneven action. The solutions need to be constantly shaken to try to mix the ingredients as best as possible.

The product that has been developed (Novisol) is a nonionic detergent that yields an emulsion of smaller particle size leading to a much more stable suspension. Once shaken, the ingredients mix evenly and stay in suspension during the entire course of the peel. As the solution is applied, the concentration is unchanged across the gauze and ultimately it is an improved product.

The ingredients are arranged in glass bowls in the order they will be added, and this routine should be repeated every time to prevent confusion. Once prepared, the acids can be stored in opaque bottles with leak-proof caps for extended periods of time.

The original Baker formulas were based on drops of croton oil. Droppers have the disadvantage of variability in the volume of drops and limiting the possible concentrations by the inability to split a drop. Hetter simplified the process of creating a standard phenol–croton oil solution

TABLE 7.1 Formulas With 35% Phenol Concentration				
	0.2%	0.4%	0.8%	1.2%
Water	5.5 mL	5.5 mL	5.5 mL	5.5 mL
Surfactant (i.e., Novisol)	0.5 mL	0.5 mL	0.5 mL	0.5 mL
USP phenol 88%	3.5 mL	3.0 mL	2.0 mL	1.0 mL
Stock solution (containing phenol and croton oil)	0.5 mL	1.0 mL	2.0 mL	3.0 mL
Total volume	10 mL	10 mL	10 mL	10 mL

Stock Solution:
24 mL USP 88% Phenol + 1 mL croton oil (0.04 mL croton oil/1 mL stock solution or 4% croton oil)
Dilute formulas with 35% phenol concentration:
    0.1%: 1 mL of 0.4% solution + 1.2 mL phenol + 1.8 mL water (total 4 mL)
    0.05%: 1 mL of 0.2% solution + 1.2 mL phenol + 1.8 mL water
    0.025%: 1 mL of 0.1% solution + 1.2 mL phenol + 1.8 mL water
    ¼X% = 1 mL of X% solution + 1.2 mL phenol + 1.8 mL water
Phenol Solution for Preliminary Anesthesia
    50% phenol without croton oil: 10 mL 88% phenol + 7.6 mL water

using larger volumes, which would then be further diluted with the other ingredients (Table 7.1). The standard solution, or "stock solution," is prepared by mixing 24 mL of 88% phenol and 1 mL of croton oil. Eighty-nine percent phenol can be used without appreciable difference. Using larger volumes allows easy measurement with standard syringes and avoids the awkwardness of drops.

Standard tables further delineate the specific volumes of each ingredient needed to arrive at a specific croton oil concentration. The phenol concentration in these formulas as devised by Hetter is approximately 35% in contrast with the Baker formula that was 50%.

In the croton oil concentration of 0.2%, 0.4%, 0.8%, and 1.2% listed in Table 7.1, the volumes of water and surfactant remain constant at 5.5 mL and 0.5 mL, respectively. The values that change are the relative volumes of phenol and stock solution (which contains phenol and croton oil). The sum of the volumes of phenol and stock solution is 4 mL in each of the formulas.

To better understand the basis of these formulas, it is valuable to examine them more closely. The stock solution consists of 24 mL of phenol and 1 mL of croton oil. Each 1 mL of stock solution has 0.04 mL of croton oil, or a 4% croton oil solution. For example, the formula for 0.8% croton oil is made up of 5.5 mL of water, 0.5 mL of surfactant, 2.0 mL of phenol, and 2.0 mL stock solution. The 2.0 mL of stock solution contains 0.08 mL of croton oil (2 x 0.04 mL). As the total volume of the solution is 10 mL, the final concentration of croton oil is 0.08 mL of croton oil in 10 mL total volume, or 0.8%. By comparing the volume of stock solution in any of the formulas with the known content of croton oil in the stock solution, the final concentration of croton oil can easily be determined. It is important to note that the concentration of croton oil in the stock solution is extremely high at 4% and should never be applied to the skin without further dilution.

To make weaker concentrations, 0.4% or 0.2% are first mixed and these are further diluted using the formulas in Table 7.1. The final volume is 4 mL and the phenol concentration is kept at 35%. Whatever starting concentration is used with this dilution formula will be diluted by one fourth, or 1ml X% solution + 1.2 mL phenol + 1.8 mL water will yield 0.025% solution.

ANESTHETIC TECHNIQUE

The Baker peel was traditionally done under general anesthesia followed by a painful early recovery. The addition of sensory nerve blocks is helpful in decreasing the intense stimulation from the caustic croton oil, but it is not complete. A serendipitous personal observation has led to a useful addition to the peeler's armamentarium.

While experimenting with different solutions on my own hands, I noticed that a dilute phenol solution (i.e., 50%) caused an initial stinging that lasted 10 to 15 seconds after which the skin appeared insensate. Testing with a needle, there was no sensation, even to the point of bleeding.

Utilizing this information, I began peeling by applying a first pass of 50% phenol to one segment of skin (such as one-half of the forehead). The patient would experience definite stinging for 10 to 15 seconds, after which the discomfort dissipated completely. At this point, the skin treated with phenol is numb and can be comfortably peeled. If the entire face is to be peeled, it is first gradually treated with 50% phenol for the anesthetic effect and then peeled. The addition of oral sedation significantly improves the overall experience. The degree of sedation depends on the practitioner's comfort and experience, but it does not have to be so deep as to require oxygen supplementation.

To perform a full-face peel as described can be challenging; therefore the addition of intramuscular pain medication, if regulations allow, is very helpful. Small segmental peels, such as eyelids, are easily done with these techniques as an informal office procedure. A more recent addition is the use of an apparatus that delivers 50% oxygen and 50% nitrous oxide on demand by the patient (Pro-Nox CAREstream Medical LTD, Altamonte Springs, FL). This concentration of nitrous oxide is not anesthetic, but it is a potent anxiolytic that clears very quickly when stopped. A lower eyelid peel can be completely done with this alone to soothe the preliminary stinging of the phenol.

MEDICATION

The possibility of a herpetic breakout must always be considered; therefore antiviral prophylaxis is routinely prescribed. Valacyclovir hydrochloride, 500 mg two times per day, is begun 3 days before the procedure and continued for 7 days after peeling. Although the recovery is not particularly painful, narcotic pain medication is prescribed along with ibuprofen 800 mg three times daily. Sleep medication is prescribed along with a mild sedative to help deal with the inconvenience of the recovery.

SURGICAL ROUTINE

Traditionally, deep chemical peels are performed under general anesthesia or intravenous sedation because of the intense stimulation of the chemical burn. After the induction of anesthesia, local sensory nerve blocks with bupivacaine 0.25% without epinephrine are performed. The skin is carefully degreased with acetone, and a preliminary pass of 50% phenol is done for the anesthetic effect.

Ophthalmic ointment and corneal protection are not used because the phenol can dissolve in the ointment and prevent flushing out if necessary.

The fear of cardiac toxicity has been historically associated with phenol, and recent personal experience has provided some elucidation. There had been speculation that arrhythmias seen with Baker peels were due to catecholamine release caused by the intense stimulation. The addition of sensory blocks and performing the peel in no less than 45 minutes appeared to have resolved the problem. When I used 50% phenol as a first pass under oral sedation, I had to proceed slowly by necessity. When I first used the technique under intravenous sedation and did it faster, I saw transient tachyarrhythmias. Simply slowing down the application while monitoring the electrocardiogram (ECG) took care of this issue.

A small handheld fan is used to dissipate the fumes, and gauze should always be available in case rapid drying is needed. A calm, focused, deliberate manner is important.

JUDGING PEEL DEPTH

Any resurfacing modality involves a controlled injury with healing that results in improved appearance and quality of the skin. Success is defined by choosing and safely reaching the appropriate endpoint. Phenol–croton oil peels go deeper than the epidermis, with medium-depth peels reaching the papillary dermis. To significantly improve wrinkles, deep peels must injure the upper to middle reticular dermis. The price to pay for a deeper peel is a longer and more involved recovery. Procedures with minimal downtime also yield minimal results.

As the peel progresses, the degree of opacity of the frost is constantly evaluated to gauge the depth. A thin, transparent frost with a pink background indicates that the peel has passed through the epidermis into the dermis. The translucent quality of the frost reveals the dermal vessels—hence the pink color. Depending on the circumstance and location, this may be the correct endpoint. With more passes, the peel proceeds to the upper and middle dermis. The frost forms a solid, opaque, even white frost. The pink hue is lost because the acid has destroyed the intradermal vessels and the opacity hides the deeper subdermal plexus. Without further peeling, the frost is gradually lost in about 15 minutes ("defrosting"), and the skin turns into a red-brown or

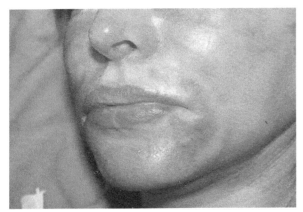

Fig.. 7.1 Red-tan appearance is indicative of reaching the reticular dermis.

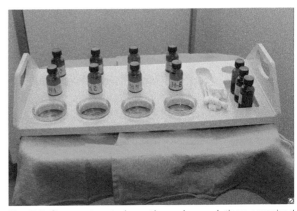

Fig. 7.2 Custom tray to keep the various solutions organized during peeling.

tan color (Fig. 7.1). This is a reliable sign that the upper to midreticular dermis has been reached. Further peeling after a solid white frost results in a gray-white color indicative of reaching the lower reticular dermis, which is not advisable.

The progression from superficial to deep is orderly, slow, and easily recognizable. The experienced peeler can control the process by peeling slow enough to recognize the visual cues and stop at the chosen depth and go no deeper. The all-or-none phenomenon attributed to the Baker peel was simply that the croton oil concentration was so high that it instantly went to a depth that resulted in hypopigmentation.

Another sign to evaluate depth of peeling is epidermal sliding. This occurs when the peel reaches the papillary dermis and the normal bonds between epidermis and dermis are broken and the epidermis can now slide as a thin independent sheet. This sliding disappears when the peel reaches the reticular dermis and a solid protein block is formed. Epidermal sliding is best seen in thin-skinned areas such as the eyelids and lateral forehead and is a reliable sign that the papillary dermis has been reached.

Defrosting times are also an indicator of depth but not as practical because it is already after the fact.

APPLICATION AND PRACTICAL RECOMMENDATIONS

Of primary importance is to always be mindful and protective of the eyes. As corneal protectors and ophthalmic ointment are not used, extreme care is necessary. The head of the bed is gently elevated to prevent acid running into the eye, never using an applying sponge so wet that it can drip, and never crossing over the eye with an applying gauze in hand. To keep the operator's hands dry, a surgical towel can be clipped to the shoulder of the scrub skirt and draped over the front to easily wipe the hands. Clearly labeled containers are lined up with glass bowls and arranged in ascending strength in a consistent manner to prevent confusion (Fig. 7.2).

The applying materials include 2-inch by 2-inch gauze (preferably synthetic fiber, which is less abrasive), large cotton-tipped applicator, small cotton-tipped applicator, and toothpicks. The solution is shaken before being poured into the bowl, and as described before, the new surfactant ensures that the mixture will not separate during the length of the peel. The gauze is folded twice to decrease the area of contact and carefully wrung out. This gauze should be moist and not so saturated that it can drip. The gauze is set down, and the hands are dried with the aforementioned towel. This is very important in segmented peels, where errors are obvious.

As the gauze is passed over the skin, the effect of the acid is seen in 10 to 15 seconds, depending on the concentration of the solution and the wetness of the gauze. The specific action of the acid is to precipitate and coagulate the protein of the skin, forming a "frost," of varying degrees of white appearance. The frosting becomes progressively more dense and opaque as the peel passes through the papillary dermis into the upper and midreticular dermis. Once the acid is applied the effect is irreversible, because there is no neutralizing agent available. As will be explained later, the process is slow enough to give the operator adequate control.

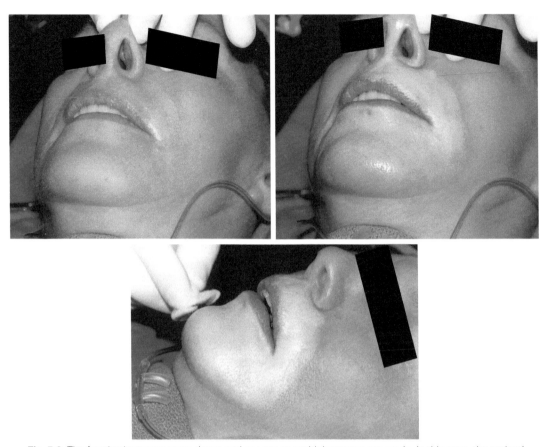

Fig. 7.3 The frosting becomes more dense and opaque as multiple passes are made. In this case, the perioral area and commissures were peeled to the reticular dermis.

The key concept is that with weaker concentrations (0.8% and 1.2% versus 2.1% of the Baker formula), the main factor of the depth reached is the application technique, which is directly controlled by the surgeon. Nuance in the technique can involve how wet the gauze is, how many passes are made, and how much pressure is applied. The same depth can be reached using different techniques or even different concentrations.

The key to chemical peeling is that the correct depth is reached, and although various concentrations will be recommended, the visual endpoint is what is important, and each area must be visually assessed. Similar depths can be reached with different concentrations and application techniques. The main advance of modern deep chemical peels is that the process is slow, giving the operator ample time to gauge the depth, with the various concentrations and application techniques being the means to getting there.

After degreasing with acetone, sensory nerve blocks can be performed if the patient is anesthetized, and a preliminary pass of 50% phenol is performed with caution, monitoring the ECG for increasing heart rate. If seen, slow down.

My routine is to start on the upper lip with 0.4% or 0.8%. The progressive degrees of frosting are easily seen on this thick skin. A light frost appears, and as further passes are made, the frost becomes denser and more organized. Continuing with the peel, redipping the gauze as needed, the frost becomes denser, whiter, and more opaque as the pink background is lost when the upper reticular dermis is reached. This process is slow and predictable, giving the operator the opportunity to stop at any point if a lesser peel is chosen. The speed at which a specific depth is reached depends on how wet the gauze is, what concentration is used, how many passes are made, and how hard one rubs.

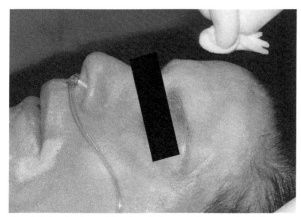

Fig. 7.4 In the lateral forehead the peel has reached the papillary dermis, denoted by a transparent frost with a pink background. The frost in the glabella is dense and more opaque, indicating that the peel has crossed into the reticular dermis.

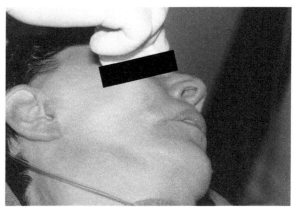

Fig. 7.5 The midface has been peeled to the papillary dermis; translucent frost with a pink background is visible.

Wrinkles in the perioral area are stretched to allow even penetration of the acid. The commissures can also be stretched and peeled deeply. The vermilion itself can be peeled with 0.2% or 0.4% solution. A lighter peel is continued onto the submandibular border to prevent a line of demarcation (Fig. 7.3).

The glabella and nose are addressed next because they often mimic the thickness and wrinkling of the perioral area and are typically peeled to the upper to midreticular dermis. The rational for the described sequence is to let some time pass while other areas are peeled, and after 15 to 20 minutes, the appearance of reddish-brown overtone will confirm having reached the reticular dermis. If this color is absent or faint, the area can be repeeled.

The forehead, which is next, is an area of variable thickness. The central area is thickest and thins out laterally, with the temporal area being especially delicate. Generally speaking, the forehead does not have significant wrinkles, except for transverse lines and oblique sleep lines laterally. A common approach is to peel centrally with 0.4% and 0.2% laterally to the papillary dermis. Deeper glabellar and transverse lines can be specifically targeted later. The peel is carried to the hairline to avoid a demarcation line and does not affect hair growth (Fig. 7.4).

The lateral face is peeled with 0.2%, with particular attention to the preauricular area, which is delicate. The peel should continue into the sideburn, the tragus, and the earlobe. The medial face is usually peeled with 0.4%, and dominant wrinkles are specifically targeted later. The inferior corridor between the mandibular angle and

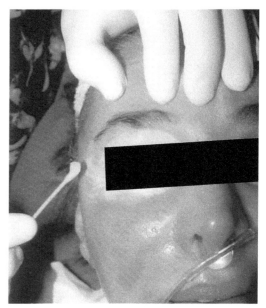

Fig. 7.6 The thin eyelid skin responds well to dilute solution such as 0.1% croton oil and possible 0.05% for the upper lids depending on the laxity.

the geniomandibular groove is delicate and rarely wrinkled, and therefore should be peeled with care (Fig. 7.5).

The eyelids are an excellent area for peeling because they show remarkable improvement and are rarely troublesome despite their thinness. A 0.1% solution is applied with one or two cotton-tipped applicators that have been dipped into the solution then touched to a gauze or cloth to lightly dry them. The peeling proceeds from inferior to superior, gradually approaching the ciliary margin (Fig. 7.6). The relative dampness of

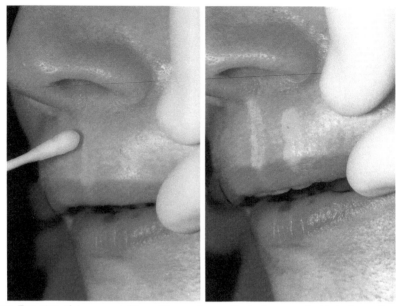

Fig. 7.7 Targeting of deeper wrinkles with a wetter applicator is very valuable in the perioral area.

the applicator and the number of passes made determine the depth. Epidermal sliding will become evident, and the frost will be an even white. After the other lid is peeled, the original lid is assessed and possibly repeeeled at midheight with 0.05% where dominant wrinkles and redundancy are seen. Some tension may be present in the lower lids early on, but it responds well to massage.

The upper lids respond to peeling by shrinking of the skin, possibly even resembling an upper blepharoplasty. Depending on the degree of laxity, the upper lids are peeled with 0.05% or 0.1%. If there is laxity below the tarsal fold, a light peel is possible. A minor inconvenience of peeling the upper lids is that the eyes may swell shut for a day or less, but it is well worth it.

The peel can be extended onto the neck to prevent a line of demarcation, but extreme caution is necessary. The neck skin is delicate and does not have the recuperative potential of facial skin. The purpose is not to improve wrinkles, because this would result in hypopigmentation or even scarring. The neck should be peeled with 0.025% or weaker with very light, wispy strokes leaving minimal or no frosting. If the practitioner is familiar and more comfortable with trichloroacetic acid, this is an option. "Less is more" is good advice.

Now is the time to examine deeper wrinkles in the lips, glabella, forehead, and midface. Precise deeper peeling of individual rhytids is a most valuable advantage of phenol–croton oil peels. The technique is to use a wetter cotton-tipped applicator to paint the individual line and quickly dry it as dense frost is seen. This is repeated until the desired endpoint is reached (Fig. 7.7). An alternative is to saturate a toothpick, wooden end of an applicator, or fine artist's brush and fill the valley of the wrinkle, leave it for a few seconds, then dry it. In the perioral and glabellar area, 1.2% solution may be used as described previously depending on severity. Lesser concentrations are used in the midface and crow's feet; an intact or splintered wooden end of an applicator are useful tools in these instances. If there is obvious demarcation between areas peeled with different concentrations a weak concentration such as 0.1% or 0.2% can be used to blend them.

The case has been made that these peels are very valuable and should be embraced by any practitioner involved in facial rejuvenation. The impediment may be that this is unknown, intimidating territory. If the inherent value is accepted, my advice is to begin gradually. The crux and nuance of these peels is visual, making it difficult to teach. Good-quality photographs and videos are available that are very useful. Live surgery workshops are an excellent way to advance rapidly in the practice. One way to gain experience is to deliberately underpeel a cooperative patient with the

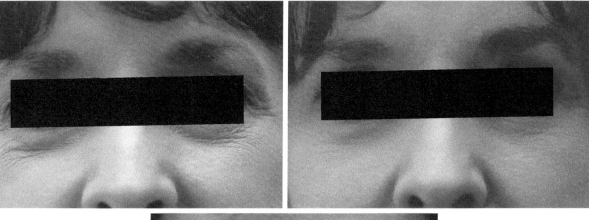

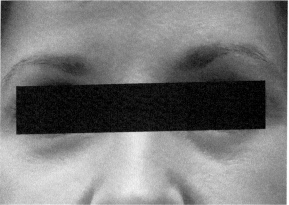

Fig. 7.8 Increased results are possible with multiple peels. Upper left, preoperatively; upper right; after one peel; below, center, after a second peel

thought of repeeling. Another approach is to downgrade the recommended concentrations by half (i.e., 0.8% to 0.4% to 0.2%, etc.) and gain experience with the mechanism and appearance of the peel. I believe that if the interested practitioner will accept this new territory in the spirit of learning, he or she will quickly advance into seasoned peelers, giving their patients results heretofore unattainable. The rewards over a career in appearance and skin health are unparalleled.

SEGMENTAL PEELS

Partial or segmental peels are possible if care and good judgment are exercised. Patients with widespread solar damage are at an increased risk for demarcation; therefore a full-face peel is preferable. An isolated perioral peel to a medium depth is possible, and the color will take 8 to 12 weeks to blend without camouflage makeup. In select patients with isolated upper lip lines, a mustache peel can give excellent results.

Eyelid skin responds particularly well to chemical peeling, making this an excellent area for segmental peeling. If the peel is kept within the boundaries of the orbital rim, the skin color change is well tolerated and easily managed with makeup or glasses. The peel can be extended to the crow's feet, but the erythema will last longer and be more noticeable. The lower eyelid skin is often the first place to show aging, usually in the early to mid-40s. This is a frustrating situation for patients, and the myriad creams and treatments are not particularly satisfactory. A simple peel, usually without anesthesia, can take care of the situation.

Lower eyelid peeling has significant advantages. If the peel is repeated, additive results are seen, and lower eyelids can usually be treated to the patient's satisfaction (Fig. 7.8). Because these changes are so common, it opens up treatment to a very large population. At whatever point there is further deterioration, the lid can be repeeled and therefore keep up with aging.

Treatment of the lower lids is relatively easy and predictable; problems with healing are a rarity. This is a good place to start peeling, and in fact, any practitioner that does not want to undertake the complexity of a full-face peeling will benefit many patients by peeling the eyelids. Upper lid peeling can result in a very natural, refreshed look.

POSTPEEL CARE

Caring for the patient after a peel can be the most challenging aspect of the entire process. The peel creates a wound, and the goal is to guide reepithelialization comfortably and without problems. There are many options

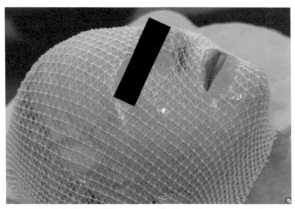

Fig. 7.9 Zinc oxide tape applied to all areas peeled.

available in the field of resurfacing, and there is not a clear consensus.

In the first part of my peeling experience, I treated the skin open by mixing triple antibiotic ointment and lidocaine jelly to all peeled areas. The patient continued applying this over the next 10 to 12 days as the skin recovered. This approach works but is messy, and problems with sensitization to the antibiotic can occur, leading to breakouts and rashes. Milia and intense erythema related to the occlusive nature are also problems.

In an attempt to improve the patient experience, a variation of an older technique has become the preferred routine. At the end of the peel, all frosting is allowed to subside, and no further action is taken; the peeled areas are then covered with zinc oxide tape, and a dressing net is applied to stabilize the tape (Fig. 7.9). If the upper lids are peeled and tape applied, opening of the lids may be impeded the first night. Petrolatum jelly is applied to the brows and hairline to prevent pulling hair during removal. A bouffant surgical cap overlaps the hairline tape and is taped in place.

The patient returns the next day and the mask is removed from inferior to superior, typically without pain. The peeled skin is washed with saline and gently debrided with the edge of a tongue depressor (Fig. 7.10).

Following this, a paste of bismuth subgallate powder and saline is mixed and applied to all peeled areas with a tongue depressor or makeup brush (Fig. 7.11). The paste is allowed to dry to a solid crust and from

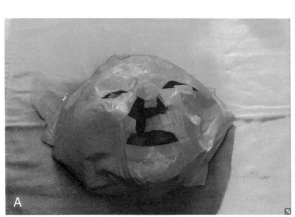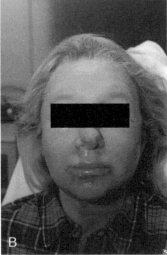

Fig. 7.10 A, Tape mask after removal on postpeel day 1. B, Appearance after tape mask removal.

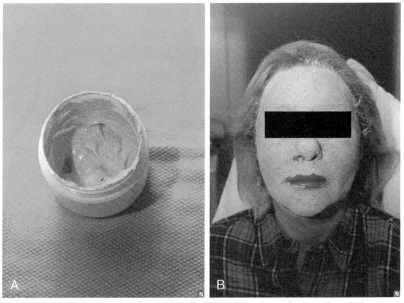

Fig. 7.11 A, Bismuth subgallate paste. B, Bismuth paste applied to all peeled areas.

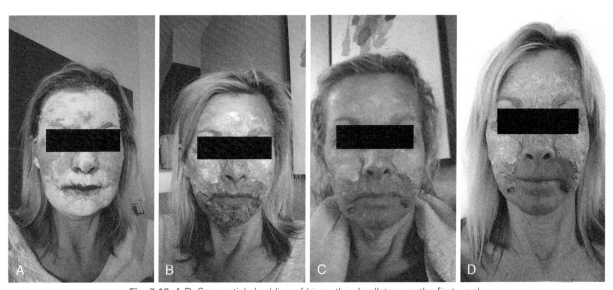

Fig. 7.12 A-D, Sequential shedding of bismuth subgallate over the first week.

this point, the patient does nothing and does not touch the face. Over the next 7 to 12 days, the healing skin underneath the mask will reepithelialize and shed the crust. The patient is strongly advised not to pick or touch the face. The patient is usually seen at day 7, and a heavy balm or petrolatum is applied to any crust that remains attached. This is allowed to seep in, and they can gently shower the next day. The process is repeated, and the bismuth is usually shed between days 10 and 12.

The exposed skin, which will be pink to red, is treated with a nonfragrant moisturizer or postprocedure cream such as Epidermal Repair (SkinCeuticals, Garland, TX) (Figs. 7.12 and 7.13).

The surprising reaction has been overwhelming acceptance of this bizarre appearance and appreciation of the hands-off approach. Patients have shown remarkable good humor and great ingenuity for covering up (Fig. 7.14). They are much more at peace with this technique,

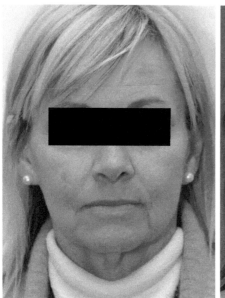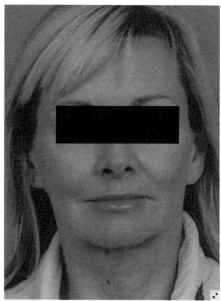

Fig. 7.13 63-year-old woman seen in Fig. 7.12. Before and 4 months after peel.

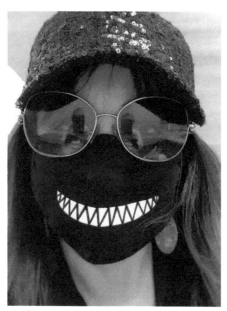

Fig. 7.14 Example of clever cover-up.

and it has significantly cut down on worried calls and visits. The typical care results in less irritated skin and decreased erythema. Postpeel erythema lasts 8 to 12 weeks, fading gradually and easily managed with makeup.

RESULTS

Croton oil peels, like other resurfacing modalities, injure the skin and elicit a healing response that stimulates the deposition of collagen. A significant difference is that new elastin is also stimulated, and the layer of collagen is thick, orderly, and remarkably stable over many years. The result is a modification in the skin anatomy with improvement of wrinkles and histologically skin that looks younger because, in essence, younger skin has been created. Light penetrates this new skin and is reflected back brightly, doing away with the dull, ashen look of sun-damaged skin. No surgical procedure can do this. The peeled skin not only looks better, it is actually healthier. Histological studies show eradication of actinic keratoses and early cancer cells. The peels reach the depth where these nests of cells exist, and it is cumulative impression of experienced peelers that patients who have been peeled do not develop facial basal cell or squamous cell cancers. This is an important observation that warrants further investigation and confirms the common intuition that beautiful skin is healthy skin.

Figs. 7.15 through 7.23 chronicle the dramatic improvement that can be obtained with phenol–croton oil peels.

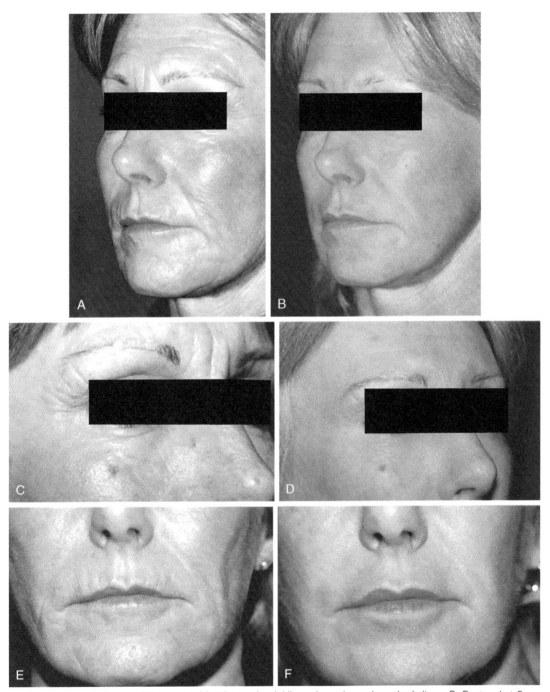

Fig.. 7.15 A, A 49-year-old woman with advanced wrinkling, elastosis, and smoker's lines. B, Postpeel at 8 months. Notable improvement in the quality of the skin and abatement of dominant wrinkles are evident. C, Prepeel and, D, postpeel of orbital and glabellar area. Visible shrinking of upper lid skin and improvement of deep wrinkles are evident. E, Prepeel and, F, postpeel views of the perioral area.

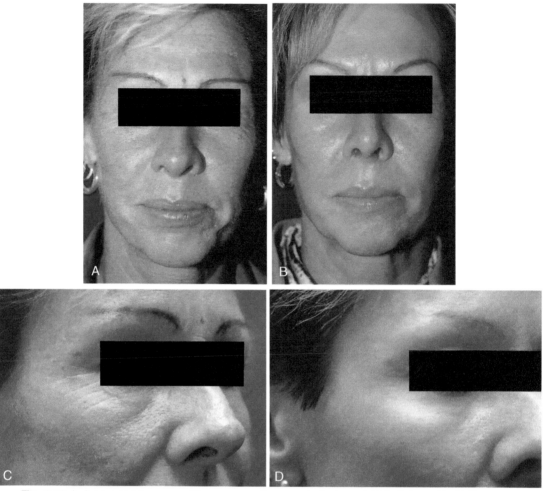

Fig.. 7.16 A, A 47-year-old woman with severe sun damage, elastosis, and thick, lifeless skin. B, Four years postpeel. Overall improvement in the quality of the skin and even pigmentation. C, Prepeel. D, One year post-peel with evident softening of the brittle, unnatural skin and improvement of the lids.

COMPLICATIONS

As with any resurfacing technique, treating too deep can result in scarring (see Chapter 16). Any skin thickening is suspicious and should be treated with topical steroids. If an early scar forms, intralesional injection of 5-fluorouracil (5-FU) is recommended. This is an off-label use. A newer approach is microneedling with nanofat, which shows great promise.

Hypopigmentation can occur if the peel goes too deep. A patient with very pronounced wrinkles may need to be peeled to a depth that causes hypopigmentation. Even if this is the case, it tends not to have the unnatural appearance seen with older peels.

Hyperpigmentation is usually the result of early sun exposure; therefore prevention is the key. Hyperpigmentation responds to tretinoin and hydroquinone 4%.

Herpetic infection is always a possibility, and all patients are treated 3 days before the peel and continued for 7 days after.

Other, lesser complications include mild ectropion, which resolves with massage, milia, and prolonged erythema.

CONCLUSION

A missing piece in facial rejuvenation is an effective technique for skin resurfacing. Modern phenol–croton oil

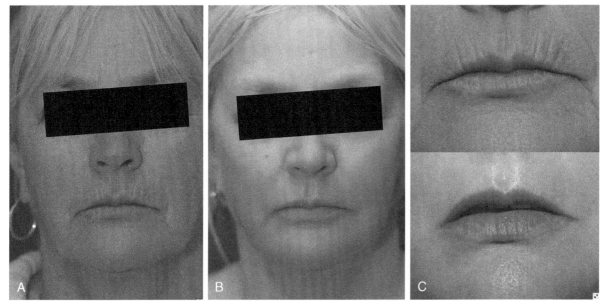

Fig.. 7.17 A, A 59-year-old woman with ashen, dull look of sun damage and pronounced lines of the upper lip. B, One year postpeel showing overall improvement and, C, dramatic effacement of perioral radial lines.

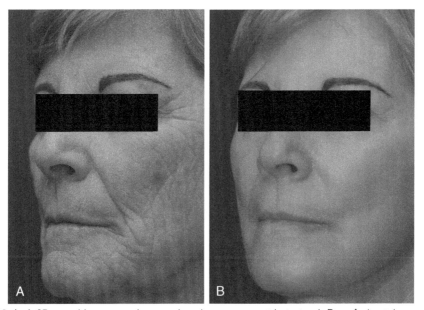

Fig.. 7.18 A, A 65-year-old woman whose main aging component is textural. Resurfacing takes precedent over surgical correction. B, One year postpeel with greatly improved appearance and normal pigmentation.

peels are a new tool that provide impressive, long-lasting results without hypopigmentation. Newer techniques make the peel more convenient and the recovery more tolerable for the patient. By manipulating the formulas and application technique, the peels are available to younger patients and are a means to keep up with aging. Phenol–croton oil peels are an excellent alternative to expensive lasers.

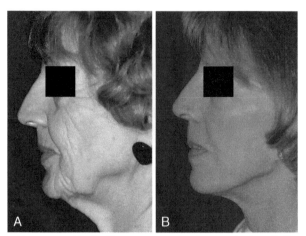

Fig.. 7.19 A, A 75-year-old woman with significant structural and textural aging. B, Results at age 81 years, 5 years after a facelift and 1 year after a peel, demonstrating the value of correcting both aspects.

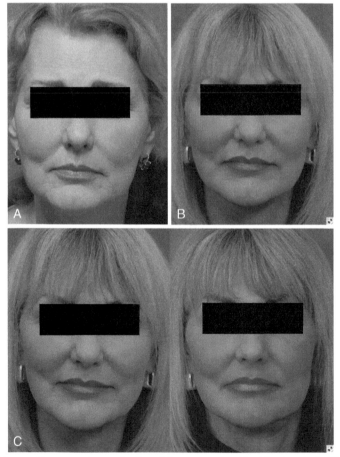

Fig.. 7.20 A, A 63-year old woman demonstrating all three aspects of facial aging: typical laxity, jowling, and wrinkling. B, One year after facelift and fat transfer with noticeable structural and volume improvements. C, One and a half years postpeel. The improvement of texture and wrinkling is the final component that ties everything together in a comprehensive result.

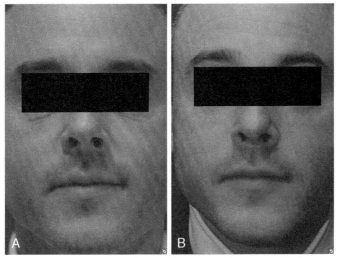

Fig.. 7.21 A, A 44-year-old man whose dominant aging change is the wrinkled and crepey appearance of the lower lid skin. B, Six months after a segmental peel of the lower lids alone. The improvement of the lower lid has been achieved without altering the shape of the lateral canthus.

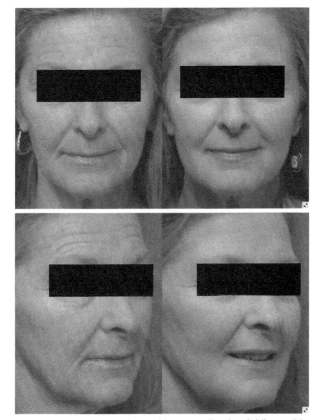

Fig.. 7.22 Left, A 61-year-old woman, smoker, with generalized wrinkling, widespread sun damage, pigment changes, and obvious aging appearance. Right, Six months postpeel without surgery. This case demonstrates the considerable power that a phenol–croton oil peel alone can have in overall rejuvenation. The postpeel appearance is that of a much younger, vital person.

continued

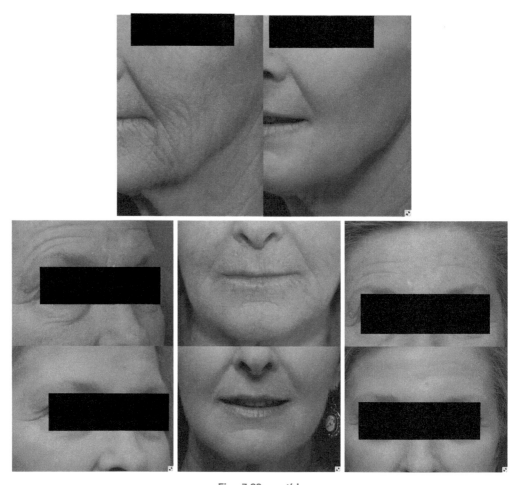

Fig.. 7.22, cont'd

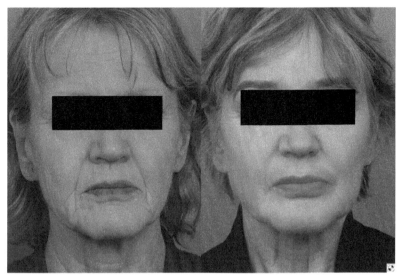

Fig.. 7.23 Left, A 69-year-old woman with advanced wrinkling and general deflation of face not wishing sur-gery. Right, At 14 months after complete face lipofilling with microfat and nanofat plus peeling at the same time. This is an example of impressive centrofacial rejuvenation without surgery.

FURTHER READING

Baker TJ. Chemical face peeling and rhytidectomy for facial rejuvenation. *Plast Reconstr Surg.* 1962;29:199–207.

Baker TJ. Is the phenol-croton oil peel safe? *Plast Reconstr Surg.* 2003;112:353–354.

Baker TJ, Stuzin JM, Baker TM. *Facial Skin Resurfacing.* St Louis: Quality Medical Publishing; 1998.

Bensimon RH. Croton oil peels. *Aesthet Surg J.* 2008;28:33–45.

Demas PN, Bridenstine JB. Diagnosis and treatment of postoperative complications after skin resurfacing. *J Oral Maxillofac Surg.* 1999;57:837–841.

Demas PN, Bridenstine JB, Braun TW. Pharmacology of agents used in the management of patients having skin resurfacing. *J Oral Maxillofac Surg.* 1997;55:1255–1258.

De Rossi-Fattaccioli D. Histologic comparison between deep chemical peels (modified Litton's formulae) and extreme pulsed laser CO_2 resurfacing. *Dermatol Peru.* 2005;15:181–184.

Dinner MI, Artz JS. The art of trichloroacetic acid chemical peel. *Clin Plast Surg.* 1998;25:53–62.

Edison RB. Lighter phenol peels allow faster recovery and less discomfort. *Aesthet Surg J.* 1996;16:239–240.

Hantash BM, Stewart DB, Cooper ZA, et al. Facial resurfacing for non-melanoma skin cancer prophylaxis. *Arch Dermatol.* 2006;142:976–982.

Hetter GP. An examination of the phenol-croton oil peel: part I. Dissecting the formula. *Plast Reconstr Surg.* 2000;105:227–239.

Hetter GP. An examination of the phenol-croton oil peel: part II. The lay peelers and their croton oil formulas. *Plast Reconstr Surg.* 2000;105:240–248.

Hetter GP. An examination of the phenol-croton oil peel: part III. The plastic surgeon's role. *Plast Reconstr Surg.* 2000;105:752–763.

Hetter GP. An examination of the phenol-croton oil peel: part IV. Face peel results with different concentrations of phenol and croton oil. *Plast Reconstr Surg.* 2000;105:1061–1083.

Johnson JB, Ichinose H, Obagi ZE, et al. Obagi's modified tri-chloroacetic acid (TCA)-controlled variable-depth peel: a study of clinical signs correlated with histological findings. *Ann Plast Surg.* 1996;36:225–237.

Kligman AM, Baker TJ, Gordon HL. Long-term histologic follow-up of the phenol face peels. *Plast Reconstr Surg.* 1985;75:652–659.

Landau M. Cardiac complications in deep chemical peels. *Dermatol Surg.* 2007;33:190–193.

Obagi ZE. *Obagi Skin Health Restoration and Rejuvenation.* New York: Springer-Verlag; 2000.

Rubin MG. *Chemical Peels: Superficial and Medium Depth.* Philadelphia: Lippincott Williams & Williams; 1995.

Stagnone JJ, Stagnone GJ. A second look at chemabrasion. *J Dermatol Surg Oncol.* 1982;8:701–705.

Stegman SJ. A comparative histologic study of the effects of three peeling agents and dermabrasion on nor-mal and sun-damaged skin. *Aesthetic Plast Surg.* 1982;6:123–125.

Tonnard PL, Verpaele AM, Bensimon RH. *Centrofacial Rejuvenation.* New York: Thieme Medical Publishers; 2018.

Truppman ES, Ellenby JD. Major electrocardiographic changes during chemical face peeling. *Plast Reconstr Surg.* 1979;63:44–48.

8

Deep Chemical Peels

Marina Landau

The results of phenol–croton oil peeling, also known as deep chemical peeling, are considered the gold standard in the treatment of the aged face. Historically, in the "pre-energy-based devices era," it was almost the only option for radical facial skin rejuvenation. The main advantages of a deep peeling procedure are its efficacy, predictability, and longevity of results. The dissection of phenol–croton oil formulas discloses that more than one formula is safe and effective. The success of the procedure depends on the surgeon's qualification, the patient's education, and adhering to safety standards.

HISTORY

Almost all the modern formulas for deep peeling contain phenol and croton oil. The early use of phenol peel was documented by two dermatologists, George Miller MacKee and Florentine Karp, in their publication on treating patients with postacne scars.[1] The first time that croton oil was mentioned as an ingredient of deep peeling solution was by Adolph M. Brown, in his 1959 patent application entitled "Skin Treating Method and Composition."[2] Among other contributors to the medical development of phenol–croton oil peels at that time were Bames,[3] Urkov,[4] Combes et al.,[5] Brown et al.,[6] and Litton.[7]

The final revival of deep chemical peeling is attributed to two American plastic surgeons, Thomas J. Baker and Howard L. Gordon, who during the 1960s legitimized this procedure by discussing it in national meetings and demonstrating their impressive results.[8,9] The scientific landmark breakthrough in phenol–croton oil peeling came from a publication of Gregory Hetter, who showed that by varying the amount of croton oil in the peel solution the strength of the peel can be modified.[10] Other authors, such as Stone and Lefer,[11] Spira et al.,[12] and Fintsi,[13] contributed to the procedure, allowing it to emerge from semiobscurity to its respectable and valued place in a field of aesthetic surgery.

CHEMICAL BACKGROUND

The active ingredients in the solution for deep peeling are a combination of croton oil and phenol.

Phenol (C_5H_5OH), or carbolic acid, is an aromatic hydrocarbon derived originally from coal tar, but prepared synthetically in a process that uses monochlorobenzene (Fig. 8.1). After this process, 98% phenol appears as transparent crystals, and the liquefied phenol consists of 88% USP solution of phenol in water.

Croton oil is an extract of the seed of the plant *Croton tiglium* and has been commercially prepared as croton resin since 1932. Its activity on the skin is related to free hydroxyl groups, which cause skin vesiculation even in low doses.

Other ingredients in deep chemical peel formulas include Septisol or Novisol, water, and vegetable oils (glycerin, olive, sesame).

Formulations

The concentration of phenol in different formulations ranges between 45% and 80%, whereas croton oil is between 0.16% and 2.05%. The role of Septisol is to reduce the skin surface tension and to improve solution penetration. Despite this, Septisol is not included in all of the formulas. Some of the formulas contain oils. The role of the oils in the formula has not been clarified yet. Our personal experience shows that oily phenol

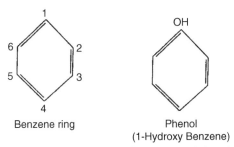

Fig. 8.1 Chemical formulas of benzene and phenol.

solutions penetrate the skin in a more controllable fashion.

Few dogmas regarding phenol-based peeling solutions have been challenged in the last two decades. The concept of the "all-or-none" effect of the Baker-Gordon formula on the skin was confronted by Gregory Hetter,[10] who showed that depth of the penetration and clinical outcomes of the peel can be manipulated by a change in the amount of croton oil. A major advantage of this concept is that by decreasing the croton oil concentration, the surgeon is able to accommodate the depth of the peel according to the skin type, area treated, or expected clinical outcome, by changing the amount of the solution applied and the number of coats.[14,15]

Histology

Biopsies obtained 48 hours after phenol peeling demonstrate necrosis of the epidermis, extending through the papillary dermis, surrounded by a marked inflammatory reaction.[6] Epidermal regeneration is completed within 7 days, whereas dermal healing usually lags behind. Histological changes in human skin induced by deep chemical peeling include a newly formed band of dermis found directly beneath the epidermis consisting of horizontal compact bundles of collagen and a dense network of fine elastic fibers, as well as even and uniformly shaped keratinocytes in epidermis. Although peeled skin tends to be hypopigmented, melanocytes are present.[16] These changes are evident even as long as 20 years after the peel.[17]

INDICATIONS AND PATIENT SELECTION

The main indications for deep chemical peels include dyschromia, especially solar lentigines; wrinkles; solar keratosis; and acne scars. Deep peels can be used to treat periorbital melanosis, benign skin growths, or deposits,

such as xanthelasma or epidermal nevus. Recently, the efficacy of phenol–croton oil peels was shown for lip enhancement.[18]

Thick male skin is usually less responsive to deep peels, but men with severe actinic damage or acne scarring benefit significantly from the procedure.

Deep peeling can be performed on the eyelids to improve excess eyelid laxity, periorbital pigmentation, or wrinkling or as an adjunct procedure to surgical or micropunch blepharoplasty.[19,20]

A combination of deep peeling performed on one cosmetic unit with a medium-depth peel performed on the rest of the face is called a *segmental peel*. Segmental peeling is a procedure of choice if a limited area (usually perioral or periorbital) is significantly more wrinkled than others (Fig. 8.2). Use of deep chemical peels on an area smaller than 1% of the body area does not require cardiac monitoring.[21]

Contraindications

There are few absolute contraindications for deep peeling, mainly physical or mental instability. Originally, the ideal patient for a deep chemical peel was a blond, blue-eyed, fair-complexioned woman. Our experience shows that phenol-based peels can be safely performed on olive- and dark-skinned patients with dark eyes and hair.[22] As long as a patient is aware and cooperative in using a skin-lightening preparation (see Chapter 3) and potent sunscreens during the postpeel period, the procedure is equally effective and safe for dark skins.[23]

During pregnancy and lactation, any cosmetic intervention is considered to be undesirable. Although patients with controlled hypertension, diabetes mellitus, and thyroid malfunction can be peeled safely, any preexisting heart condition requires special precautions. All patients are required to have an electrocardiogram before the procedure. Medications prolonging QT interval should be stopped or switched before the procedure, because QT interval prolongation has been reported during phenol–croton oil peels.[24] It is always recommended to work in cooperation with a patient's cardiologist.

Systemic isotretinoin (Accutane) used to be an absolute contraindication to any cosmetic intervention. This approach has been recently challenged.[25] We feel that minimal interval to peeling after stopping this medication can be shortened from the traditional 6 months, especially when performing a procedure on a patient with thick sebaceous skin.

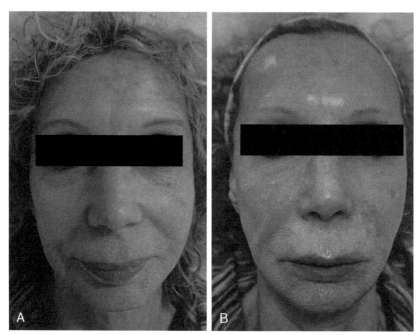

Fig. 8.2 Segmental peel. A, Candidate. B, Peeling procedure: perioral phenol–croton oil peel combined with Jessner's trichloroacetic acid 35% peeling elsewhere.

According to our experience, smoking does not adversely affect the postpeel healing or the extent of the results. We suggest adding frontal fibrosing alopecia (FFA) as a relative contraindication for the procedure. Once a rare disease, FFA has recently become a prevalent condition. Inflammation and fibrosis of the hair follicles in facial skin, as happens in this disease, may affect the healing process after deep peeling.[26]

Prepeeling Preparation

Honest dialog with the patient is important before any cosmetic intervention, and its value cannot be overestimated for a deep chemical peel.

It should be verified that the patient completely understands the following points:

1. Until reepithelization is accomplished, the patient should expect to look extremely "unattractive." Pictures of real patients during this phase are shown to make the idea more concrete (Fig. 8.3). Supportive family significantly eases this phase for the patient.
2. Full rehabilitation of the skin, including complete fading of the redness, takes a few months. Strict compliance with postprocedural instructions, including sun avoidance, is necessary for an uneventful postpeel course.
3. Complying with the strict and frequent follow-up visits is necessary to assure that any developing adverse reaction is addressed in a timely manner.

Prophylactic acyclovir, valacyclovir, or famciclovir is given to patients with a history of recurrent herpes simplex, starting a day before the procedure and continuing for 10 days or until full reepithelialization is achieved.

Standard photography is performed and a consent form is signed before the procedure.

Preparation of the Skin

It is still debatable whether preparation of the skin is required for deep chemical peeling. Topical application of retinoic acid cream for 3 to 6 weeks before the procedure may create better and more even penetration of the peeling solution, especially in thick sebaceous skin.

Monitoring and Pain Control

Phenol-based peels can be performed as a full-face or a segmental procedure. When conducting full-face peels, intravenous fluids should be administered throughout the procedure to reduce cardiac complications related to phenol toxicity. For segmental peels, patients are instructed to drink a minimum of 1 L of water throughout the procedure.

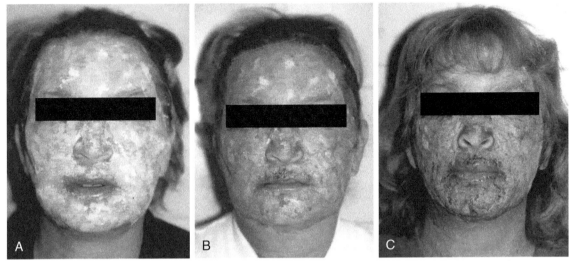

Fig. 8.3 A–C, Post–full-face peel course, used for patient consultation and preparation for the procedure.

The critical period of procedure-related discomfort is during the peeling and up to 4 hours after it. Variations of oral and intravenous anesthesia as well as regional nerve blocks can be used. Although full cardiopulmonary monitoring is required during full-face peeling, no cardiopulmonary monitoring is needed during segmental peel.

PREPARATION OF THE PEELING SOLUTION

The formulation of the peeling solution is of uppermost importance for the efficacy, safety, and reproducibility of the results. Experienced peelers prepare their own solutions, altering the solution strength by changing the concentration of croton oil, according to Hetter's principles.[10]

For less experienced or beginner peelers, commercial formulas with fixed croton oil concentration might be a better and safer choice. In this case, the depth is controlled mainly by the number of passes performed.

The first step in preparing the peeling solution is to mix 1 mL of croton oil in 24 mL of 88% phenol to create a stock solution, to be further diluted following Hetter's protocols (Table 8.1). *This stock is not a peeling solution and should not be used on the skin.*

From the stock solution light to very strong peeling solutions are prepared according to the clinical indication and treatment area (Table 8.2).

To make a strong solution containing 1.2% croton oil, 3 mL of stock solution is mixed with 1 mL phenol 88%,

TABLE 8.1 **Hetter's Stock Solution[a]**	
24 mL phenol 88% USP	1 mL croton oil

[a]Used for mixing the other peel solutions and NOT for use directly on skin.

5.5 mL water, and 0.5 mL Septisol. For medium-strength solution, 2 mL of stock is mixed with 2 mL of phenol 88%, 5.5 mL water, and 0.5 mL Septisol (Table 8.3).[27]

If left nonagitated, the solutions tend to separate into two phases. Repetitively mixing the phases is necessary during the application.

PEELING TECHNIQUE

On the day of the procedure, a patient is required to avoid using any cosmetics or creams. Before the peeling, meticulous cleaning of the skin is performed. While a patient is on the operating table, the skin is degreased by acetone-soaked gauze sponges. This step is imperative to obtain an even penetration of the solution into the skin.

Cotton-tipped applicators (CTAs) or 4-inch by 4-inch gauzes are used to apply the peeling solution. The ready-to-use applicators come in different sizes, but usually a CTA is too dense and has only limited absorption ability. Therefore, we suggest adding regular cotton to soften the tip (Fig. 8.4).

The volume of peeling solution, pressure of the application, and number of strokes are the main technical variables to control the depth of penetration. To control

TABLE 8.2   Hetter's Standard Solutions and Indications

	Very Strong	Strong	Medium	Light
Croton oil %	1.6%	1.2%	0.8%	0.4%
Indications	Deep wrinkles	Moderate wrinkles	Mild wrinkles	Laxity
Areas	Perioral, nose	Forehead, cheeks	Temples	Eyelids and neck

TABLE 8.3   Hetter's Standard Solutions Preparation to Make 10 mL of Peeling Solution

	Very Strong	Strong	Medium	Light
Hetter's stock	4 mL	3 mL	2 mL	1 mL
Phenol 88%	-	1 mL	2 mL	3 mL
Water	5.5 mL	5.5 mL	5.5 mL	5.5 mL
Septisol	0.5 mL	0.5 mL	0.5 mL	0.5 mL

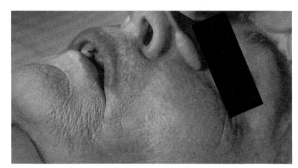

Fig. 8.5 Application of the peeling solution. Ivory-white color of the skin is the endpoint of the application.

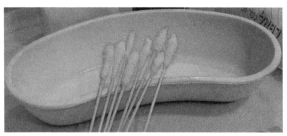

Fig. 8.4 Cotton tips are used to apply the peeling solution.

the amount of the peeling solution, semidry applicators or gauze are used. In the most sensitive areas, such as the periorbital skin, barely wet applicators should be used, and only a single layer of the solution is applied.

The procedure starts on the forehead, and the solution is feathered into all hair-bearing areas, including the scalp and eyebrows. Peeling solution does not affect hair growth. All the cosmetic units are gradually covered, including the earlobes and a "hidden" triangle above the ears. The usual endpoint is ivory-white to gray-white color of skin (Fig. 8.5). In the most wrinkled facial areas additional application of peeling solution is advisable, after the frosting fades. It is important to keep the final volume of the solution used on the face at no more than 5 mL.

Full-face peels should be carried out under full cardiopulmonary monitoring with intravenous sedation and hydration throughout the procedure.

Air circulation and safety pauses are recommended to allow phenol to be metabolized and excreted from the circulation. In addition to central ventilation, an electric fan to vent the phenol fumes out or masks with activated carbon are recommended for the comfort of the staff.[28]

Postpeel occlusion of the most wrinkled areas deepens the penetration of the solution. In an animal study, no difference in terms of depth of necrosis and neutrophilic infiltrate was noted when comparing occlusion by adhesive tape, petrolatum, or bacitracin ointment and nonoccluded areas.[29] However, the study was performed using the traditional Baker's solution, for which the "all or none" principle is applicable, as previously discussed.

The most wrinkled areas are occluded using short strips of waterproof zinc oxide nonpermeable tape applied in an overlapping fashion (Fig. 8.6). Overlapping allows slight motion and flexibility between the strips; therefore the swelling of the face during the postoperative period does not cause separation of the tape from the skin surface.

AFTERCARE

After 24 hours, the tape is easily removed, because the exudate separates it from the skin. Analgesia is not required, because the procedure is almost painless. After removing the tape mask, the exudate is cleaned by sterile saline. We cover the face with bismuth subgallate

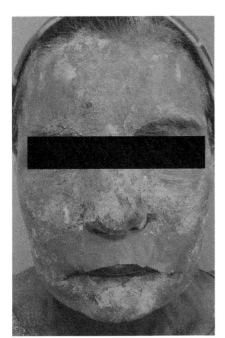

Fig. 8.6 Waterproof zinc oxide nonpermeable tape is applied to the most wrinkled areas to deepen the penetration of the solution to enhance the effect of the procedure.

antiseptic powder for seven days (see Fig. 8.6). Other options include occlusive moisturizers, antibiotic ointments, and biosynthetic occlusive dressings, such as Meshed Omiderm (ITG-Medev, San Francisco, CA).

We prescribe regular painkillers to be taken every 4 hours for the first 2 postoperative days. Some physicians administer systemic corticoids to reduce the swelling and inflammation after the peel. Neck swelling is expected after a deep peel. It resolves after 4 to 6 days.

Bismuth subgallate powder acts as regenerative mask and absorbs skin exudate and gradually creates a firm and rigid mask. It may crack in some areas, usually around the mouth and eyes. Some patients experience itching and can be helped by oral antihistamines. On the eighth day, wet soaking with tap water while standing in the shower is used to soften the powder mask. Repeated applications of petroleum jelly enhance the detachment of the "second mask" from the newly formed skin.

After the procedure, the patient is advised to use water-based lotion creams and potent sunscreens. The erythema is extremely intense the first 6 weeks and gradually resolves over a period of 3 to 6 months (Fig. 8.7). During this time, patients are encouraged to wear makeup with a green foundation and to resume all daily activities. In males, faster disappearance of erythema is expected. In cases of darker-skinned patients (Fitzpatrick skin type III or IV), application of retinoic acid–hydroquinone preparation is recommended to prevent reactive hyperpigmentation.

Immediate and long-term results of phenol–croton oil peels for various indications in patients of different skin phototypes, as well as segmental peeling, are shown next (Figs. 8.7–8.14).

COMPLICATIONS

Complications occur with any type of skin resurfacing. Understanding the risks and identifying the complications early allows for quick intervention with little long-term consequences (see also Chapter 16).

Cardiac Arrhythmias

The most important potential complication of phenol-based peels is cardiotoxicity. Phenol is directly toxic to myocardium. Studies in rats showed a decrease in myocardial contraction and in electrical activity after systemic exposure to phenol.[30] Because fatal doses ranged widely in these studies, it seems that individual sensitivity of myocardium to this chemical exists. In humans neither sex, age, nor previous cardiac history or blood phenol levels are accurate predictors for cardiac arrhythmia susceptibility.[31] The arrhythmias include tachycardia, premature ventricular beats, bigeminy, and atrial and ventricular tachycardia.[32]

After the application of the peeling solution, there is a quick absorption of phenol from the skin surface into the circulation.[33] Approximately 75% of phenol is excreted directly through kidney or detoxified by the liver. The other 25% is metabolized to CO_2 and water.

Phenol blood levels measured after application of 3 mL of 50% solution of phenol is 0.68 mg/dL, whereas in patients who survived an accidental oral ingestion of phenol a blood level of 23 mg/dL was found. Application of phenol to one cosmetic unit is equivalent to the application of phenol into a nail matrix for matrixectomy.

In a recent study, cardiac arrhythmia was recorded in 6.6% of the patients during the procedure, but not afterward. Cardiac arrhythmia was more common in patients taking medication for diabetes, hypertension, and depression, probably related to the medications prolonging the QT interval.[34]

If an arrhythmia occurs, the application of the solution should be stopped until normal sinus rhythm

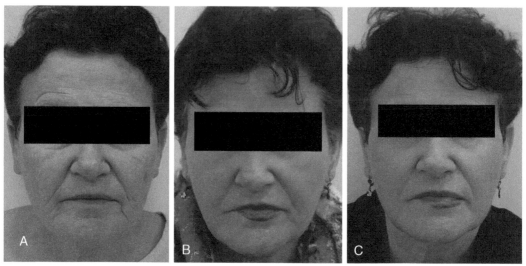

Fig. 8.7 A 69-year-old patient before (A), 10 days after (B), and 3 month after (C) the procedure.

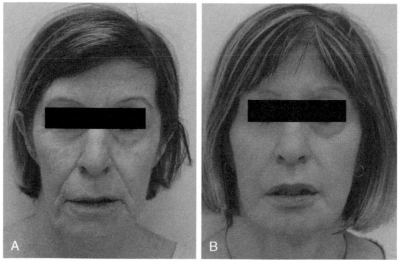

Fig. 8.8 A 72-year-old patient before (A) and 2 weeks after (B) the peel. The patient is wearing makeup with a green foundation to conceal redness.

returns. Medications are sometimes needed to control arrhythmias. Ensure the patient received adequate intravenous hydration during the phenol peel.

No hepatorenal or central nervous system toxicities have been reported in the literature with properly performed chemical peels.[35]

Pigmentary Changes

Delayed hypopigmentation is a reason some doctors disliked the long-term results of the traditional, high

croton oil concentration in the Baker-Gordon peel. Hypopigmentation after phenol peels is proportional to the depth of the peel, amount of the solution used, inherent skin color, and postpeel sun-related behavior.

Reactive hyperpigmentation can occur after any chemical peel. Usually lighter-complexion patients have a lower risk for hyperpigmentation. Retinoic acid– and hydroquinone-based creams are reintroduced to prevent or treat postpeel pigmentation. The return of pigment in previously existing intradermal nevi is a well-known

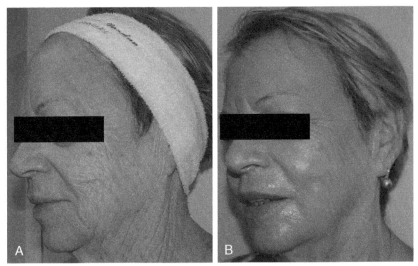

Fig. 8.9 An 82-year-old patient before (A) and 4 weeks after (B) the peel.

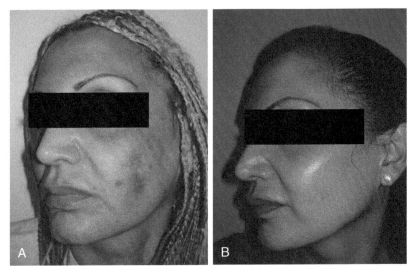

Fig. 8.10 A dark-skinned patient before (A) and 6 months after (B) the peel.

phenomenon and should not alarm the physician or patient.

Scarring

Scarring remains the most dreadful complication of chemical peels. The contributing factors are not well defined yet. The incidence of scarring with a traditional Baker's formula is less than 1%, whereas with less aggressive phenol–croton oil peels, the incidence is even lower.[34] The most common location of the scars is in the lower part of the face, probably related to more aggressive treatment in this area or to the greater tissue movement, because of eating and speaking, during the healing process. Delayed healing and focal persistent redness are important alarming signs for forthcoming scarring. Topical or intralesional steroids together with vascular laser treatments should be introduced as soon as this diagnosis is made.

Infection

Bacterial and fungal complications in deep chemical peels are rare, because phenol is bactericidal

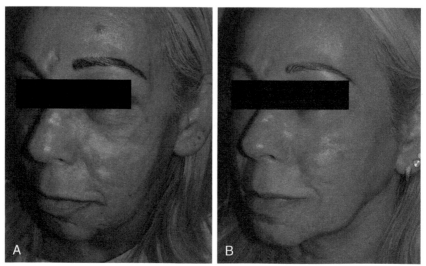

Fig. 8.11 A 50-year-old patient with severe postacne scarring before (A) and 6 months after (B) a deep peel.

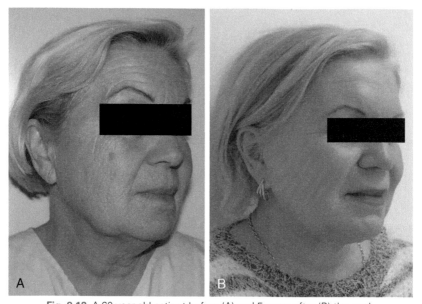

Fig. 8.12 A 60-year-old patient before (A) and 5 years after (B) the peel.

and fungicidal. Patients with a positive history of herpes simplex infection should be prophylactically treated.

Milia

Milia can appear 6 to 8 weeks postresurfacing in up to 20% of patients. Electrosurgery is a simple and effective method to treat this postpeel complication.

Acneiform Dermatitis

Acneiform eruption after deep chemical peels is a common phenomenon appearing immediately after reepithelialization. Its etiology is multifactorial and is related to either exacerbation of previously existing acne or the overgreasing of newly formed skin. Short-term systemic antibiotics together with discontinuation of any oily preparations will usually provide a satisfactory resolution.

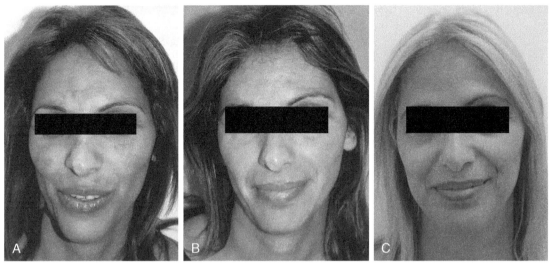

Fig. 8.13 A dark-skinned patient before (A), 3 months after (B), and 12 years after (C) the peel.

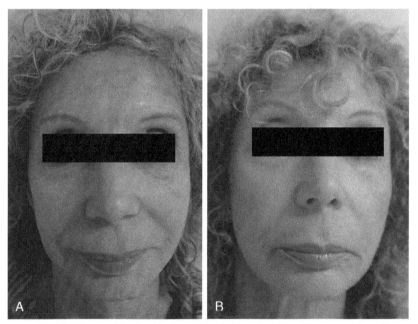

Fig. 8.14 A 70-year-old patient before (A) and 6 months after (B) segmental peeling.

SUMMARY

The main advantage of phenol–croton oil peels is in treating photodamaged skin with wrinkles, dyschromia, and precancerous lesions. In general, a deep peel is the most powerful and legitimate tool in the hands of practicing dermatologists for facial skin rejuvenation. Perioral

wrinkling is a condition in which a deep peel has an obvious advantage over other medical and surgical methods. Facial scars, such as acne scars, especially of atrophic character, may be significantly improved by deep chemical peels.

The main disadvantage of a deep peel is the special setup needed for the procedure, because of the potential risk of cardiotoxicity with phenol. Segmental peels are easier to adopt as a first step to learn the technique.

REFERENCES

1. Mackee GM, Karp FL. The treatment of post acne scars with phenol. *Br J Dermatol.* 1952;64:456–459.
2. Brown AM. Inventor; mount Sinai Hospital Corp; Foundation for Prosthetic Research, assignee. Skin treating method and composition. *US Patent.* 1959;3:067–106. Issued April 7.
3. Bames HO. Truth and fallacies of face peeling and face lifting. *Med J Record.* 1927;126:86–87.
4. Urkov JC. Surface defects of the skin: treatment by controlled exfoliation. *Ill Med J.* 1946;89:75.
5. Combes FC, Sperber PA, Reisch M. Dermal defects: treatment by a chemical agent. *NY Physician Am Med.* 1960;56:36.
6. Brown AM, Kaplan LM, Brown ME. Phenol induced histological skin changes: hazards, techniques and users. *Br J Plast Surg.* 1960;13:158.
7. Litton C. Chemical face lifting. *Plast Reconstr Surg.* 1962;29:371.
8. Baker TJ. Chemical face peeling and rhytidectomy. *Plast Reconstr Surg.* 1962;29:199.
9. Baker TJ, Gordon HL. The ablation of rhytids by chemical means: a preliminary report. *J Fla Med Assoc.* 1961;48:541.
10. Hetter G. An examination of the phenol-croton oil peel: Part I. Dissecting the formula. *Plast Reconstr Surg.* 2000;105:239–248.
11. Stone PA, Lefer LG. Modified phenol chemical face peels: recognizing the role of application technique. *Clin Facial Plast Surg.* 2001;9:351–376.
12. Spira M, Dahl C, Freeman R, et al. Chemosurgery: a histological study. *Plast Reconstr Surg.* 1970;45:247.
13. Fintsi Y. Exoderm—a novel phenol-based peeling method resulting in improved safety. *Am J Cosm Surgery.* 1997;14:49–54.
14. Larson DL, Karmo F, Hetter GP. Phenol-croton oil peel: establishing an animal model for scientific investigation. *Aesthet Surg J.* 2009;29:47–53.
15. Bensimon RH. Croton oil peels. *Aesthet Surg J.* 2008;28:33.
16. Baker TJ, Gordon HL, Seckinger DL. A second look at chemical face peeling. *Plast Reconstruc Surg.* 1966;37:487.
17. Baker TJ, Gordon HL, Mosienko P, et al. Long-term histological study of skin after chemical face peeling. *Plast Reconstr Surg.* 1974;53:522.
18. Wambier CG, Neitzke IC, Lee KC, et al. Augmentation and eversion of lips without injections: the lip peel. *J Am Acad Dermatol.* 2019;80:e119–e120.
19. Sterling JB. Micropunch blepharopeeling of the upper eyelids: a combination approach for periorbital rejuvenation—a pilot study. *Dermatol Surg.* 2014;40:436–440.
20. Gatti JE. Eyelid phenol peel: an important adjunct to blepharoplasty. *Ann Plast Surg.* 2008;60:14–18.
21. Lee KC, Sterling JB, Wambier CG, et al. Segmental phenol-Croton oil chemical peels ortreatment of periorbital or perioral rhytides. *J Am Acad Dermatol.* 2019. https://doi.org/10.1016/j.jaad.2018.11.044.
22. Fintsi Y, Landau M. Exoderm: phenol-based peeling in olive and dark skinned patients. *Int J Cosm Surgery Aesthet Dermatol.* 2001;3:173–178.
23. Park JH, Choi YD, Kim SW, Kim YC, Park SW. Effectiveness of modified phenol peel (Exoderm) on facial wrinkles, acne scars and other skin problems of Asian patients. *J Dermatol.* 2007;34:17–24.
24. Wambier CG, Wambier SPDF, Pilatti LEP, Grabicoski JA, Wambier LF, Schmidt A. Prolongation of rate-corrected QT interval during phenol-croton oil peels. *J Am Acad Dermatol.* 2018;78:810–812.
25. Mysore V, Mahadevappa OH, Barua S, et al. Standard guidelines of care: performing procedures in patients on or recently administered with Isotretinoin. *J Cutan Aesthet Surg.* 2017;10:186–194.
26. Bomar L, McMichael A. Frontal fibrosing alopecia. *Br J Dermatol.* 2017;177:e58–e59.
27. Wambier CG, Lee KC, Soon SL, et al. Advanced chemical peels: phenol-croton oil peel. *J Am Acad Dermatol.* 2019. https://doi.org/10.1016/j.jaad.2018.11.060.
28. Wambier CG, Beltrame FL. Air safety and personal protctve equipment for phenol-croton oil peels. *Dermatol Surg.* 2018;44:1035–1037.
29. Zukowski ML, Mossie RD, Roth SI, Giese S, McKinney P. Pilot study analysis of the histologic and bacteriologic effects of occlusive dressings in chemosurgical peel using a minipig model. *Aesthetic Plast Surg.* 1993;17:53–59.
30. Stagnone GJ, Orgel MB, StagnoneJJ. Cardiovascular effects of topical 50% trichloroacetic acid and Baker's phenol solution. *J Dermatol Surg Oncol.* 1987;13: 999–1002.
31. Litton C, Trinidad G. Complications of chemical face peeling as evaluated by a questionnaire. *Plast Reconstr Surg.* 1981;67:738–744.
32. Truppman F, Ellenbery J. The major electrocardiographic changes during chemical face peeling. *Plast Reconstr Surg.* 1979;63:44.
33. Wexler MR, Halon DA, Teitelbaum A, et al. The prevention of cardiac arrhythmias produced in an animal model by topical application of a phenol preparationin common use for face peeling. *Plast Recontsr Surg.* 1984;73:595–598.
34. Landau M. Cardiac complications in deep chemical peels. *Dermatol Surg.* 2007;33:190–193.
35. Brody HJ. *Chemical Peeling and Resurfacing.* 2nd ed. Mosby; 1997:188–189.

Peels in Men: Special Considerations

Jeave Reserva, David Surprenant, Rebecca Tung

INTRODUCTION

The low cost and reliable results of chemical peeling have made it a staple procedure in aesthetic medicine. The American Society of Plastic Surgeons ranked chemical peels as the third most popular cosmetic minimally invasive procedure in 2018, with an annual total of 1,384,327 chemical peel procedures performed. Based on estimates by the American Society for Aesthetic Plastic Surgery, consumers spent over $64.5 million on chemical peel procedures in 2017. Men account for only 5.5% and 9.3% of all chemical peel procedures performed in the United States and worldwide, respectively, but the aesthetic market for men is continually growing. The modern aesthetic practitioner understands men's top cosmetic concerns and can effectively address them using chemical peels as monotherapy or in combination with surgical or minimally invasive procedures.

INTRINSIC GENDER-LINKED SKIN DIFFERENCES RELEVANT TO CHEMICAL PEELING

Basic background information about the different parts of a chemical treatment plan (e.g., pretreatment, preparation, peel technique, etc.) are discussed in detail in the previous chapters. Because chemical peeling can be very operator-dependent and requires careful consideration of many variables, practical knowledge of gender-linked skin differences may increase the likelihood of achieving excellent peeling outcomes. The Obagi Skin

Classification assesses skin variables such as color, oiliness, thickness, laxity, and fragility to systematically create a chemical treatment plan. Although the literature on chemical peels in men is scant, an understanding of how intrinsic (cutaneous biology) and extrinsic (psychology/sociology) skin variables differ between genders provides a solid foundation to effectively execute chemical peeling in men. Table 9.1 summarizes male-specific intrinsic and extrinsic skin variables and relevant peeling considerations.

Based on intraethnic group comparative studies of skin tone, men display darker and less reflective complexions, possibly because they have more epidermal melanin and a more highly vascularized superficial dermis. Men's constitutive and sun-induced facultative pigmentation states are more robust with longer pigment retention than women. Given these inherent features, men may benefit from relatively longer pretreatment and more aggressive photoprotection than their female counterparts within individual geneticoracial skin groups. When evaluating postprocedural erythema, it may be important to consider that chromacity studies, which assess color differences between erythema and normal skin, have demonstrated higher basal values in men because of a relatively more vascularized dermis.

The androgenic stimulation in men causes higher sebum production with resultant pore enlargement and predisposition to acne vulgaris and impaired barrier function. Sebum-induced alterations in intercellular lipid structure and poor corneocyte maturation

TABLE 9.1   Intrinsic and Extrinsic Skin Variables in Men and Relevant Peeling Considerations

	Gender-Specific Skin-Related Variables	Peeling Considerations in Men
Intrinsic	Elasticity • Lower eyelid sagging presents much earlier Thickness • Increased dermal collagen in men due to androgen receptor activation • Thicker epidermis Color • Robust facultative pigmentation after sun exposure Oiliness • Higher sebum production • Predisposition to acne vulgaris Pain perception • Ablative CO_2 laser-evoke potentials are lower in amplitude than females suggesting better pain tolerance Reepithelialization rate • Slower wound healing due to androgens Histamine response • More robust response in men and increasing age	• Discuss the efficacy of segmental peels in periorbital rejuvenation and synergistic aesthetic outcomes when combined with other minimally invasive procedures • May require longer pretreatment and more aggressive degreasing • Commonly need higher volumes and higher concentrations of peeling agent • Firmer peel application pressure • Additional treatment sessions may be necessary • May require longer pretreatment • Higher risk for PIH → need more aggressive photoprotection • May require longer pretreatment and more potent topical retinoids • Must aggressively degrease (hard "scrub" as opposed to "wipe") • Better candidates for lipophilic peeling agents (e.g., salicylic acid) • High risk for postpeel acne flare → consider continuing or restarting oral acne meds • May require less aggressive pain management (although individual variations likely) • Set realistic expectation regarding postprocedural downtime • Aggressive antihistamine prophylaxis and/or systemic steroids to mitigate postprocedural edema especially in periorbital rejuvenation with medium or deep peeling agent
Extrinsic	Ultraviolet radiation exposure • Higher occupational risks • Inadequate photoprotective behavior • Reduced skin antioxidant capacity Smoking • More prevalent in men (25%) than women (5%) Facial skin care habits • Aggressive scrubbing quite common • Avoidance of face products due to fear of worsening tacky skin sensation from sebum Skin care product preferences • Cleansers: thin, clear blue or green-tinged • Emollients: preference for less occlusive vehicles	• Increased skin cancer risks → Discuss benefits of chemical peeling for actinic keratosis reduction/skin cancer prevention • May need additional counseling on photoprotective behavioral modification • Discuss resultant accelerated aging, poor wound healing, and increased scarring risks → counsel on smoking cessation • For deep peels, at least 1-year cessation recommended • Counsel on gentle skin care practices • Emphasize high risks for scarring and PIH if aggressive exfoliation is performed postpeel • Poor skin barrier function → need more counseling on consistent daily skin regimen • Always consider vehicle preferences when recommending pretreatment or other skin conditioning medication (e.g., adapalene 0.3% gel may be preferred than tretinoin 0.1% cream) • For medium- or deep-peel postprocedure emollients, explain the barrier function rationale for using occlusive vehicles which may help ensure adherence

cause transepidermal water loss that can be further worsened by behavioral tendencies related to excess sebum. Men with excess sebum tend to avoid skin care products because of the perceived fear of exacerbating their already tacky-feeling skin. Because of men's relatively oilier skin, a longer or more aggressive pretreatment (e.g., more potent retinoid, gel versus cream vehicle) and/or more aggressive degreasing may be warranted. Postprocedure acne flares may also be more likely.

Conversely, men's significantly higher average number of appendageal structures (e.g., sebaceous glands, dermal blood vessels) may dampen their rate of rhytid development, particularly in the perioral area. Their higher sebaceous gland density may also render lipophilic peels (e.g., salicylic acid [SA], Jessner's solution) more effective. For example, sebum production, which is critical in the growth of *Malassezia restricta* and *Malassezia globosa*, may be improved by these peels, thus preventing flares of seborrheic dermatitis. Facility in performing focal deep peels for sebaceous hyperplasia may also be of value, because men may be more likely to seek treatment for this condition.

The heterogeneity of study design, research instruments, sample size, and genetic background likely played a role in some studies' conflicting findings regarding gender differences in skin thickness. Although the extent of differences varies by anatomical region, dermal thickness is greater in men, particularly on the forehead and neck, as a result of increased dermal collagen, resulting in part from androgen receptor activation. Similarly, epidermal thickness is greater in men's cheeks and back than that in women. Thus to achieve the intended depth of peel penetration in men, greater peel application pressure, larger volumes, and higher concentrations of peeling agent are required. The relatively thicker male skin may also entail a need for longer pretreatment to ensure that the peeling agent penetrates evenly.

Although there are no significant differences in skin elasticity between men and women, lower eyelid sagging is significantly more severe in men starting middle age. Indeed, the periorbital area, among all facial features, is of most concern to men and is their top treatment priority. Counseling men about the efficacy of segmental (targeted peeling of a specific cosmetic unit) combination (use of multiple peeling agents) chemical peeling can guide their selection from among the various resurfacing modalities available to address their most common cosmetic concerns.

In general, higher skin perfusion is observed in men than in women. Studies investigating susceptibility of the male skin to persistent erythema is lacking. This complication is thought to result from angiogenic factors stimulating vasodilation and is a sign of a prolonged phase of fibroplasia that may lead to scarring. In theory, the larger number of microvessels in the male face could predispose men to these complications.

Although men may be more likely to tolerate pain from chemical resurfacing, androgen-associated decelerated reepithelialization may extend their expected postprocedural downtime. Furthermore, more robust histamine response is observed in men and older age. Men's propensity for postprocedural edema should be kept in mind, especially when performing periorbital rejuvenation, during which significant edema may cause the eyes to swell shut, but may be mitigated by aggressive prophylaxis and treatment with antihistamines and systemic corticosteroids.

EXTRINSIC GENDER-LINKED SKIN DIFFERENCES RELEVANT TO CHEMICAL PEELING

As previously alluded to, men may be more likely to avoid healthy skin care practices. Higher prevalence of smoking (tobacco and nicotine-containing electronic cigarettes) and ultraviolet (UV) light exposure are also observed in men and contribute significantly to skin aging. Patients who fail to modify these behaviors should be thoroughly counseled on their higher risks for suboptimal peeling outcomes and worse complications and hence are generally not candidates for chemical peeling.

Tobacco exposure–related mechanisms of skin aging include vasoconstriction, increased oxidative damage, inhibition of fibroblastic activity, and upregulation of matrix metalloproteinases. Given the higher prevalence of daily smoking in men (25%) than women (5%) and smoking's association with disastrous resurfacing complications, tobacco exposure assessment and smoking cessation are crucial in chemical peeling. This caution extends to the use of nicotine-containing vaping solution or electronic cigarettes.

TABLE 9.2 Peeling Considerations in Sexual-Minority Men	
Skin-Related Variables in Sexual-Minority Men	Peeling Considerations
Transgender Men on Cross-Hormone Testosterone therapy • Acne vulgaris on face and trunk peak after 4 to 6 months of therapy **Gay and Bisexual Men** UV exposure • Indoor tanning six times more prevalent than heterosexual counterpart Anabolic Androgenic Steroid Use • More prevalent among ethnic minority gay and bisexual men and adolescents • Unlikely for many to openly discuss steroid misuse	• Consider serial salicylic acid peels as adjunct to standard acne treatment. • For body peeling: Consider salicylic acid in polyethylene glycol vehicle given lower absorption and decreased risks for salicylism. • Photoprotective behavior counseling should focus on concepts of UV-associated accelerated aging/wrinkle formation. • Serial chemical peeling may circumvent the need and associated risks from using oral antibiotics to improve acne in patients concomitantly on anabolic steroids.

Outdoor occupations overwhelmingly comprise men. To make matters worse, men, including those with personal history of skin cancer, are less likely to practice sun-protective behaviors. On a cellular level, such a nonchalant approach can compound UV damage because of male skin's reduced antioxidant capacity and increased tendency for UV-induced immunosuppression. These behaviors place men at a higher risk for postinflammatory hyperpigmentation (PIH) after a peel. Apart from UV-exposure behavior modification, aggressive and/or prolonged skin conditioning may be necessary to prevent pigmentary complications. Moreover, chemical peeling can be of unique benefit to those seeking cosmetic resurfacing but who also have medical conditions such as actinic keratoses or history of keratinocyte carcinoma. Trichloroacetic acid medium-depth peels can be used to prevent and reduce the incidence of these UV-induced disorders.

Peeling practitioners should also be familiar with current research on men's preferences regarding skin care products. Men's adherence to various aspects of a chemical treatment plan may be augmented by catering to some extent to their preferences toward particular skin care products (e.g., blue/green-tinged cleansers, emollients in "lighter" vehicles). Familiarity with new and existing skin care products that conform to men's preferences but also fulfill their necessary role in the chemical peeling process may improve peeling outcomes by virtue of improving patient experience and treatment adherence.

PEEL CONSIDERATIONS IN SEXUAL-MINORITY MEN

About 3.9% of men in the United States identify as a sexual minority (gay, bisexual, or transgender). The literature specifically addressing chemical peel considerations in sexual-minority men appear even more sparse than that in heterosexual men. This section aims to synthesize known epidemiological, behavioral, and physiological data pertaining to sexual-minority men that are relevant to chemical peeling procedures (Table 9.2).

Homosexual men engage in riskier UV-exposure behaviors, with rates of indoor tanning reported up to six times more than that observed in heterosexual men. Additional counseling on photoprotection may be necessary for peel candidates who are light skinned but whose perceived ideal skin tones are darker, as these individuals are more likely to engage in indoor and outdoor tanning. UV-exposure behavior modification among sexual-minority men whose cultures value lighter skin may be much less of a challenge, although this remains to be investigated. Although they have a higher prevalence of skin cancer than their heterosexual counterparts, photoprotection counseling in sexual-minority men may be most effectively relayed by emphasizing wrinkle and skin aging prevention. Knowing that homosexual men are more likely to consider noninvasive and invasive cosmetic procedures, those who present to the clinic with expressed interest in chemical peels should be explicitly forewarned that inadequate photoprotection can jeopardize their candidacy and/or the outcomes of their chemical peeling procedure.

Up to 94% of transgender men undergoing cross-sex hormone treatment with testosterone develop acne vulgaris on their face, chest, and back, with symptoms peaking 4 to 6 months after testosterone initiation. Although the majority improve in severity after 12 months and respond adequately to standard acne management, some cases may be severe and/or persistent. Face or body peeling using serial SA and other peels should be considered, because they can offer immediate and reliable improvement of comedonal and inflammatory acne. Severe cases may require treatment with isotretinoin, which requires nuanced comprehension of the complexities surrounding contraception and pregnancy testing in this population. Superficial peels such as SA or Jessner's solution (JS) may still be safely performed in patients concomitantly on isotretinoin and may serve as an effective adjunctive treatment.

A higher prevalence of anabolic androgenic steroid (AAS) use is reported among sexual-minority men compared with their heterosexual counterparts. These behaviors may start early in life, because AAS misuse among sexual-minority adolescent boys is three to four times higher than in heterosexual boys, especially among Black and Hispanic males. Although addressing misuse of AAS in these populations is well beyond the scope of this chapter, similar peeling recommendations as discussed in transgendered men applies to this group and may improve self-esteem in this population known to have a pervasive unhealthy body image. The potential role of chemical peels in acne management in cisgender and transgender men undergoing testosterone therapy is an area in need of research.

OVERVIEW OF TREATMENT STRATEGY

Indications

Indications for chemical peeling in men (Table 9.3) are very similar to those for women. As with any aesthetic procedure, proper patient selection, preoperative consultation, and procedural planning are tantamount to desirable outcomes. The histopathological changes present in the condition to be treated and the depth at which they occur dictates which peeling agent(s) may be used. However, peel agent selection must also incorporate patient preferences, such as those regarding postprocedural downtime and postpeel skin regimen. For example, although the outcomes of phenol–croton oil peel rivals that of fully ablative CO_2 laser resurfacing and would produce outstanding improvement of the very deep static rhytids that can be seen in men, full-face phenol–croton oil peels may not be realistic options for some men given the expected postprocedure erythema that is difficult to camouflage without makeup.

Prepeel Consultation

A comprehensive prepeel consultation is crucial to ensure that both the physician and patient have communicated their expectations and that risks and benefits are appropriately discussed. Few differences exist in the approach to the prepeel consultation between men and women. Aspects of the prepeel consultation most relevant to men's cosmetic preferences and men's behavioral tendencies are discussed.

As covered in prior sections, gender-specific extrinsic factors relevant to peeling, such as UV radiation (recreational outdoor, occupational, or indoor tanning) exposure, should be thoroughly assessed. Ideal peel candidates should be both willing to be and actually adherent to prepeel and postpeel care regimen. Poor adherence to prepeel skin conditioning could be a tell-tale sign of inability to closely follow postoperative instructions. Men who work or regularly exercise outdoors may present a relative contraindication depending on the patient's ability and/or willingness to avoid sun exposure of the treated area postpeel.

Although superficial chemical peels may be safely performed during or within 6 months after isotretinoin therapy, current evidence precludes recommendation on the use of medium or deep chemical peels while on isotretinoin. Hence the reported and potential risks of concomitant isotretinoin and medium or deep peels should be discussed thoroughly with the patient. Patients with acne concurrently taking oral antibiotics such as doxycycline may continue therapy, although photosensitivity should be emphasized during counseling. Similarly, potential increased risk for hyperpigmentation should be discussed in patients taking minocycline. Concurrent exogenous testosterone use may portend the need for ongoing serial chemical peeling procedures.

A broad knowledge of men's cosmetic concerns may allow peeling practitioners to identify peeling regimens

TABLE 9.3 Summary of Chemical Peel Indications for Men and Corresponding Peel Selection

Indication	Example of Peel Selection	Practical Considerations
Acne vulgaris and scarring		Combine with other modalities: microneedling, PDL, subcision, Erb:Glass laser
Comedonal and mild/moderate inflammatory	Salicylic acid (20%–30%) Glycolic acid (70%)	
Truncal acne or skin of color patients (Fitzpatrick Skin Types IV, V, and VI)	Salicylic acid (30%) in polyethylene glycol	Polyethylene glycol vehicle may decrease risk of salicylism and PIH-prone "hot spots"
Rolling acne scars	Salicylic acid (30%) + TCA (10%–20%)	CROSS via phenol–croton oil contraindicated in skin phototype VI
Ice-pick and/or box-car acne scars	Combination medium-depth TCA peels (e.g., Brody combination) CROSS method TCA (50%–100%) CROSS method phenol–croton oil (88%/4%)	
Rosacea Erythrosis	Salicylic acid (20%)	1 application
Papulopustular	Salicylic acid (20%–30%)	2–3 applications
Keratosis pilaris	Glycolic acid (50%–70%)	Daily maintenance therapy with glycolic acid lotion (12–20%) 48 hours postpeel
Melasma/PIH	Salicylic acid (20%–30%) ± TCA (10%) Glycolic acid (50%–70%) TCA (10%–30%) Phenol–croton oil peels (light or very light Hetter formulation for resistant cases)	Perform at 2-week intervals May start at lower glycolic acid concentrations (30%) for PIH
Actinic keratosis	Salicylic acid (30%) + TCA (10%–35%) Jessner's solution + spot TCA (35%) Glycolic acid (70%)	May pretreat with 5-FU (5%) cream for 1 week or perform as "pulse peels"
Sun damage/periorbital rejuvenation		
Mild photoaging	Jessner's solution Glycolic acid (70%) Salicylic acid (30%) + TCA (10%)	Use in combination with other minimally invasive procedures including neurotoxins, fillers, microneedling, and/or skin tightening devices
Moderate to severe photoaging	Jessner's-TCA (35%) Solid CO_2-TCA (35%) Glycolic acid (70%)-TCA (35%) Hetter phenol–croton oil Phenol (88%) in micropunch blepharopeeling	Segmental peeling (not full face) recommended when using phenol–croton oil in men due to difficulty camouflaging postprocedural erythema without makeup Always perform "snap-back" test when treating lower eyelid with medium/deep peel.
Pseudofolliculitis barbae	Salicylic acid (30%) Glycolic acid (50%–70%) Jessner's solution	Repeat every 2–4 weeks as needed.

PIH, Postinflammatory hyperpigmentation; *TCA,* trichloroacetic acid.

Data from Reserva J, Champlain A, Soon SL, et al. 2017. Chemical peels: Indications and special considerations for the male patient. *Dermatological Surgery* 43 Suppl 2:S173.

best suited for those indications. The periorbital region (crow's feet, tear troughs, dark circles and bags under the eyes) as well as dyschromias, acne scars, and pseudofolliculitis are among the most common cosmetic concerns in men. Because men tend to be more direct when discussing their desired outcomes and have very specific self-perceived cosmetic flaws, evaluation of each cosmetic unit and selecting peels best suited to treat the pathology in that specific facial area can be very effective (e.g., combination segmental peeling).

Similar absolute and relative contraindications to chemical peels apply to men as they do in women. Because of smoking prevalence in men, it is important to note that some authors recommend smoking cessation for at least 12 months before proceeding with any deep peeling procedure. Although there are no absolute contraindications for periorbital peeling, unless corrected before the chemical peel, preexisting ectropion or moderate to severe lower lid laxity are relative contraindications for lower eyelid peeling. If a lag or ectropion is observed after the lower lid is pulled down and away from the globe for several seconds (snap-back test), deep resurfacing of the lower eyelid with phenol–croton oil or ablative fractionated laser should be avoided because it can lead to an ectropion.

Skin type assessment is an integral part of the prepeel consultation. Common classification has been primarily based on degree of skin pigmentation and tanning/burning susceptibility. Similar to the Obagi skin classification, another reliable skin type classification for chemical peeling has been proposed by Fanous and Zari. that uses a genetico-racial category (Table 9.4). Inhabitants from the three ancient continents—Europe, Africa, and Asia—exhibit predictably lighter, thinner skin and smaller features as one moves north, and gradually display darker, thicker skin with larger features as one moves south. A useful peeling guideline that incorporates this genetico-racial classification is as follows: (1) medium to deep peels for mid-Europeans and southern Europeans (Mediterraneans), (2) medium and light to medium peels for northern Europeans (Nordics) and Asians, (3) light peels for southern Caucasians (Indo-Pakistanis), and (4) very light peels for Africans.

Prepeel Skin Conditioning

Skin priming (pretreatment and preparation) facilitates uniform peeling agent penetration, prevention of postinflammatory dyspigmentation, and predictable and more rapid reepithelialization. Because of various intrinsic and extrinsic factors previously discussed, men may require a longer pretreatment regimen as well as more aggressive skin preparation. Agents used during the pretreatment phase can include topical retinoids (tretinoin, retinaldehyde, adapalene, or tazarotene), keratolytics (lactic acid, SA, kojic acid, or glycolic acid), and lightening agents (hydroquinone or azelaic acid) (Table 9.5). Because men gravitate toward simple, quick therapeutic strategies, their adherence to regimens that entail multistep daily routines may be dismal. Because men typically value convenience and simplicity, agents already commercially available in combination or an individually compounded topical prescription may be more ideal. For genetico-racial groups at risk for postpeel hyperpigmentation, as well as those with history of dyschromia, expert consensus recommends cessation of topical retinoid 1 week before chemical peel to prevent potential peel overpenetration.

Pretreatment of the entire face should be performed, including the upper eyelids, which should be treated once to twice a week, especially if periorbital rejuvenation is planned. Pretreatment feathering into the hairline, jawline, and preauricular areas is also recommended, noting that the hairline may extend significantly into the scalp in some men due to androgenetic alopecia. The daily regimen should include a broad-spectrum UVA/UVB sunscreen with a minimum SPF 30. Visible light protection, present in tinted sunscreens, should be strongly considered in skin of color patients (Fitzpatrick Skin Types IV, V, and VI) and is a must for those with dyschromia, because visible light has been shown to induce pigment darkening in these individuals. Men with facial hair in the areas to be treated should shave the day before (except in pseudofolliculitis barbae) or trim to a length (approximately 3 mm or shorter) that does not interfere with even peel application.

Regarding skin preparation, no difference in efficacy has been found among degreasers (alcohol, acetone, or chlorhexidine gluconate). In general, men will require more vigorous scrubs given the higher sebaceous quality of their skin and higher prevalence of deeper rhytids. Skin preparation may also involve application of topical anesthesia and/or administration of a mild sedative. Nonsedating antihistamines should be administered before the procedure to minimize edema and be continued after the procedure to minimize pruritus. Antiviral prophylaxis for medium and deep peels is identical in men and women. In addition, for patients undergoing

TABLE 9.4   Genetico-Racial Skin Classification Categories and Trichloroacetic Acid[a] Peel Outcomes

	Central and Southern Africans	Southern Caucasians/Indo-Pakistanis (e.g., Saudi Arabian, Indian, or Egyptian)	Northern, Central, and Southern Asians (e.g., Chinese, Japanese, or Filipino)	Northern Europeans/Nordics (e.g., Irish, Scandinavian, or Scottish)	Southern Europeans/Mediterraneans (e.g., Spanish, Greek, Italian, or Turkish)	Mid-Europeans (e.g., English, French, or German)
Geographic Origin	Central and Southern Africa	Northern Africa and Western Asia	Eastern Asia	Northern Europe	Southern Europe, Northern Africa, and Western Asia	Central Europe
Recommended Maximum TCA Peel Depth	Very light	Light	Light to medium	Medium	Medium to deep	Deep
Facial Features	Large	Moderately large	Moderately large	Fine	Slightly large	Medium
Skin Characteristics	Thick, with black to deep black	Thick, with a deep tan to dark brown	Thick, with light medium, or dark brown	Thin white, with a pink element	Slightly thick, with a medium tan	Average thickness, white, or light tan
Hyperpigmentation	+++	+++	++	+/-	++	+
Hypopigmentation	(If deep peel)	(If deep peel)	(Rare with deep peel)	-	-	-
Erythema	+/-	+/-	++ (later turns into hyperpigmentation)	+++	++	+

TCA, Trichloroacetic acid.

[a]Very light peels with TCA is less than 30%; light is 30%–35%; medium is 35%–40%; and deep is 40%–45%.

Data from Fanous N, Zari S. 2017. Universal trichloroacetic acid peel technique for light and dark skin. *JAMA Facial Plastic Surgery* 19(3):219.

TABLE 9.5 **Pretreatment Regimen**[a]

Indication	Medication and Dosing
PIH prevention and peel absorption optimization	*Topical retinoids:* Start at least 4–6 weeks before peel (8–12 weeks in skin of color); stop 1–2 weeks if treating PIH or melasma; 1–2 days for photoaging. Tretinoin 0.02%–0.1% cream or gel QHS Adapalene 0.3% gel QHS *For more sensitive skin, consider:* Glycolic acid 8%–10% lotion/cream Adapalene 0.1% lotion or cream *For patients with moderate to severe acne scars, consider:* Tazarotene 0.05% cream QHS *Lightening agents:* Start 4–6 weeks before peel; stop 1–2 days before peel Hydroquinone 4%–10% BID Azelaic acid 15% gel or 20% cream BID
Preexisting melasma or PIH	Fluocinolone cream (0.01%–0.025%) twice a day for 2–12 weeks Tinted sunscreen for visible light protection
UV radiation protection	Broad-spectrum SPF (titanium dioxide and zinc oxide–based sunscreen preferable)

BID, Twice daily; *QHS,* nightly; *PIH,* postinflammatory hyperpigmentation; *SPF,* sun protectant factor; *UV,* ultraviolet.
[a]Consider commercially available combination products or having pretreatment agents compounded together to potentially improve adherence.
Data from Rullan P, Karam AM. 2010. Chemical peels for darker skin types. *Facial Plastic Surgery Clinics of North America* 18(1):111–131.

medium and deep peels, the authors prefer empiric doxycycline 100 mg twice daily for 7 to 10 days beginning the day of the procedure, with the patient understanding that photoprotection becomes even more crucial.

Postpeel Skin Care

Immediate postpeel skin care, which occurs up until full reepithelialization, may vary based on chemical peel depth but is identical in both genders, with a few caveats. Men should avoid shaving the treated area until fully reepithelialized. The postpeel skin care regimen should be initiated immediately upon full reepithelialization, which may begin as early as 3 days for superficial peels to as late as 14 days for deep peels. Once again, keeping regimens simple may promote better adherence in men; hence restarting the same pretreatment combination topical formulation that the patient previously used may be a wise recommendation.

TREATMENT TECHNIQUES

It is best to contain one's peeling repertoire to a select number of agents. This way, one becomes intimately familiar with all aspects and nuances of such peeling agents, which in turn increases the likelihood of

delivering outstanding outcomes, as opposed to only possessing a limited experience using a broad variety of peels. Similar peeling agents and techniques can be used in men and women. Key points relevant to men's chemical peeling are discussed within each peeling agent.

Salicylic Acid Peel

SA, a lipophilic beta-hydroxy acid, is known for its efficacy in treating inflammatory and noninflammatory acne lesions and its safety profile in all skin types. The most commonly used formulations are SA 20% to 30% in ethanol, which crystallizes upon ethanol evaporation. This leaves a pseudofrost that can be a visual aid that facilitates uniform peel application (Fig. 9.1). SA peels should be repeated in 2- to 4-week intervals, with optimal results seen after a series of three to six sessions.

SA 30% in a polyethylene glycol (SA-PEG) vehicle is a newer SA formulation that is associated with minimal to no discomfort after application and has shown superior results in improving acne compared with SA in ethanol. SA-PEG causes minimal desquamation and little to no risk of the PIH often associated with "hot spots" of ethanolic SA overpenetration. Because of minimal peel absorption beyond the cornified layer, salicylism risks for SA-PEG may be clinically insignificant even

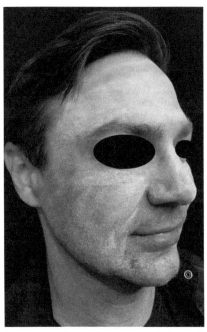

Fig. 9.1 Even pseudofrost after two applications of ethanolic salicylic acid (30%).

with use over large surface areas. This may be of clinical value when performing body peeling in those with a propensity to develop truncal acne, such as cisgender or transgender men on exogenous testosterone therapy. SA-PEG must have at least 5 minutes of contact time and requires thorough rinsing after application because of its occlusive vehicle. When performing body peeling for truncal acne, three to five sessions of ethanolic SA or SA-PEG peels may be performed at 2- to 4-week intervals for optimal results.

Glycolic Acid Peel

Glycolic acid (GA) is the most commonly used alpha-hydroxy acid, applied as a single peeling agent. Combining topical 5-fluorouracil (5-FU) (5%) with GA (70%) peel increases 5-FU's efficacy for treating actinic keratosis (AK) when performed as "pulse peels" every 1 to 2 weeks. GA (70%) is applied evenly to the treatment areas and left on until even erythema is achieved for up to 2 minutes before neutralization. The area is cleansed with a gentle cleanser before application of a thin layer of 5-FU, which is left on for at least 12 hours and up to a maximum of 24 hours as tolerated before washing off thoroughly.

Trichloroacetic Acid, Combination Medium-Depth Peels, and Chemical Reconstruction of Skin Scars Technique

Trichloroacetic acid (TCA) is a reliable and versatile peeling agent that can be used in superficial, medium, or deep peeling. TCA (35%) alone or preceded by solid CO_2, GA (70%), or JS can be repeated every 12 weeks as needed to achieve desired results (Fig. 9.2). The chemical reconstruction of skin scars (CROSS) method involves the firm and focal application of TCA at high concentrations (50%–100%) deep into the depressed area of atrophic acne scars (Fig. 9.3) or enlarged pores. This method is discussed in detail in a separate chapter. Boxcar and icepick acne scars are the acne scar types most responsive to CROSS technique.

Phenol–Croton Oil Peel

The role of phenol–croton oil peels in men tends to revolve primarily around segmental peeling techniques for specific indications such as periorbital rejuvenation. This is because the postpeel erythema from phenol–croton oil can be expected to last for 3 to 6 months after the procedure. Segmental single cosmetic unit deep peels can address the most bothersome facial cosmetic concerns in men and circumvent the need for cardiac monitoring or intravenous hydration typical of phenol–croton oil peeling of larger surface areas. Other indications for phenol–croton oil peel in men include acne scars by CROSS technique, actinic keratosis, actinic cheilitis, and lip rejuvenation.

Newer formulations by Hetter have allowed for phenol-croton oil peels to be used in the treatment of mild to moderate photoaging and acne scarring. The light (35%–0.4%) and very light (27.5%–0.12%) phenol–croton oil Hetter's Heresy formulas are considered appropriate for the periorbital areas. For example, in men who are not yet seeking surgical interventions and only have lower eyelid textural changes and minimal fat protrusion, a single session using the very light formulation can provide significant tightening of the anterior lamella. Light or very light phenol–croton oil peeling may also be performed as a "touch-up" procedure after a lower eyelid transconjunctival blepharoplasty to improve persistent skin wrinkling.

Alternatively, periorbital rejuvenation may be achieved by micropunch blepharopeeling performed using straight phenol (89%). This procedure has shown excellent aesthetic outcomes in treating periocular

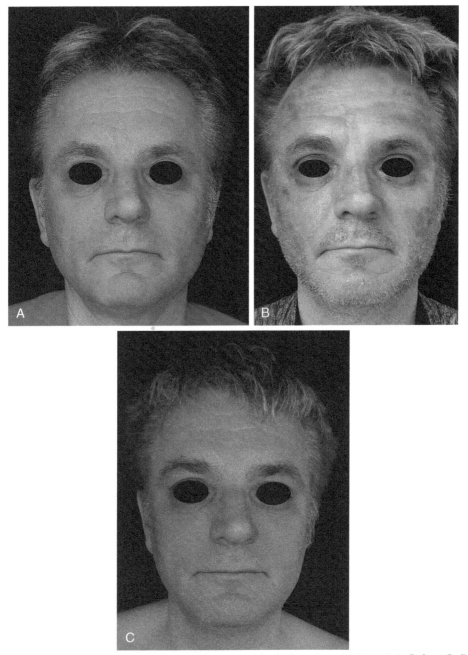

Fig. 9.2 Solid CO_2–trichloroacetic acid (35%) (Brody combination) medium-depth peel. A, Before. B, Four days after the procedure. C, Eight days after the procedure.

rhytides without the associated volume loss and linear scarring seen in conventional surgical blepharoplasty. Phenol (89%) is applied to the area between the upper eyelid's superior tarsal plate border and the eyebrow's inferior border, as well as within 1 to 2 mm of the lower eyelid margin. Immediately after frosting, multiple (5–20) 3- to 5-mm snip excisions arranged in a random grid-like pattern are performed on the central and lateral areas of the upper eyelid, which are left to heal by secondary intention.

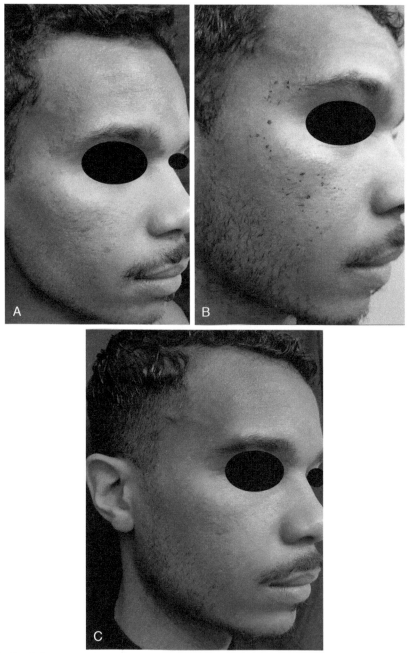

Fig. 9.3 A, Postinflammatory hyperpigmentation, comedonal acne, and mild atrophic acne scarring in a Fitzpatrick phototype V male. B, After two sessions of ethanolic salicylic acid (30%) and one session of trichloroacetic acid (TCA) (100%) CROSS (5 days postpeel) performed at 2-week intervals. C, After an additional session of salicylic acid (30%) and TCA (100%) CROSS.

Similar safety precautions are used in men and women when performing a phenol–croton oil peel, including continuous electrocardiographic monitoring and hydration (orally or intravenously) when total body surface area to be peeled exceeds 1%. Because phenol can penetrate into latex and nitrile gloves, neoprene gloves must be worn when performing phenol peeling, especially if gauze pads will be used to apply the agent or catch any inadvertent drip. Use of activated carbon-containing masks is also recommended.

Combination of Chemical Peeling With Other Minimally Invasive Procedures

Combining chemical peels with other minimally invasive procedures can optimize aesthetic outcomes. Performing a TCA (20%) peel, extensive subcision, and fractional CO_2 laser in a single session has shown excellent improvement of rolling acne scars. Prepeel treatment with botulinum toxin and/or hyaluronic acid filler has also shown synergistic effects in the treatment of rhytides. In patients previously treated with neurotoxin, some authors recommend neurotoxin injection 2 to 3 weeks before a medium or deep chemical peel, which may also facilitate healing due to diminished facial movement. For treatment-naïve patients, neurotoxin injection 10 to 14 days after a phenol–croton oil peel may prolong desired neuromuscular blockade. Although same-day neurotoxin treatment and chemical peeling is generally not recommended (due to potential neurotoxin diffusion from edema), soft tissue augmentation may be performed on the same day if superficial or medium-depth peels are used or different areas are treated. Otherwise, filler treatment should be performed 4 to 6 months after a deep chemical peel.

COMPLICATIONS

As previously discussed, intrinsic and extrinsic male skin variables can predispose men to slower reepithelialization rates, more exuberant postprocedural edema, and bruising. Chemical peeling complications are discussed in detail in a separate chapter. Although early identification, treatment, and prevention of chemical peel complications are not gender-specific, special circumstances are worthy of discussion. In an atrophic bald scalp with multiple actinic keratoses, chemexfoliated areas showing delayed reepithelialization may be a consequence of diminished adnexal structures or actinically damaged

skin itself. In these patients, adherence to postoperative wound care should be further emphasized while maintaining a high index of suspicion for infection or erosive pustular dermatosis of the scalp. Certain areas are prone to hypertrophic scarring from medium or deep peels and should be peeled less vigorously, even in men. These areas are the medial upper eyelids, lateral lower eyelids, zygomatic arch, preauricular area, and neck. Medium-depth peels have unpredictable outcomes on the neck and a tendency to cause scarring; superficial peels in combination with skin-tightening devices, neurotoxin, and/or biostimulatory fillers should be considered instead.

CONCLUSION

Chemical peels are a mainstay of aesthetic medicine and an increasingly popular cosmetic procedure performed in men. The approach to chemical peels in men includes consideration of intrinsic and extrinsic skin variables that affect various aspects of the peeling process. Because of the increased sebaceous quality of their skin and thicker dermis, male patients, in general, may require a greater number of treatments, larger volumes of peeling agent, more aggressive degreasing and peel application, and/or higher concentration of peeling agent to achieve optimal results. Patient selection is of utmost importance, because poor photoprotective behavior and nonadherence to prepeel and postpeel regimens could jeopardize clinical outcomes. Facility in performing chemical peels and understanding gender-specific nuances of this technique may be well rewarded in today's growing aesthetic market.

FURTHER READING

Bagatin E, Teixeira SP, Hassun KM, Pereira T, Michalany NS, Talarico S. 5-fluorouracil superficial peel for multiple actinic keratoses. *Int J Dermatol.* 2009;48(8):902–907.

Brody HJ. Commentary on chemical peels in men. *Dermatol Surg.* 2017;43(suppl 2):S175.

Crudele J, Kim E, Murray K, Regan J. The importance of understanding consumer preferences for dermatologist recommended skin cleansing and care products. *J Drugs Dermatol.* 2019;18(s1):75.

Dainichi T, Ueda S, Imayama S, Furue M. Excellent clinical results with a new preparation for chemical peeling in acne: 30% salicylic acid in polyethylene glycol vehicle. *Dermatol Surg.* 2008;34(7):9; discussion 899.

Fanous N, Zari S. Universal trichloroacetic acid peel technique for light and dark skin. *JAMA Facial Plast Surg.* 2017;19(3):219.

Giacomoni PU, Mammone T, Teri M. Gender-linked differences in human skin. *J Dermatol Sci.* 2009;55(3):144–149.

Handler MZ, Goldberg DJ. Cosmetic concerns among men. *Dermatol Clin.* 2018;36(1):5–10.

Hantash BM, Stewart DB, Cooper ZA, Rehmus WE, Koch RJ, Swetter SM. Facial resurfacing for nonmelanoma skin cancer prophylaxis. *Arch Dermatol.* 2006;142(8):976–982.

Jagdeo J, Keaney T, Narurkar V, Kolodziejczyk J, Gallagher CJ. Facial treatment preferences among aesthetically oriented men. *Dermatol Surg.* 2016;42(10):1155–1163.

Keaney TC. Aging in the male face: intrinsic and extrinsic factors. *Dermatol Surg.* 2016;42(7):797–803.

Landau M, Bensimon RH. Chemical peels. In: Cantisano-Zilkha M, Haddad A, eds. *Aesthetic oculofacial rejuvenation.* New York, NY: Elsevier; 2010:29–37.

Lee KC, Wambier CG, Soon SL, et al. Basic chemical peeling-superficial and medium-depth peels. *J Am Acad Dermatol.* 2018. https://doi.org/S0190-9622(18)33049-4 [pii].

Mancuso JB, Maruthi R, Wang SQ, Lim HW. Sunscreens: an update. *Am J Clin Dermatol.* 2017;18(5):643–650.

Marrero GM, Katz BE. The new fluor-hydroxy pulse peel. A combination of 5-fluorouracil and glycolic acid. *Dermatol Surg.* 1998;24(9):973–978.

Montes JR, Santos E. Evaluation of men's trends and experiences in aesthetic treatment. *J Drugs Dermatol.* 2018;17(9):941–946.

Rahrovan S, Fanian F, Mehryan P, Humbert P, Firooz A. Male versus female skin: what dermatologists and cosmeticians should know. *Int J Womens Dermatol.* 2018;4(3):122–130.

Reserva J, Champlain A, Soon SL, Tung R. Chemical peels: indications and special considerations for the male patient. *Dermatol Surg.* 2017;43(suppl 2):S173.

Rullan P, Karam AM. Chemical peels for darker skin types. *Facial Plast Surg Clin North Am.* 2010;18(1):111–131.

Sterling JB. Micropunch blepharopeeling of the upper eyelids: a combination approach for periorbital rejuvenation—a pilot study. *Dermatol Surg.* 2014;40(4):436–440.

Wambier CG, de Freitas FP. Combining phenol-croton oil peel. In: Issa MCA, Tamura B, eds. *Chemical and physical procedures.* Cham: Springer International Publishing; 2018:101–113.

Wambier CG, Lee KC, Soon SL, et al. Advanced chemical peels: phenol-croton oil peel. *J Am Acad Dermatol.* 2018. https://doi.org/S0190-9622(18)33051-2 [pii].

10

Combination Therapy in Acne: Peels as Adjuvant Therapy

David Surprenant, Jeave Reserva, Rebecca Tung

INTRODUCTION

Acne vulgaris is an exceedingly common inflammatory condition with a lifetime prevalence approaching 80%. Acne has been associated with depression, anxiety, and low self-esteem; untreated or poorly managed acne often has major effects on patient quality of life and has significant associated socioeconomic and healthcare costs. This underscores the importance of an effective and cost-conscious approach to acne treatment.

An accurate understanding of the disease process is essential to formulating a therapeutic plan for acne. The pathogenesis of acne is multifactorial and begins with corneocyte adhesion (Box 10.1). As corneocytes collect and obstruct the pilosebaceous unit, sebum is simultaneously produced by sebaceous glands, in part because of hormonal stimulation. This combination of follicular obstruction and continued sebum production creates an environment that is conducive to the growth of bacteria, namely gram-positive *Propionibacterium acnes (Cutibacterium acnes)*. The resulting inflammatory response results in clinically visible acne: comedones, pustules, inflammatory papules, and cysts. If severe, this inflammatory process can result in significant and permanent scarring. There are several approaches to treating acne, and various treatments target specific steps in the disease process: decreasing corneocyte adhesion,

minimizing sebum production, and lowering bacterial counts. Management is often approached in a stepwise fashion: topical retinoids and topical antibiotics for primarily comedonal acne, adjunctive systemic antibiotics and/or antiandrogens for inflammatory acne, and systemic retinoids for severe or recalcitrant cases. There are also several adjuvant therapies available for both active acne and acne scarring, including light-based therapies (photodynamic therapy, pulsed dye laser, CO_2 laser) and mechanical-based therapies (microneedling, microdermabrasion). Chemical peels represent an additional effective, well-tolerated, and economical adjuvant treatment option for acne and acne scarring. As an often under utilized acne treatment modality, this chapter aims to reintroduce chemical peels as a valuable tool worthy of consideration when approaching the acne patient. Chemical peels are low cost, have minimal side effects, and are an effective method for treating acne and acne scarring. For patients with severe inflammatory acne, the adjuvant use of chemical peels should be considered only after first improving the condition with a systemic medication. Nonetheless, even these patients can frequently benefit from chemical peels.

ACNE: WHY CHEMICAL PEELS?

Broadly speaking, chemical peels work by inducing controlled cutaneous damage and fostering dermal and epidermal regeneration. The mechanism of action and characteristics of many chemical peels make them well suited for the treatment of active acne and acne scarring. Many chemical peels exhibit keratolytic and comedolytic effects, especially helpful for noninflammatory comedonal acne. Chemical peels may also decrease sebum production and pore size, and many have

---

BOX 10.1 Pathogenesis of Acne Vulgaris: A Disease of the Pilosebaceous Unit

Abnormal follicular keratinization → microcomedo formation → comedo rupture → release of keratin and sebum → inflammatory papule/pustule → nodule/cyst

---

TABLE 10.1   Selected Peeling Regimens for Mild to Moderate Comedonal and Inflammatory Acne

Peel	Properties	Regimen	Contact Time	Considerations
Salicylic acid	Keratolytic, comedolytic, antibacterial, antiinflammatory	30% salicylic acid every 2–4 weeks for 3–6 sessions	~6 minutes	Safer for darker skin types
Glycolic acid	Keratolytic, comedolytic, antibacterial, antiinflammatory	30%–70% glycolic acid every 2 weeks for 3–5 sessions	~3–5 minutes	Requires neutralization Safe in pregnancy
Mandelic acid	Keratolytic, comedolytic, antibacterial, antiinflammatory	10% mandelic acid + 20% salicylic acid every 2 weeks for 6 sessions	~3–5 minutes	Requires neutralization May help with skin lightening
Trichloroacetic acid (lower strength)	Desquamation induced via protein denaturation, antibacterial	25% trichloroacetic acid every 2 weeks for 4 sessions	N/A	Higher risk of procedure-related dyspigmentation
Jessner's Solution	Keratolytic, comedolytic, antibacterial	Jessner's every 2 weeks for 3–6 sessions	N/A	May help with skin lightening
Pyruvic acid	Keratolytic, comedolytic, antibacterial	50% pyruvic acid every 2 weeks for 5 sessions	~3–5 minutes	Requires neutralization

antibacterial and antiinflammatory properties useful in decreasing bacterial counts on acne-prone skin. Additionally, the controlled cutaneous damage induced by chemical peels promotes the absorption of other topical acne medications, augmenting their pharmacological effect. By increasing the efficacy of topical medications, systemic medications and their associated health risks and economic costs may be avoided. Although chemical peeling can be an excellent adjuvant modality in the treatment of mild and moderate comedonal and inflammatory acne, chemical peels are not appropriate for the treatment of severe inflammatory or nodulocystic acne. Severe inflammatory or nodulocystic acne must first be improved with other medications before initiating a peeling regimen.

PEELING AGENTS AND PATIENT CONSIDERATIONS

A variety of chemical peel formulations and treatment regimens exist. When treating active acne vulgaris, the most commonly used peels are superficial or light peels (Table 10.1; see also Chapter 4). Peel depth depends on type of peel agent and concentration used, skin preparation technique, and skin contact time. Superficial chemical peels induce controlled cutaneous damage limited primarily to the epidermis. Their limited depth

of penetration affords notable clinical improvement with minimal (if any) patient discomfort or downtime. Salicylic acid (SA) (5%–30%) and glycolic acid (GA) (20%–70%) are the most commonly used agents for the treatment of mild to moderate comedonal and inflammatory acne. Additional agents used include lactic acid (LA), mandelic acid (MA), trichloroacetic acid (TCA), and Jessner's solution (JS). Unique qualities of each agent, coupled with practitioner confidence and patient characteristics, help guide chemical peel selection. Furthermore, the use of combination chemical peel treatments—treating patients in a sequential manner with one peeling agent followed by a different agent—can be considered when developing a treatment plan.

Salicylic Acid

SA is a beta-hydroxy acid commonly used for the treatment of acne vulgaris. Its strong keratolytic and comedolytic properties make it particularly suitable as an acne treatment. SA promotes desquamation of the upper lipophilic layers of the stratum corneum, resulting in superficial desquamation and rejuvenation. SA also penetrates pores and has antibacterial and antiinflammatory properties. SA may also decrease sebum production in acne-prone patients. In clinical studies, SA peels have been shown to reduce the number of inflammatory and noninflammatory lesions in patients

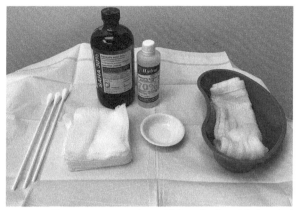

Fig. 10.1 The typical setup for a 30% salicylic acid chemical peel for acne treatment is quite simple. A degreasing agent, the peeling agent, cotton-tipped applicators (CTAs), and some gauze should be on hand. A handheld fan and/or ice packs should also be available to help minimize patient discomfort.

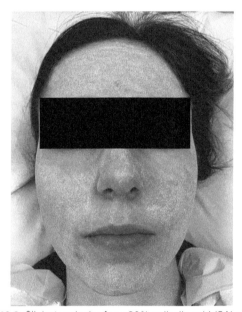

Fig. 10.2 Clinical endpoint for a 30% salicylic acid (SA) chemical peel. Application yields pseudofrosting as SA crystalizes. Typically, one to three layers are applied until a uniform pseudofrost is achieved. The face is then washed with water after approximately 6 minutes.

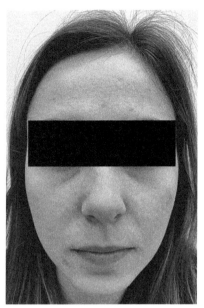

Fig. 10.3 Three days after 30% salicylic acid chemical peel. There is very minimal superficial peeling resulting in minimal to no downtime.

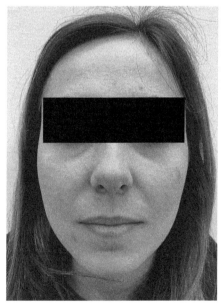

Fig. 10.4 One week after 30% salicylic acid chemical peel.

with active acne. Although several concentrations and treatment regimens exist, the most commonly utilized concentrations for treatment of acne is 30% SA. A common regimen includes 30% SA applied every 2 to 4 weeks for a total of three to six sessions (Figs. 10.1–10.4). Lower concentrations can be used but typically require a greater number of treatment sessions to achieve an equivalent treatment effect. SA peels are self-neutralizing and generally very well tolerated. Patients occasionally note minimal procedural discomfort (i.e., tingling and burning) that is easily mitigated with the use of a

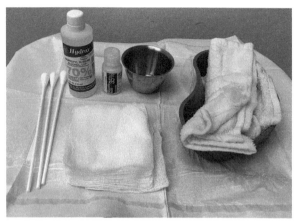

Fig. 10.5 The typical setup for a 35% glycolic acid chemical peel. One must ensure that a neutralizing agent (either water or 10%–15% sodium bicarbonate) is readily available when using GA.

handheld fan. Downtime is minimal, with postprocedural erythema and desquamation often resolving in 1 to 3 days and with reepithelialization complete in 7 to 10 days. SA peels represent a safe peeling agent even in darker-skinned patients, because postprocedural dyspigmentation is rare.

Glycolic Acid

GA is an alpha-hydroxy acid that shares many beneficial qualities with SA. In particular, GA reduces corneocyte adhesion and keratinocyte plugging. GA also has proven antibacterial efficacy against *P. acnes*. The only published randomized-controlled clinical trial comparing a chemical peel to placebo in the treatment of acne vulgaris demonstrated statistical improvement in both inflammatory and noninflammatory lesions with GA. GA acne treatment outcomes are largely comparable to outcomes with SA. One clinical study found a patient preference for GA over SA (41% versus 35%), but the underlying reason and clinical significance of this preference was unclear and has not been replicated in additional studies. GA does require neutralization with an alkaline solution to halt exfoliative effects, which should be considered when selecting this agent. A longer application time interval prior to neutralization results in increased penetration of the chemical peel. Treatment regimens typically use 30% to 50% GA every 2 weeks for 3 to 5 minutes for three to six sessions (Figs. 10.5–10.8). Higher concentrations typically require shorter treatment times and fewer

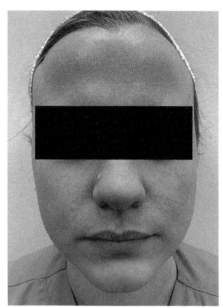

Fig. 10.6 Clinical endpoint for 35% glycolic acid chemical peel. The peel is typically neutralized after a predetermined period of time, usually 3 to 5 minutes. Erythema or a grayish-white appearance of the skin should prompt more rapid neutralization.

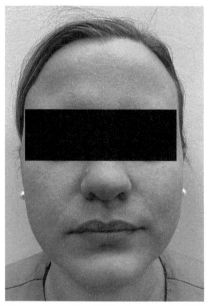

Fig. 10.7 Three days after 35% glycolic acid (GA) chemical peel. Superficial GA chemical peels do not usually induce any visible peeling or erythema and consequently cause minimal to no downtime.

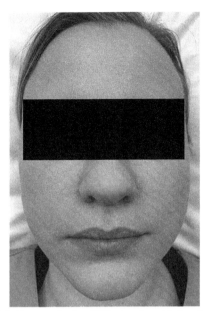

Fig. 10.8 One week after 35% glycolic acid chemical peel.

sessions but are likely to result in increased patient discomfort and carry a higher risk of complications. Generally, GA peels are safe and well tolerated, with common adverse effects limited to transient procedural burning and erythema and postprocedural desquamation. Although safety data are limited, GA is generally considered safe for pregnant patients given its limited dermal penetration.

Trichloroacetic Acid

TCA is a crystalline inorganic compound that induces controlled tissue damage through epidermal and dermal protein denaturation. Various concentrations of TCA cause varying degrees of tissue damage. Although higher concentrations are frequently used for resurfacing and rejuvenation, 20% to 25% TCA can be used to treat acne vulgaris. Published literature suggests 25% TCA applied every 2 weeks for four sessions has the same efficacy as 30% SA applied every 2 weeks for four sessions in treating active acne vulgaris. Higher concentrations of TCA are associated with a higher risk of potential postpeel dyspigmentation and should be used cautiously in patients with dark skin types or in any individuals prone to hyperpigmentation. Although self-neutralizing, neutralization with an alkaline solution is recommended to avoid unintentional overtreatment. Focal TCA, in concentrations of 90% to 100%, is particularly useful in addressing acne scarring, especially with the chemical reconstruction of skin scars (CROSS) technique, described later.

Jessner's Solution

JS is a superficial peeling agent composed of 14% SA, 14% resorcinol, and 14% LA in 95% ethanol. JS is commonly used to augment the penetration and efficacy of medium-depth peeling agents for resurfacing but can be used alone to treat acne vulgaris. JS is well tolerated, and adverse effects are limited to procedural discomfort (i.e., burning or stinging), erythema, and postprocedural desquamation. Dyspigmentation is rare. JS is commonly applied every 2 weeks for three to six sessions. Modified JS (17% LA, 17% SA, and 8% citric acid in 95% ethanol) can also be considered for the treatment of acne. Modified JS lacks resorcinol, an ingredient that can occasionally result in unwanted side effects such as allergic reactions and syncope.

Lactic Acid

LA is another alpha-hydroxy acid frequently used in combination with other peeling agents to treat acne. LA decreases corneocyte adhesion and also has a moisturizing effect on the skin. This latter effect can be particularly helpful because many topical acne treatments, such as retinoids and benzoyl peroxide, are particularly drying. In vitro analysis has demonstrated the ability of LA (300 µg/mL) to suppress tyrosinase and inhibit melanogenesis. Thus the addition of LA may help with skin lightening and may decrease the risk of procedural hyperpigmentation. Several premixed peeling products containing lactic acid are available commercially including Vitalize Peel (Allergan Plc) and Ultra Peel Forte (PCA SKIN). There is no published data investigating the use of LA monotherapy for the treatment of active acne vulgaris, although the use of high-concentration (46%–92%) LA has demonstrated benefit for superficial acne scars. LA has a lower pH than glycolic acid, and thus lower concentrations of LA can generally be used to achieve a similar treatment effect. Just as with glycolic acid, neutralization is required with lactic acid.

Mandelic Acid

MA is a large-molecule alpha-hydroxy acid with slow epidermal penetration. Similar to the other alpha-hydroxy acids described, MA decreases corneocyte adhesion and is keratolytic. Aside from acne treatment,

MA is often used for skin rejuvenation and lightening. MA can be combined with SA for the treatment of acne vulgaris. One clinical study found combination therapy with 10% MA and 20% SA (every 2 weeks for six sessions) superior to 35% GA (every 2 weeks for six sessions) for reducing comedones, pustules, inflammatory papules, and total acne score. The combination of MA and SA induced more visible postprocedural peeling compared with GA alone. As monotherapy, MA is less aggressive than glycolic acid, and shorter treatment intervals may be used. Some sources recommend limiting MA contact time to 5 minutes. Neutralization is required at the conclusion of the peel.

Pyruvic Acid

Pyruvic acid (PA) is an α-ketoacid used to induce superficial peeling. With keratolytic, antibacterial, and sebostatic properties, PA can also be used for active acne vulgaris. Fifty percent PA can be applied every 2 weeks for approximately five sessions to augment the treatment of acne vulgaris. Typical treatment contact time is 3 to 5 minutes, and acid neutralization with an alkaline solution is required. PA is a well-tolerated peeling agent with adverse events similar to those associated with salicylic acid.

Commercially Available Peeling Blends

There are numerous skin care companies with commercially available proprietary chemical peel products that can be used as adjuvant therapy for acne vulgaris. These products often contain blends of a variety of different agents and come with manufacturer-suggested treatment protocols. Many of the premixed products contain a combination of lower-concentration TCA (6%–20%) or salicylic acid (14%) mixed with a combination of one or several other ingredients such as lactic acid (12%–20%), Kojic acid, azelaic acid, L-ascorbic acid, retinol, citric acid, etc. These additional ingredients aim to add to or augment peel benefits such as skin lightening, hydration, and exfoliation.

ACNE SCARRING

Chemical peels are commonly used for skin resurfacing and to improve texture and scarring. Although skin resurfacing with chemical peels can in general improve texture and dyspigmentation, the CROSS technique can be particularly helpful for the treatment of atrophic or "icepick" acne scars. First described by Lee et al. in 2002, this technique involves focal application of high-concentration TCA (50%–100%) directly to acne scars using a precise applicator, commonly a sharp wooden-tipped applicator or even a needle. This technique can be repeated every 4 to 6 weeks for typically five or more sessions. CROSS has demonstrated significant improvement, especially in correcting icepick scarring secondary to acne. Efficacy is a result of stimulated collagen production and dermal thickening induced by high-concentration TCA. The focal application of TCA to only scarred areas limits the risk of procedural dyspigmentation. Studies in darker skin types (particularly the Asian population) have demonstrated an excellent safety profile. Focused TCA application to acne scars spares normal surrounding skin and results in minimal down time. Patients should nevertheless be counseled on the possibility, although rare, of hyperpigmentation should the TCA inadvertently contact normal skin.

THE AUTHORS' APPROACH

When approaching a patient with mild to moderate inflammatory acne, the authors introduce the idea of using chemical peels as adjuvant therapy early in the treatment course. For the typical patient with mild to moderate acne requiring systemic medication in addition to topical modalities, chemical peels can be initiated as soon as desired by the patient. Chemical peels should be not be reserved as a last resort, because they can hasten improvement and potentially avoid the need to advance up the "therapeutic ladder" of topical and oral prescription medications. Although chemical peels are relatively affordable, they almost always represent an out-of-pocket expense for patients, which can be a barrier to implementation. Without dermatologic guidance, many patients fail to recognize the financial and clinical value of chemical peels for the treatment of their acne. It is important for clinicians to present patients with all treatment options and guide patients through the decision-making process.

For patients who proceed with chemical peel treatments, adherence to prepeel and postpeel care regimens is imperative (Table 10.2). Strong emphasis is placed on regular broad-spectrum sunscreen use both before and after a peel. Mineral-based sunscreens are often preferred in the postpeel period. The authors do not recommend chemical peels in patients who tan or will be in an environment where they anticipate greater than normal

TABLE 10.2   Approaching the Use of Chemical Peels as Adjuvant Therapy for Mild to Moderate Inflammatory and Comedonal Acne

Prepeel Treatment	Immediately Prepeel	Chemical Peel	Immediately Postpeel	Postpeel Care	Treatment Interval
Topical or systemic therapies as medically indicated for acne vulgaris	Low-dose antihistamine (i.e., loratadine 10 mg)	Consider less-aggressive degreasing with only alcohol versus acetone in darker skin types or patients with sensitive skin	Application of topical corticosteroid in the office to minimize procedural discomfort and erythema	Expect erythema and peeling for 3–7 days following peel (longer with deeper peels)	Repeat treatment depending on peeling agent used and patient response to therapy (typically 2–4 week intervals).
Discontinue topical acne medications 48 hours before chemical peel (consider longer for darker skin types)	Consider concomitant pulsed dye laser to complement peel results with minimal downtime	Peeling agent based on patient considerations, physician preference, and product availability	Application of sunscreen	Daily photoprotection with sunscreen and sun avoidance	Consider maintenance therapy with chemical peels every 4–12 weeks once acne is controlled.
			+/– Application of manufacturer recommended topicals if using proprietary peel blends	+ Topical corticosteroids if inflammation and discomfort intolerable (+ short course of systemic corticosteroids if needed) Resume topical acne medications once acute peeling and erythema resolve (usually day 5–7)	

sun exposure (i.e., a tropical vacation)—even with the use of "low-risk" superficial peels such as low-concentration salicylic acid. Immediately before the chemical peel, we pretreat all patients with an antihistamine (i.e., 10 mg of loratadine). This helps reduce procedural swelling and erythema. Patients with Fitzpatrick skin type I and II are typically instructed to hold their topical retinoid for at least 2 days before the procedure. Patients with darker skin (Fitzpatrick type III and greater) are instructed to stop retinoids and any other potentially irritating topicals a week before the peel. In patients with darker skin types, we also perform a less-aggressive pretreatment skin degreasing using only 70% alcohol in place of acetone and alcohol. Less aggressive degreasing can decrease the efficacy of the peel by limiting peel penetration, but the risk of procedural dyspigmentation is minimized.

In patients with significant erythema or who desire more rapid results, we offer combination therapy of laser and chemical peeling. Erythematous papules and macular scars are first lasered with 595 nm pulsed-dye laser (PDL) (VBeam Perfecta, Syneron-Candela, Inc, Irvine, CA) at settings of 7 mm spot size, energy 8 to 10 Joules, 6- to 10-millisecond pulse duration, cooling setting 2, before peel application. Laser settings will vary by laser manufacturer. If a PDL laser is unavailable or if a patient has darker skin, an Nd:YAG laser (1064 nm), Alexandrite laser (755 nm), or long-wavelength Nd:YAG laser (1320 nm) can be used, because these lasers either target the *P. acnes* bacteria or heat the underlying sebaceous glands to reduce oil production. This combination laser and chemical peel regimen has minimal downtime and can also result in enhanced acne clearance compared with chemical peels alone.

The authors prefer SA given its low side-effect profile, its ease of use, and its well-established efficacy for acne vulgaris. Typically, two to three coats of the 30% SA peel are applied to the entire face and left to sit for approximately 6 minutes. As SA precipitate first appears, cool compresses are applied. A handheld fan is used to mitigate any procedural burning or discomfort. This treatment is performed every 3 to 4 weeks as tolerated by the patient and as directed by clinical response. The typical patient requires three sessions of treatment.

After a peel, patients are counseled to expect some degree of erythema and desquamation for 3 to 5 days (longer if stronger peeling agents are used). Topical triamcinolone 0.1% cream is typically applied after the peel to help minimize postprocedure discomfort and inflammation—this is not continued beyond the single application in the office. Should a patient have an extreme inflammatory reaction to their chemical peel, additional topical corticosteroids can be considered to mitigate inflammation. In the rare patient, a short course of oral steroid taper (methylprednisolone dose pack) may be used to help with an exuberant or intolerable peel reaction. For all patients, fastidious sun protection and sun avoidance are mandatory. Patients are continued on their topical acne medications after their acute peeling is completed (3–7 days after the peel). Patients are generally very satisfied with their peel treatments, and many patients choose to continue with intermittent superficial chemical peels every 4 to 12 weeks for maintenance therapy once their acne is controlled.

ADVERSE EVENTS AND SPECIAL CONSIDERATIONS

Clinicians should be aware of several potential adverse events and special considerations when using chemical peels as adjuvant therapy for acne. First, peeling is not indicated for individuals with severe inflammatory or nodulocystic acne. Chemical peels are not helpful for these patients because they can induce an exacerbation of acne. Although chemical peels have proven efficacy in treating mild to moderate inflammatory acne, they are particularly helpful in addressing comedonal, noninflammatory acne.

Often patients with facial acne will additionally have issues with acne on their chest and/or back. Superficial chemical peels may also be used off the face in areas such as the neck, chest, and back. However, the authors caution against the use of medium-depth or deep peels off of the face, because the regenerative capacity in these areas is not equivalent to facial skin and complications are more likely to arise. The authors suggest using superficial peels to treat acne on the neck, chest, and back in individuals of all skin types.

Many patients with acne are taking medications that should be considered before initial treatment with chemical peels. Doxycycline is a common oral antibiotic with antiinflammatory properties used in patients with acne vulgaris. The photosensitizing effect of doxycycline further underscores the importance of fastidious photoprotection before and after a peel procedure to minimize the risk of potential adverse effects—particularly postinflammatory hyperpigmentation. For many adult women with cyclical acne, oral contraceptives and/or spirono-lactone may be used safely alongside intermittent chemical peels to control symptoms. Topical tretinoin and other retinoids can augment the effects of a chemical peel if used nightly for 6 weeks before the procedure. We have patients discontinue their retinoid at least 48 hours before the peel to limit the risk of dyspigmentation and scarring related to enhanced penetration of the peeling solution. Darker-skinned patients stop their retinoid 7 days before the procedure. When using oral isotretinoin for the treatment of acne, the shrinking of the pilosebaceous unit theoretically could impede regeneration and healing following a chemical peel. Historically, a general recommendation was to avoid any procedural intervention, such as chemical peels, for 6 to 12 months after completion of isotretinoin. However, a recent systemic review and consensus recommendation concluded there was no evidence to suggest peeling needs to be delayed and that performing superficial peels on patients taking isotretinoin is likely safe.

Finally, do not peel in patients with active facial herpes simplex virus (HSV) infections. In patients with frequent HSV outbreaks, prophylactic antiviral medications should be given for 1 week, starting on the day of the peel.

CONCLUSION

Chemical peels represent an effective, safe, and low-cost adjuvant therapy for patients with acne vulgaris. The unique qualities of chemical peels make them well suited to address the underlying pathogenic mechanisms of acne vulgaris. Their ability to augment the effect of topical acne medications may allow patients to avoid the adverse effects associated with systemic acne medications and could in fact help reduce the cost burden of acne treatment on the healthcare system. Clinicians should familiarize themselves with the use of chemical peels as adjuvant therapy for acne so they can offer their patients a low-risk, efficacious, and cost-effective option to achieve clear skin.

FURTHER READING

Al-Talib H, Al-Khateeb A, Hameed A, Murugaiah C. Efficacy and safety of superficial chemical peeling in treatment of active acne vulgaris. *An Bras Dermatol.* 2017;92(2):212–216. https://doi.org/10.1590/abd1806-4841.20175273. Review. PubMed Central PMCID: PMC5429107 28538881.

Atzori L, Brundu MA, Orru A, Biggio P. Glycolic acid peeling in the treatment of acne. *J Eur Acad Dermatol Venereol.* 1999;12(2):119–122. PubMed PMID: 10343939.

Castillo DE, Keri JE. Chemical peels in the treatment of acne: patient selection and perspectives. *Clin Cosmet Investig Dermatol.* 2018;11:365–372. https://doi.org/10.2147/CCID.S137788. eCollection 2018. Review. PubMed PMID: 30038512; PubMed Central PMCID: PMC6053170.

Chen X, Wang S, Yang M, Li L. Chemical peels for acne vulgaris: a systematic review of randomized controlled trials. *BMJ Open.* 2018;8(4):e019607. https://doi.org/10.1136/bmjopen-2017-019607. PubMed Central PMCID: PMC5931279 29705755.

de Vries FMC, Meulendijks AM, Driessen RJB, van Dooren AA, Tjin EPM, van de Kerkhof PCM. The efficacy and safety of non-pharmacological therapies for the treatment of acne vulgaris: a systematic review and best-evidence synthesis. *J Eur Acad Dermatol Venereol.* 2018;32(7):1195–1203. https://doi.org/10.1111/jdv.14881. Epub 2018 Mar 6. Review 29444375.

Dréno B, Fischer TC, Perosino E, et al. Expert opinion: efficacy of superficial chemical peels in active acne management—what can we learn from the literature today? Evidence-based recommendations. *J Eur Acad Dermatol Venereol.* 2011;25(6):695–704. https://doi.org/10.1111/j.1468-3083.2010.03852.x. Epub 2010 Oct 3. Review. PubMed PMID: 21029205.

Jae J, Dong Ju H, Dong Hyun K, Yoon MS, Lee HJ, eds. Comparative study of buffered 50% glycolic acid (pH 3.0) + 0.5% salicylic acid solution vs Jessner's solution in patients with acne vulgaris. *J Cosmet Dermatol.* 2018;17(5):797–801. https://doi.org/10.1111/jocd.12445. Epub 2017 Nov 21. PubMed PMID: 29164826.

Jartarkar SR, Gangadhar, et al. Single-blind, active controlled study tocompare the efficacy of salicylic acid and mandelic acid chemical peel in the treatment of mild to moderately severe acne vulgaris. *Clin Dermatol Rev.* 2017;1(1):15–18.

Kaminaka C, Uede M, Matsunaka H, Furukawa F, Yamomoto Y. Clinical evaluation of glycolic acid chemical peeling in patients with acne vulgaris: a randomized, double-blind, placebo-controlled, split-face comparative study. *Dermatol Surg.* 2014;40(3):314–322. https://doi.org/10.1111/dsu.12417. Epub 2014 Jan 21. PubMed PMID: 24447110.

Kessler E, Flanagan K, Chia C, Rogers C, Glaser DA. Comparison of alpha- and beta-hydroxy acid chemical peels in the treatment of mild to moderately severe facial acne vulgaris. *Dermatol Surg.* 2008;34(1):45–50; discussion 51. Epub 2007 Dec 5. PubMed PMID: 18053051.

Kim RH, Armstrong AW. Current state of acne treatment: highlighting lasers, photodynamic therapy, and chemical peels. *Dermatol Online J.* 2011;17(3):2. Review. PubMed PMID: 21426868.

Kim SW, Moon SE, Kim JA, Eun HC. Glycolic acid versus Jessner's solution: which is better for facial acne patients?

A randomized prospective clinical trial of split-face model therapy. *Dermatol Surg*. 1999;25(4):270–273. PubMed PMID: 10417580.

Kontochristopoulos G, Platsidaki E. Chemical peels in active acne and acne scars. *Clin Dermatol*. 2017;35(2):179–182. https://doi.org/10.1016/j.clindermatol.2016.10.011. Epub 2016 Oct 27. PubMed PMID: 28274356.

Lee HS, Kim IH. Salicylic acid peels for the treatment of acne vulgaris in Asian patients. *Dermatol Surg*. 2003;29(12):1196–1199; discussion 1199. PubMed PMID: 14725662.

Lee JB, Chung WG, Kwahck H, Lee KH. Focal treatment of acne scars with trichloroacetic acid: chemical reconstruction of skin scars method. *Dermatol Surg*. 2002;28(11):1017–1021; discussion 1021. PubMed PMID: 12460296.

Lekakh O, Mahoney AM, Novice K, et al. Treatment of acne vulgaris with salicylic acid chemical peel and pulsed dye laser: a split face, rater-blinded, randomized controlled trial. *J Lasers Med Sci*. 2015;6(4):167–170. https://doi.org/10.15171/jlms.2015.13. Epub 2015 Oct 27. PubMed PMID: 26705462; PubMed Central PMCID: PMC4688384.

Nofal E, Nofal A, Gharib K, Nasr M, Abdelshafy A, Elsaid E. Combination chemical peels are more effective than single chemical peel in treatment of mild-to-moderate acne vulgaris: a split face comparative clinical trial. *J Cosmet Dermatol*. 2018;17(5):802–810. https://doi.org/10.1111/jocd.12763. Epub 2018 Sep 10. PubMed PMID: 30203434.

Soleymani T, Lanoue J, Rahman Z. A Practical approach to chemical peels: a review of fundamentals and step-by-step algorithmic protocol for treatment. *J Clin Aesthet Dermatol*. 2018;11(8):21. PubMed PMID: 30214663.

Trivedi MK, Kroumpouzos G, Murase JE. A review of the safety of cosmetic procedures during pregnancy and lactation. *Int J Womens Dermatol*. 2017;3(1):6–10. https://doi.org/10.1016/j.ijwd.2017.01.005. eCollection 2017 Mar-PubMed Central PMCID: PMC541895428492048.

11

Treatment of Acne Scars With a Combination of Chemical Peels and Microneedling

Jaishree Sharad

INTRODUCTION

Postacne scarring is the most important sequelae for acne and can be psychologically traumatic to the patient. It can occur even in patients with milder degrees of acne. The pathogenesis of atrophic acne scarring is most likely related to inflammatory mediators and enzymatic degradation of collagen fibers and subcutaneous fat.[1] Picking at acne lesions adds to scarring. Postacne pigmentation and pigmented scars are very common in acne patients with darker skin types. The pathogenesis of such hyperpigmentation is complex and seems to be related to many factors, including skin color and lesion trauma, and may also be related to the acne disease itself, especially the severity of inflammation.[2] Scars following acne are usually atrophic and sometimes hypertrophic. Atrophic acne scars have been best described by

Fabbrocini et al. as rolling scars, icepick scars, and superficial and deep boxcar scars[3] (Fig. 11.1). Icepick scars are narrow, sharply demarcated, V-shaped tracts, less than 2 mm in diameter, that extend into the deep dermis or even subcutaneous layer. Boxcar scars are wider (1–4 mm in diameter), U-shaped tracts, with sharp, vertical edges that extend 0.1 to 0.5 mm into the dermis. Rolling scars are characterized by tethering of the dermis to the subcutis. They are generally at least 4 mm in diameter, irregular, with a rolling or undulating appearance. Rolling scars are best visualized with indirect lighting to cast a shadow upon the skin, thus highlighting the scars. This classification helps in planning a treatment protocol for the scars. From simple excision; subcision; and a variety of punch techniques such as punch excision, punch grafting, and punch elevation, we have come a

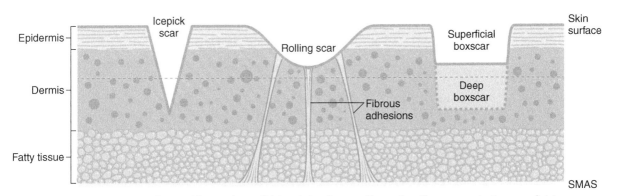

Fig. 11.1 Icepick, rolling, and boxcar (superficial and deep) scars. The *yellow line* represents the superficial musculoaponeurotic system to which fibrous bands adhere, creating rolling scars. *SMAS,* superficial musculoaponeurotic system.

long way. Chemical peels, fractional and nonfractional ablative and nonablative lasers, microneedling, radiofrequency microneedling, fat grafts, and filler injections are other modalities of treatment for acne scars. Because one individual may have various forms of scars, no single modality of treatment helps all the scars. It is always a combination treatment that gives the best treatment outcome. Treatments also depend on the severity of acne scars. The most commonly used acne scar severity grading scale has been proposed by Goodman and Baron.[4] Most techniques induce collagen remodeling to improve the scars. The degree of collagen remodeling seems to be proportional to the severity of the injury, and the result is hard to judge prospectively. The final result may not manifest until 4 to 6 months after treatment, and multiple therapies are often required.[5]

A combination of microneedling and chemical peels can be done for the treatment of atrophic acne scars in dark skin with promising results. Although microneedling helps reduce atrophic boxcar and rolling scars, chemical peels will help in reducing postinflammatory hyperpigmentation (PIH). This combination has minimum risk of PIH or scarring in patients with dark skin.

MICRONEEDLING

Pioneered in 1995, Orentreich and Orentreich described subcision or dermal needling for scars.[6] This approach involves pricking or puncturing the skin and then subcising the dermis with the needle to build up connective tissue beneath the scars. In 1997, Camirand and Doucet used a tattoo gun to "needle abrade" scars.[7] Based on these principles, Fernandes and Signorini developed a new technology called microneedling or percutaneous collagen induction therapy to initiate the natural posttraumatic inflammatory cascade.[8]

The Instrument

The manual drum-roller, also known as a dermaroller, is a handheld device equipped with medical-grade solid steel microneedles, projecting from a cylindrical roller. There are 24 circular arrays of eight needles, each located on the roller for a total of 192 needles. The needles vary in length ranging from 0.2 to 3 mm. The microneedles are synthesized by reactive ion etching techniques on silicon or medical-grade stainless steel. For adequate and uniform penetration, the needles are arranged at an angle of 15 degrees to the center of the instrument. The

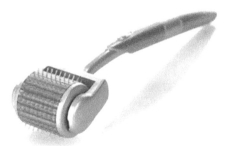

Fig. 11.2 Manual dermaroller.

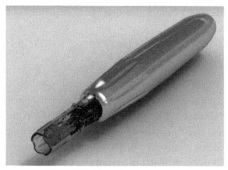

Fig. 11.3 Electric Dermapen.

most preferred needle length for treating acne scars is 1.5 to 2 mm. The depth of penetration varies from 0.1 to 1.3 mm depending on the pressure and extent of skin stretching. The instrument is presterilized by gamma irradiation (Fig. 11.2).

The other microneedling device that is gaining more popularity now is the electric-powered pen, which can be either operated with a battery pack or an alternating current power cord. When used with corded power, the device speed can be adjusted, ranging from 10,250 to 23,750 rpm. With battery power, the device speed is fixed at 13,500 rpm. Sterile disposable needle cartridges are made of 12 array count/32 gauge and 36 array count/30 gauge. Skin on the forehead is treated with needle depths ranging from 0.5 to 1.0 mm, whereas on the rest of the face, needle depths of 1.5 to 3.0 mm are preferred. Thicker or more fibrotic skin is usually treated with deeper needle depths[9] (Fig. 11.3 and Box 11.1).

Mechanism of Action

Microneedling involves the use of a handheld rolling instrument or electric-powered pens with tiny needles that create multiple superficial puncture wounds in the skin until fine pinpoint bleeding is achieved. The tiny microinjuries in the upper dermis release numerous growth factors, such as fibroblast growth factor, platelet-derived growth factor, and transforming growth factors alpha and beta, which all facilitate the production and propagation of intercellular matrix proteins. The fibroblasts line up along the axis of the fibronectin matrix, and it is here that they synthesize collagen and elastin. Collagen type III is the dominant form in the early wound-healing phase. Fibroblast collagen synthesis causes tissue remodeling over the next few months. Collagen type III is gradually replaced by collagen I over a period of 1 year or more. Scar collagen synthesis related to thermal injury involves upregulation of TGF-β1 and β2, whereas natural collagen synthesis after microneedling is related to upregulation of TGF-β3.[10]

Liebl et al. have proposed another hypothesis to explain how microneedling works. When new wounds are formed in microneedling, the cells create a "demarcation current" that is further increased by the needles' own electric potential.[11] This demarcation current (also called *bioelectricity*) triggers a cascade of growth factors that stimulate the healing phase and help in the proliferation and synthesis of collagen fibers.

Histopathology After Microneedling

In a study done by Fernandes et al., histological examination showed thicker skin, with greatly increased collagen type I and type III deposition and significantly more elastin, but otherwise was unremarkable from normal skin.[12] Type VII collagen, which is the main component of anchoring fibrils, also increases significantly. The collagen bundles are laid down in a normal lattice pattern rather than in parallel arrangement.

Aust et al. reported a considerable increase in collagen and elastin deposition at 6 months postprocedure.

The epidermis showed 40% thickening of the stratum spinosum and normal rete ridges at 1 year postoperatively.[12]

CHEMICAL PEELS

Chemical peels are applied on the skin to even skin pigmentation, exfoliate, and revitalize through promotion of the fibroblasts, glycosaminoglycans, and remodeling of the elastin and collagen fibers. Superficial and medium-depth peels are very safe in dark skin and have been established in the treatment of acne scars.

The following peels can be combined with microneedling for the treatment of atrophic acne scars:

- Glycolic acid (GA) is an alpha-hydroxy acid peel that in high strength and acidic pH has keratolytic properties. The peel causes enzymatic degradation at the corneocyte surface and facilitates peeling. Subsequent regeneration results in a thin stratum corneum and compact epidermis. There is dispersion of epidermal melanin and thus evening of skin color.
- Because of its small molecular size, GA penetrates through the horny layer rapidly, increases the density of collagen by increasing collagen synthesis, and improves the quality of elastin, thus helping improve scars. Glycolic acid peels can be done in the same session as microneedling safely. Concentrations of 20% to 35% GA are preferable for dark skin.
- Mandelic acid is an alpha-hydroxy acid with a slow penetration rate, thus reducing the chances of skin irritation. It causes dissolution of intercellular cement substance, stimulates collagen synthesis, and promotes cellular regeneration. It has antibacterial and antiinflammatory properties. A concentration of 20% to 50% mandelic acid is also known to improve hyperpigmentation. Hence it can be used to treat hyperpigmented atrophic acne scars in people with sensitive skin or a history of PIH or in people who have scars as well as a few comedones. Mandelic acid peels can be done in the same session as microneedling, but there are no studies supporting it yet.
- Salicylic acid (SA) is a beta-hydroxy acid with keratolytic properties. It exfoliates pigmented keratinocytes and accelerates cell cycle turnover, thus reducing new pigment transfer. A 20% SA peel can be done in combination with microneedling in alternate sessions in patients with seborrhea or in those who have a mild, active acne along with scars. It is not suggested to

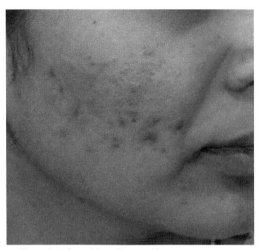

Fig. 11.4 Atrophic rolling and boxcar acne scars.

perform the SA peel at the same time as microneedling in patients who have seborrhea or active acne to prevent PIH or infection.

- Trichloroacetic acid (TCA) peel in concentrations of 15% to 20% causes precipitation of epidermal protein, epidermal necrosis, dermal inflammation, and collagen remodeling. It helps in reducing pigment and aids in microneedling to reduce atrophic scars. Microneedling and TCA peel in the same session should be done with precaution and care in patients with dark skin. Although a single study has been published on same-day treatment with both modalities, the risk of PIH may be higher if the peel is done in the same session in skin types IV through VI. The peel can be done safely 2 weeks after microneedling.
- Tretinoin peels have keratolytic, sebolytic, comedogenic, and antiinflammatory properties. They can be used in dark skin when the skin is primed well. They help in smoothing the skin in those with thick skin in addition to aiding in pigment reduction and reduction of superficial scars. They should be done alternately with microneedling rather than on the same session.

Indications (Fig. 11.4)

- Atrophic rolling acne scars and boxcar scars in all skin types
- Hyperpigmented atrophic acne scars in all skin types, especially dark skin

Contraindications

1. Active infection like verrucae vulgaris, herpes labialis, and active acne
2. Keloids and hypertrophic scars
3. Uncontrolled diabetes, neuromuscular disease, collagen vascular disease
4. Rosacea
5. Chronic skin condition like scleroderma, psoriasis, and eczema
6. Pregnancy
7. Skin malignancy, moles, actinic keratosis
8. Patients with blood clotting disorders (It is advisable to stop the anticoagulants a week before the procedure.)
9. Patients with unrealistic expectations

Protocol

After priming the skin (see Chapter 3 and see the following information), the patient can be scheduled for microneedling. After a session of microneedling, 20% to 35% glycolic acid is applied immediately onto the skin surface. The peel is neutralized after 5 minutes. The procedure is repeated after 3 weeks. In those with a history of postinflammatory hyperpigmentation or with a history of frequent outdoor activities, it is better to do a session of microneedling separately from the peel, which can be performed 3 weeks later. Every 3 weeks the patient can alternate microneedling with light peels. The cycle can continue for four to five sessions of each treatment. One may opt for 20% to 35% glycolic acid or 15% TCA peels for dark scars. If there are comedones, mandelic acid or SA is preferred. If the patient has patchy hyperpigmentation or wants an overall even skin tone, or in males with acne scars and thick sebaceous skin, tretinoin peels can also be done.

Preprocedure Preparation[13]

- Any active infection or active acne should be treated before doing the microneedling procedure. Patients should be put on topical anticomedogenic creams about 2 to 3 weeks before doing the procedure if there is a history of acne flare-ups. If there is a past history of recurrent herpes simplex, it is important to administer a prophylactic course of oral acyclovir or valacyclovir starting the night before the procedure.

- Microneedling has been found to be safe in patients who are on low-dose isotretinoin.
- Priming a patient before microneedling is very important. Topical bleaching agents such as hydroquinone, vitamin C, or Kojic acid and peeling agents such as glycolic acid or vitamin A cream can be used for priming 2 to 3 weeks before the procedure. This enhances the efficacy and prevents postprocedural pigmentation.
- Patients should also be counseled about the importance of strict sun protection and should be advised to use a broad-spectrum sunscreen regularly. Topical preparations containing hyaluronic acid help in faster healing.
- A written informed consent must be obtained before the procedure. Standardized photographs using identical patient positioning, lighting, and camera settings should be obtained. The patient should understand what the procedure(s) entails.

THE MICRONEEDLING PROCEDURE[14]

The area to be treated should be thoroughly cleansed to remove makeup and dirt. Apply a topical anesthetic in the form of a eutectic mixture of 2.5% lidocaine and 2.5% prilocaine under occlusion. After an hour, remove the anesthetic cream with acetone, and the area to be treated can be cleansed with chlorhexidine, povidone-iodine, or 70% isopropyl alcohol solutions. Clean the skin one last time with normal saline.

With one hand, stretch the skin to be treated. With the other hand, grip the roller like a pen and roll it on the skin. The needles will penetrate at a greater depth if the skin is stretched. Roll the instrument to and fro six to ten times in four directions; horizontally, vertically, and diagonally right and left, to cover an area of roughly 2-inch by 2-inch (Fig. 11.5). This ensures an even pricking pattern, resulting in about 250 to 300 pricks/cm^2. Pinpoint bleeding is considered the clinical end point. (Fig. 11.6) The movements have to be short and the pressure has to be moderate to ensure a uniform depth of penetration. The technique is operator-dependent, and therefore depth of penetration also depends on the pressure applied. Aggressive rolling or lateral pressure can lead to scarring and breakage of needles. Certain areas need special consideration. Lesser pressure is required over bony areas like the forehead and nose. When treating the orbital area, a needle length

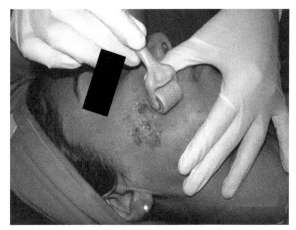

Fig. 11.5 Technique of microneedling.

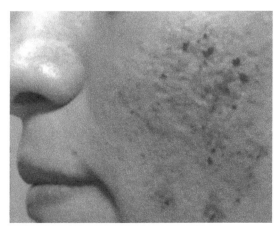

Fig. 11.6 Pinpoint bleeding (endpoint).

of 0.5 mm or less should be used to minimize the pain and also to prevent hematoma formation. The number of roller movements should also be less in the orbital region. While treating the skin around the lips, ask the patient to purse lips together so that the vermillion borders touch. Every needle initially penetrates at an angle and then goes deeper as the roller turns. Finally the needle is extracted at a converse angle, therefore curving the tracts and redirecting the path of the needle as it rolls into and then out of the skin for about 1.5 to 2 mm into the dermis.

Wipe the blood and the serous fluid using normal saline after the procedure. If performing a peel in the same session, apply the peel, such as 20% to 35% glycolic acid, sequentially all over the face (Fig. 11.7). Neutralize the peel after 5 minutes with sodium bicarbonate. Then apply an antibacterial cream and sunscreen.

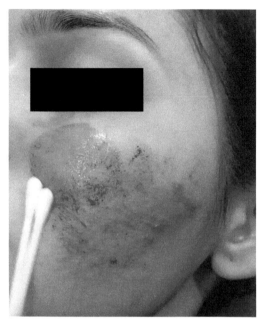

Fig. 11.7 Application of 35% glycolic acid peel.

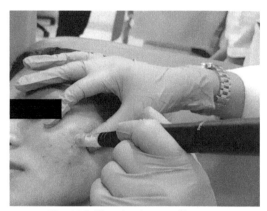

Fig. 11.8 Electric microneedling pen.

For staged procedures, once the microneedling is performed, a topical antibiotic and a sunscreen are applied. The patient should return after 2 to 3 weeks for a chemical peel. This cycle is repeated four to five times for each of the procedures.

Microneedling creates multiple microchannels in the epidermis that close within minutes of the treatment. In case of deeper scars, dermarollers with 2-mm needles are used to achieve deeper penetration and thus give better results. Also, longer needles result in better conductivity and lesser electrical resistance. Electric pens are easier to use and are gently moved sequentially on the entire face or targeted specifically on the scars (Fig. 11.8).

POSTPROCEDURE CARE

There may be erythema, edema, and mild crusting for 2 to 4 days posttreatment. The crusts usually fall off after a few days, and the patient should be instructed to avoid scratching or picking at the crusts. Patients should be advised to use a broad-spectrum sunscreen and to avoid sun exposure for a week to prevent postinflammatory hyperpigmentation. Antibacterial creams containing mupirocin should be used twice a day for 5 to 7 days. Moisturizers containing hyaluronic acid help in faster repair of the skin. A short course of an oral antibiotic and oral nonsteroidal antiinflammatory drugs may be prescribed if indicated. The patient is advised to avoid any irritant substances like chloroxylenol, astringent, or abrasive scrubs. An interval of 6 weeks is preferred between sessions of microneedling. An interval of 2 to 3 weeks in preferred between a session of microneedling and a chemical peel if they are done as two separate treatments (Box 11.2).

COMPLICATIONS

The procedure is usually well tolerated. Erythema and swelling occur a few hours after the procedure. The complications of microneedling include the following:
1. Bruising
2. Mild scabbing for a few days after the procedure
3. Hematoma on the bony areas
4. Secondary bacterial infection
5. Milia formation[6]

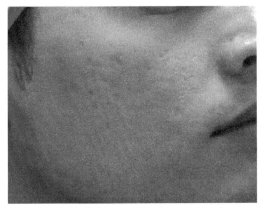

Fig. 11.9 Before combination treatment.

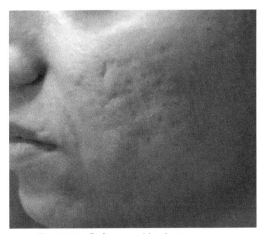

Fig. 11.11 Before combination treatment.

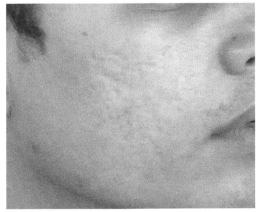

Fig. 11.10 After microneedling and 35% glycolic acid peel in alternate sessions.

6. Postinflammatory hyperpigmentation
7. Tram track effect seen mainly on bony prominences[15]
8. Allergic and foreign body granulomatous reaction[16]
9. Reactivation of herpes simplex and activation of acne

DISCUSSION

Macular hyperpigmented scars and mild boxcar scars improve with superficial and medium-depth chemical peels. However, moderate to deep boxcar and rolling scars do not disappear completely with chemical peels. Moreover, in dark-skinned individuals, deep chemical peels carry a higher risk of PIH and scarring. Microneedling helps in reducing moderate to deep boxcar and rolling scars. A combination of superficial or medium-depth chemical peels along with microneedling can be opted for in dark-skinned individuals (Figs. 11.9–11.12).

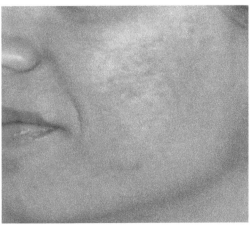

Fig. 11.12 After microneedling and 35% glycolic acid peel in the same session.

The author reported a study of 30 patients, 22 women and 8 men in the age group of 20 to 40 years, with atrophic boxcar and rolling scars. All the patients had skin type III through V by the Fitzpatrick skin type classification. Group A patients, 15 out of the 30 patients, underwent microneedling once every 6 weeks for a total of five sessions. Group B patients, 15 patients out of 30, underwent five treatments of microneedling and five sessions of 35% glycolic acid peels. They were treated every 3 weeks alternately with microneedling and 35% GA peel. Patients from both groups were assessed and photographed at the end of each treatment and again 3 months after their last treatment session. Scars were assessed and graded objectively as well as on the basis of photographs by the treating dermatologist. All the data were analyzed using SPSS 15 (Statistical Package for the Social Sciences, IBM, New York). A "t" test was used to compare the results. Three months after all the treatment sessions were completed, the mean improvement in scars in group A was 31.33%, whereas in group B it was found to be 62%. The difference was statistically significant ($P = 0.001$). Patients from group B showed better improvement compared with group A. In addition to the improvement in scars, there was an improvement in skin texture and tone. Reduction in pore size was also seen. These were more evident in group B. There was an excellent improvement in postacne pigmentation in group B.[17]

In a study by Leheta et al., 39 patients with Fitzpatrick skin types III and IV with postacne atrophic scars were randomly equally divided into three groups. Group 1 was subjected to six sessions of microneedling (2 mm) combined with 20% TCA in the same session; group 2 was subjected to six sessions of 1540 nm fractional laser; and group 3 was subjected to microneedling combined with 20% TCA in one session followed by 1540 nm fractional laser in the next session for a total of three sessions of each. It was seen that the scar severity scores improved by a mean of 59.79% (95% CI 47.38–72.21) ($P < 0.001$) in group 1, a mean of 61.83% (95% CI 54.09–69.56) ($P < 0.001$) in group 2, and a mean of 78.27% (95% CI 74.39–82.15) ($P < 0.001$) in group 3. The difference in the degree of improvement was statistically significant when comparing the three groups using the ANOVA test ($P = 0.004$). Hence they concluded that combining 1540 nm nonablative fractional laser in alternation with microneedling and chemical peel with 20% TCA was a better option for the treatment of atrophic acne scars.[18]

In another study by Garg and Baveja, 50 patients with Fitzpatrick skin types III, IV, and V with atrophic acne scars underwent subcision, after which microneedling with dermaroller (1.5 mm) was performed alternatively with 15% TCA peel at 2-week intervals for a total of six sessions of each. Grading of acne scar photographs was done pretreatment and 1 month after all six sessions. The patient's own evaluation of improvement was assessed. It was found that all the patients showed significant improvement in their scars.[19]

With microneedling, there is increased collagen deposition and significantly more elastin. This leads to improvement in the scar depth. Microneedling also helps break up collagen strands in the superficial layers of the dermis, which leads to the untethering of scars

and stimulates revascularization. Hence rolling scars, which are characterized by dermal tethering, improve with microneedling. The epidermis remains intact, so there is very little chance of infection. Aust et al. showed that microneedling does not cause any damage to the stratum corneum, other layers of the epidermis, or the basal membrane, and there is no dermabrasive reduction of epidermal thickness evident 24 hours after the procedure. The number of melanocytes neither increased nor decreased in any of the groups.[12] This explains why microneedling can be repeated safely in dark skin and is also suited in cases where laser treatments and deep peels cannot be performed.

Superficial and medium-depth chemical peels have shown good results in both postacne pigmentation and PIH in skin types III through V. The author has treated postacne pigmentation in patients with Fitzpatrick's skin types III through IV with 20% to 35% glycolic acid peels without any adverse effects and complete clearance of lesions.[20]

Wang et al. studied 35% to 50% GA peels in Taiwanese patients and saw improvement in the lesions. Only 5.6% patients reported PIH or a flareup of acne.[21] In another study, in 16 cases, there was rapid and greater improvement in postacne PIH in patients who were treated with GA peels compared with those treated with topical lightening agents.[22] Grimes studied 20% to 30% SA peels in skin of color and reported marked clearance in PIH in all patients. Some patients had mild dryness and crusting with transient hyperpigmentation.[23]

Microneedling can be combined with chemical peels either in consecutive sessions or in the same session. It is safe to do 20% to 35% GA, tretinoin peel, mandelic–SA peels, and 15% to 20% TCA peels alternately with microneedling every 2 to 3 weeks in dark skin.[24] There is one study of 20% TCA done in the same session immediately after microneedling, and there was no PIH found in this study.[25] The author also chooses to perform a 35% GA peel in the same session as microneedling with better results in rolling and boxcar scars as well as postacne pigmentation. Combining microneedling and a peel in the same session facilitates the penetration of the solution deeper into the skin without causing great epidermal damage. This allows better collagen remodeling with minimal chances of PIH or scarring in dark skin. Fresh scars or scars less than 1 year old respond best to this treatment. Old fibrosed scars may not show an excellent response (Boxes 11.3 and 11.4).

BOX 11.3 Advantages of Combination of Microneedling and Chemical Peels

Peels help in elimination of pigment and improve skin texture.

Patient tolerance and compliance are better.

Peels are synergistic to microneedling in treating atrophic scars.

Both are simple office procedures done under topical anesthesia.

Combining both treatments results in less downtime.

Both treatments are cost effective.

Microneedling is safe in dark skin (skin types III–V), because there is no thermal damage and the epidermis is not injured.

BOX 11.4 Disadvantages of Microneedling

Multiple sessions, compared with ablative CO_2 laser, because it a relatively milder procedure and less collagen is synthesized in a single sitting.

The instrument cannot be used for multiple sittings, because the needles become blunt in one sitting.

Proper aseptic precautions have to be taken to prevent any infection.

Icepick scars do not show any improvement.

CONCLUSION

Microneedling has established its place in the management of scars as a simple and affordable office procedure. It is the most useful for the improvement of boxcar and rolling acne scars. It is also an effective modality of treatment for open pores, facial rejuvenation, alopecia, transdermal drug delivery, and many more indications. It has gained popularity because of its simplicity, cost effectiveness, decreased downtime, and side effects compared with other treatment modalities. It is considered safe in treating patients with Fitzpatrick skin types IV and V because it overcomes the side effects of scarring and hyperpigmentation resulting from other procedures in which the epidermis is compromised.

Combining chemical peels and microneedling can enhance the outcome in case of atrophic boxcar and rolling scars in dark skin. There have been studies to prove the efficacy of both individually and a few studies on the combination as well. Studies need to be conducted on combining peels other than GA and TCA with microneedling for the treatment of atrophic acne scars, although the author already performs them in her practice with satisfactory results.

REFERENCES

1. Fife D. Practical evaluation and management of atrophic acne scars: tips for the general dermatologist. *J Clin Aesthet Dermatol*. 2011;4:50–57.
2. Ho SGY, Yeung CK, Chan NPY, Shek SY, Kono T, Chan HHL. A retrospective analysis of the management of acne post-inflammatory hyperpigmentation using topical treatment, laser treatment, or combination. *Lasers Surg Med*. 2011;43:1–7.
3. Fabbrocini G, Annunziata MC, D"Arco V, et al. Acne scars: pathogenesis, classification and treatment. *Dermatol Res Pract*. 2010;2010:893080.
4. Goodman GJ, Baron JA. Post acne scarring: a qualitative global scarring grading system. *Dermatol Surg*. 2006;32(12):1458–1466.
5. Goodman Greg, Van Den Broek Amanda. The modified tower vertical filler technique for the treatment of post-acne scarring. *Aus J Dermatol*. 2015;57. https://doi.org/10.1111/ajd.12390.
6. Orentreich DS, Orentreich N. Subcutaneous incisionless (subcision) surgery for the correction of depressed scars and wrinkles. *Dermatol Surg*. 1995;21:543–549.
7. Camirand A, Doucet J. Needle dermabrasion. *Aesthetic Plast Surg*. 1997;21:48–51.
8. Fernandes D, Signorini M. Combating photoaging with percutaneous collagen induction. *Clin Dermatol*. 2008;26:192–199.
9. Alster Tina, Graham Paul. Microneedling: a review and practical guide. *Dermatol Surg*. 2017;44:1. https://doi.org/10.1097/DSS.0000000000001248.
10. Fabbrocini G, Fardella N, Monfrecola A, Proietti I, Innocenzi D. Acne scarring treatment using skin needling. *Clin Exp Dermatol*. 2009;34:874–879.
11. Liebl Horst, Kloth Luther C. "Skin cell proliferation stimulated by microneedles". *J Am Coll Clin Wound Spec*. 2012;4(1):2–6. PMC. Web. 2016.
12. Aust MC, Fernandes D, Kolokythas P, et al. Percutaneous collagen induction therapy: an alternative treatment for scars, wrinkles and skin laxity. *Plast Reconstr Surg*. 2008;21:1421–1429.
13. Sharad J. microneedling. In: Venkataram Mysore, ed. *ACS(I) Ttextbook on Ccutaneous & Aaesthetic Surgery*. Jaypee medical publishers; 2012:572–579.

14. Sharad J. Microneedling. In: Khunger Nz, ed. *Step by Sstep Ttreatment of Aacne Sscars.* Jaypee Medical Publishers; 2014:102–113.

15. Pahwa M, Pahwa P, Zaheer A. "Tram track effect" after treatment of acne scars using a microneedling device. *Dermatol Surg.* 2012;38(7 Pt 1):1107–1108.

16. Soltani-Arabshahi R, Wong JW, Duffy KL, Powell DL. Facial allergic granulomatous reaction and systemic hypersensitivity associated with microneedle therapy for skin rejuvenation. *JAMA Dermatol.* 2014;1501:68–72.

17. Sharad J. Combination of microneedling and glycolic acid peels for the treatment of acne scar in dark skin. *J Cosmet Dermatol.* 2011;10:317–323.

18. Leheta Tahra M, Rania M, et al. Do combined alternating sessions of 1540 nm nonablative fractional laser and percutaneous collagen induction with trichloroacetic acid 20% show better results than each individual modality in the treatment of atrophic acne scars? A randomized controlled trial. *J Dermatol Treat.* 2014;25(2):137–141. https://doi.org/10.3109/09546634.2012.698249.

19. Garg S, Baveja S. Combination therapy in the management of atrophic acne scars. *J Cutan Aesthet Surg.* 2014;7;(1):18–23.

20. Sharad J. Glycolic acid peel therapy—a current review. *Clin Cosmet Investig Dermatol.* 2013;6:281–288. https://doi.org/10.2147/CCID.S34029. Published 2013 Nov 11.

21. Wang CM, Huang CL, Hu CT, Chan HL. The effect of glycolic acid on the treatment of acne in Asian skin. *Dermatol Surg.* 1997;23:23–29.

22. Burns RL, Prevost-Blank PL, Lawry MA, Lawry TB, Faria DT, et al. Glycolic acid peels for post inflammatory hyperpigmentation in black patients. A comparative study. *Dermatol Surg.* 1997;23:171–174.

23. Grimes PE. The safety and efficacy of salicylic acid peels in darker racial-ethnic groups. *Dermatol Surg.* 1999;25:18–22.

24. Grimes PE. Chemical peels in dark skin. In: Tosti A, Grimes P, De Padova M, eds. *Color Atlas of Chemical Peels.* Berlin, Heidelberg: Springer; 2011.

25. Leheta TM, Abdel Hay RM, El Garem YF. Deep peeling using phenol versus percutaneous collagen induction combined with trichloroacetic acid 20% in atrophic post-acne scars; a randomized controlled trial. *J Dermatolog Treat.* 2014;25:130–136.

12

The Rullan Two-Day Croton Oil–Phenol Chemabrasion Peel

Peter Rullan

INTRODUCTION

The phenol peel has been called a *chemical facelift* because it removes photodamage-related wrinkles and tightens the skin more effectively than other ablative techniques. To accomplish this, a deep croton oil–phenol peel extends to the upper to midreticular dermis (approximately 600 microns). Many physicians who perform cosmetic surgery still equate deep phenol peels with the well-known Baker-Gordon phenol peel. However, formula modifications made in the last 20 years have led to much lower croton oil concentrations, resulting in phenol peels that are much less cardiotoxic, are less melanotoxic, and have less risk of scarring, as long as published formulas and techniques are followed.

The 2-day phenol chemabrasion technique that I developed[1] is useful for deep wrinkles or acne scars. As a modified version of the chemabrasion technique introduced by Dr. Yoram Fintsi (2001)[2,3] this technique includes the use of HyTape occlusion for 24 hours, the concept of debridement, the reapplication of a phenol formula into deep scars or wrinkles on day 2, and the use of a powder mask (bismuth subgallate) to absorb the ensuing drainage for 7 days. Additionally, this technique includes intravenous (IV) titratable conscious sedation, regional nerve blocks, and variations from the published formulas. A tongue depressor and varied curettes are used on day 2 (instead of sandpaper) to perform debridement of the necrotic coagulum and the remaining epithelium lining acne scars and deep wrinkles.

BENEFITS OF THE RULLAN METHOD

1. The use of a lower croton oil concentration lowers the risk of hypopigmentation.
2. Useful for all skin types, especially among acne scar patients (44% of Dr. Rullan's patients have ethnic skin).

3. Following these methods for application, hydration and pain control have been shown to reduce the risk of cardiac arrhythmias.
4. Chemabrasion with curettes allows better removal of epithelium and inflammatory coagulum, promoting secondary healing inside scars and wrinkles.
5. Segmental croton oil/phenol is effective and does not require monitoring

SAFETY RECOMMENDATIONS

1. Follow medical screening and Advanced Cardiac Life Support (ACLS) protocols.
2. Maintain PO_2 above 90%, and prevent tachycardia.
3. Avoid pain-related adrenergic chaos by using effective sedation and analgesia.
4. Peel the neck and chest using either low percentage croton oil and phenol or TCA (15%–20%).
5. Consider peeling nonfacial regions with an intense pulsed light (IPL)/Erbium combination.

PATIENT SELECTION AND PREOPERATIVE PROTOCOL

The most common indication for deep peels is to treat moderate to severe wrinkles (Glogau scale wrinkles III through IV) in Fitzpatrick skin types I to III (Figs. 12.1 and 12.2). If a patient has facial wrinkling accompanied by significant tissue laxity or volume deficiency, dermal fillers or cosmetic surgery may also be needed to achieve optimal results. In the case of acne scars, dark skin types IV through VI can be peeled as long as the patient understands the face–neck skin color tones will be discordant for almost 2 years (Figs. 12.3 and 12.4). The patient must be willing to adopt strict avoidance of sun and the chronic use of skin lighteners

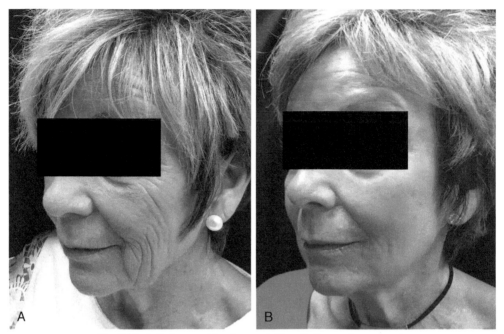

Fig. 12.1 A, Before peel for deep wrinkles. B, Six weeks postpeel.

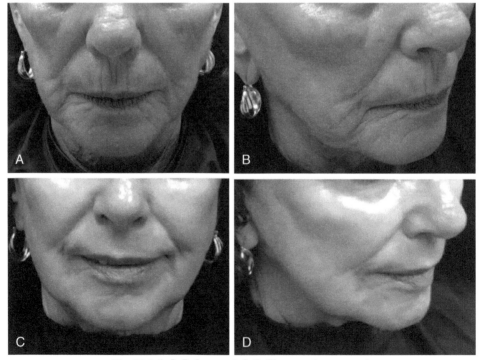

Fig. 12.2 A–B, Before peel. C–D, Five months postpeel.

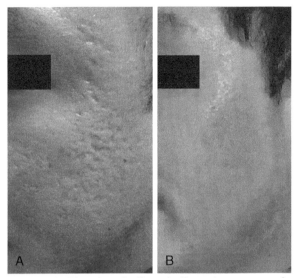

Fig. 12.3 A, Phenol peel offers significant improvement for acne scarring in skin types IV and V. B, Four weeks after 2-day chemabrasion; skin is still erythematous but will have natural color tones by 12 weeks.

on the neck during those 2 years. For patients with dark skin who do not want to make these long-term changes, a recommended alternative is to perform three to four sessions of chemical reconstruction of skin scars (CROSS), as discussed by Lee et al. (2002).[4] See Chapter 13 for further discussion on effective treatment of acne scars using CROSS.

During the initial consultation for the peel, the physician should make note of the patient's risk for demarcation lines and the tendency for postinflammatory hyperpigmentation (PIH). Assess factors that may impact the pigmentary healing process, such as the presence of a suntan or the patient's exercise habits (specifically any temperature-increasing activities). The patient's available downtime and ability or willingness to conceal lingering redness with makeup should also be taken into consideration. The patient will need to have family or nursing support for the first 3 days postpeel and must accept having a "mask" on their face for 8 days. During this time, they will only be able to eat liquefied food through a plastic bottle (provided by physician).

Patients with active acne should be treated with oral and topical antibiotics, retinoid creams, acne surgery, or isotretinoin before receiving the peel. The peel should

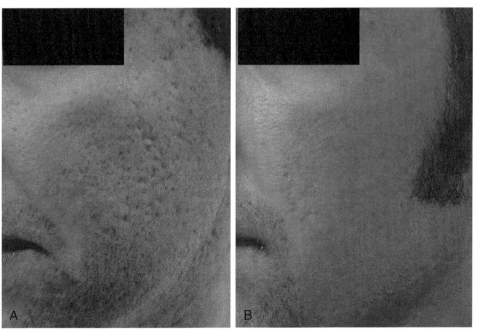

Fig. 12.4 A, Phenol peel offers significant improvement for acne scars. B, Postpeel. Scars have filled in and natural pigmentation has returned.

be delayed until the patient has discontinued isotretinoin for 6 months or until the skin has regained its normal sebaceous activity. For patients with acne scarring, photographic documentation should be obtained with direct lighting and indirect (shadow) lighting.

Most patients with an oily complexion are prescribed a low-dose, 30-day course of isotretinoin after the peel, because I (and other experienced peelers, including Zein Obagi) believe excessive sebum is an inflammatory state that can lead to PIH. However, no controlled studies have been conducted on this yet.

The preoperative procedure for this technique requires a laboratory workup with hepatic, renal, and cardiac tests (10-lead electrocardiogram). Because phenol is hepatically metabolized and renally excreted, blood levels of phenol can become cardiotoxic if the liver or kidneys are not functioning well. The patient must procure a letter from their primary physician clearing them for the peel. Patients should also be screened for risk factors of QTc prolongation before the peel. Dr. Carlos Wambier (2018)[5,6] has reported that phenol may cause a QTc prolongation, especially when other additive factors are present, such as certain medications (erythromycin, fluconazole, antimalarials, amiodarone, antidepressants, antipsychotics, terfenadine, hydrochlorothiazide, and others) or electrolytic abnormalities (hypomagnesemia, hypokalemia). When two or more of these factors are present, the risk for QTc interval prolongation occurs (dangerous if above 480 ms), triggering a potentially fatal torsade de pointe (TdP) ventricular arrhythmia during a phenol peel.

Skin Preparation

Tretinoin and hydroquinone (or similar) are used to prime the skin for 4 to 6 weeks leading up to the peel, because they are known to improve healing and reduce pigmentary complications. Tretinoin 0.05% to 0.1% should be applied thoroughly across every area of the face except the sensitive upper eyelids. Apply one pea size per cheek and apply a ceramide-based moisturizer along with it. This can also be mixed with a barrier cream if needed, to dilute and reduce irritation. Application should extend past every edge of the area to be peeled, which may include the neck. By doing this, the stratum corneum is thinned, epidermal turnover is increased, dermal collagen is stimulated, and the transfer of melanin is normalized.

Patients may experience minimal flaking skin as a side effect of this treatment, which should not be a concern. The frequency of application should be determined by skin sensitivity; it can be applied two to three times a day or nightly, as tolerated, to avoid excessive

peeling and redness. Application of tretinoin and hydroquinone is discontinued 4 to 5 days before the peel and will resume a few weeks after the peel.

PROCEDURE PROTOCOL

Anesthesia, Medications, and Monitoring

During the peripeel period, patients should be hydrated and monitored for cardiac arrhythmias. To avoid adverse effects, the peels should be administered slowly in a cosmetic subunit approach. Typically, peel administration should span 60 minutes (15 minutes per section).

Intravenous (IV) access is always required to comply with ACLS guidelines for conscious sedation and to ensure adequate hydration for the patient throughout the peel. Patient comfort is paramount to avoid an adrenergic chaos, which can lead to arrhythmias. Sedation and analgesia can be accomplished with oral (diazepam, triazolam, or hydromorphone), intramuscular (IM; ketorolac 30–60 mg), or IV agents (midazolam, fentanyl). I recommend following the oral sedation strategy popularized by Dr. Lawrence Kass (2017)[7] in which the patient takes 1 mg of Alprazolam at 4 hours, 2 hours, and 1 hour before the peel and 10 mg of Zolpidem upon arriving at the appointment for the peel. This provides real amnesia and sedation. The use of facial nerve blocks is effective at reducing the need for systemic medication. The use of epinephrine has been avoided or minimized in these blocks to reduce the risk of tachycardia and arrhythmias. Clonidine (0.1 mg) used orally as a preoperative medication also reduces this risk and provides mild sedation. General anesthesia is not recommended because of respiratory and pH issues. The PO_2 must be kept above 90% throughout the procedure, and sinus tachycardia must be brief and minimized.

The patient is discharged home with diazepam, hydromorphone, triazolam, and ondansetron for nausea. Acyclovir is started one day before the peel (400 mg three times daily for 10 days). If antibiotics are prescribed, they should not be used until the third day to avoid nausea. The IV access should be maintained overnight, and the nurse or family member must be trained in assisting with medications. Antibacterial and antiviral prophylaxis are prescribed (start 1 day before the peel and take for total of 10 days) along with vinegar compresses to prevent bacterial and yeast infections or flares of herpes simplex during the healing process. In addition, patients send daily photo updates via text message after the peel. This allows the physician to monitor their progress between office visits and promptly identify any complications.

TABLE 12.1 Hetter Peel Formulas Containing 35% Phenol

	0.2%	0.4%	0.8%	1.2%	1.6%
Water	5.5 mL	5.5 mL	5.5 mL	5.5 mL	5.5 mL
Septisol	0.5 mL	0.5 mL	0.5 mL	0.5 mL	0.5 mL
USP phenol 88%	3.5 mL	3.0 mL	2.0 mL	1.0 mL	0.0 mL
Stock solution containing phenol and croton oil	0.5 mL	1.0 mL	2.0 mL	3.0 mL	4.0 mL
Total	10 mL	10 mL	10 mL	10 mL	10 mL

Note: 0.1% = 1 mL of 0.4% + 1.2 mL phenol + 1.8 mL water.

TABLE 12.2 Alternative Way to Compound Hetter Formulas Using "Drops" to Measure Croton Oil

Hetter 35% Phenol	Croton Oil %	Phenol 88%	Water	Septisol	Drops Croton Oil
Medium light	0.35%	4 mL	6 mL	16 gtts	1
Medium heavy	0.7%	4 mL	6 mL	16 gtts	2
Heavy	1.1%	4 mL	6 mL	16 gtts	3

Note: Very Light Peel (0.1%, 28% phenol) = 3 mL of medium light formula plus 2 mL of 88% phenol and 5 mL water.

Croton Oil–Phenol Peel Formulas

The Hetter and Baker-Gordon phenol formulas (Tables 12.1 and 12.2) typically consist of 88% phenol (carbolic acid), croton oil, Septisol (hexachlorophene), and water. Alternatively, lay peelers' formulas (such as Gradé) may contain croton oil, carbolic acid, water, olive oil, and glycerin.

Phenol disrupts sulfide bonds, resulting in keratolysis and protein coagulation. Phenol is also melanotoxic. Hexachlorophene is an antiseptic with surfactant properties, which allows a more uniform and deeper penetration by decreasing surface tension. Croton oil is a vesicant (and therefore epidermolytic) that greatly enhances the absorption of phenol. Croton oil is now commonly considered the most important ingredient in phenol formulas. In some formulas, olive oil is added to slow the cutaneous absorption rate of these agents and reduce any systemic toxicity.

Commonly used phenol formulas (see Table 12.1) include Hetter's Heresy formulas, which have 35% phenol. The croton oil concentration for these formulas ranges from 1.6% (perioral and tip of nose) to 0.7% (for mid-cheeks), 0.35% (forehead, temples, upper cheeks), and 0.1% (for eyelids and neck—this concentration is also known as *very light*) (Fig. 12.5). For example, the Hetter medium light formula is made by adding one drop of croton to 4 mL phenol 88%, 6 mL water, and 16 gtts Septisol (as shown in Table 12.2). Use two drops of croton oil for the 0.7% formula, three drops for the 1.1% formula, or four drops for the 1.6% formula (see Table 12.2). Dr. Richard

Bensimon's (2008)[8] review of the newer croton oil–phenol peels emphasizes the advantage of using the range of Hetter formulas (based on varying croton oil concentrations) customized for the thickness of the skin being peeled to attain the best peel for each area. Using the right application technique is equally important to achieve appropriate endpoints with different Hetter formulas.

DR. RULLAN'S TWO-DAY CROTON OIL–PHENOL CHEMABRASION TECHNIQUE

Day 1

Ringer's lactate (1–2 L) is infused for 2 hours. The face is thoroughly cleansed and degreased using alcohol and acetone. IV sedation is given. Nerve blocks and degreasing are performed immediately before each anatomical area being peeled. A full face peel can be done using Dr. Rullan's modification of the Gradé II formula (with 0.35% croton oil and 64% phenol); Stone's Gradé II formula of 0.2% croton oil and 64% phenol with glycerin and olive oil; or Hetter's "all-around stock" formula of 0.35% croton oil and 33% phenol (Table 12.3).

These are slowly applied with regular cotton-tipped applicators, which are first rolled against the edge of the stainless-steel cup to remove excess fluid. Apply the solution slowly, one "stripe" at a time. The depth of peel is determined by the concentration used, the amount applied, and how firmly it is applied (apply gently at first, then harder if the skin is not frosting). Therefore it is crucial to recognize

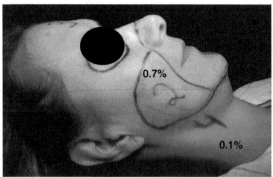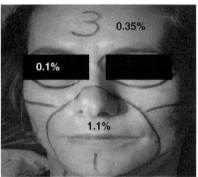

Fig. 12.5 Croton oil percentages. (Adapted from an article published in *Advances in Ophthalmology and Optometry*, Vol. 2.1, Kass L, The lost art of chemical peeling: my fifteen year experience with croton oil peel, 401, copyright Elsevier (2017), Fig. 5, with permission from Dr. Lawrence Kass.)

TABLE 12.3   Rullan's Modification of Stone's Gradé II Formula

	Rullan 0.35%	Stone 0.2%
Phenol	40 mL	40 mL
Glycerin	1.13 mL	1.13 mL
Olive oil	0.025 mL	0.025 mL
Croton oil	0.21 mL	0.1 mL
Water	18.5 mL	18.5 mL

the appropriate depth and endpoints for each area. The endpoint varies according to skin thickness and can be identified by the level of frosting. Thin eyelid or lateral forehead skin is peeled until a transparent frost with a pink background is achieved, representing a medium-depth peel down to the papillary dermis. For thicker skin, such as the perioral or glabellar regions, a thicker, solid white frost signifies that the upper to midreticular dermis has been reached. In addition, a sustained red-brown microvesiculation (called *epidermolysis*) appears as another endpoint when performing a deep peel to thick skin such as the perioral region. Medium peels should reach the papillary dermis, whereas deep peels extend to the upper or midreticular dermis. Peeling to the lower reticular dermis may cause scarring and should be avoided.

Each of the five anatomical areas (forehead, each cheek, perioral-chin, and periorbital-nose) are peeled according to these endpoints. This takes 10 to 15 minutes per area, meaning overall application of the peel takes approximately 60 minutes. Icepick scars receive an additional peel application with a fine paintbrush to ensure complete wetting of each lesion. A complete, organized frost must be achieved in each area, and a yellowish edematous appearance indicating epidermolysis should be noted

after 15 to 30 minutes (Fig. 12.6). Once complete, the face is completely taped (except the upper lids) with 1-inch to 2-inch strips of waterproof HyTape (HyTape International, Patterson, NY, USA), and covered with a surgical face net (Fig. 12.7). No rinsing is needed. See Table 12.4 for a step-by-step checklist of the peel procedure.

Day 2

The patient is usually groggy but pain-free when returning to the clinic. The HyTape is easily removed. Additional sedation and analgesia are sometimes given if the patient has severe acne scarring or deep wrinkles and aggressive abrasion is expected. The necrotic coagulum is debrided using a tongue blade or a large 6 mm Fox curette (Fig. 12.8). Icepick scars and box scars or deep wrinkles are debrided using 1 to 2 mm chalazion-type curettes to achieve punctate bleeding inside the scars and ensure deepithelialization of these types of lesions. The goal is to create a true open wound within the lesions to induce secondary healing and wound closure (Fig. 12.9). Additional phenol solution (Rullan 0.35% croton oil, 64% phenol, glycerin, water, and olive oil; see Table 12.3) is applied with a fine paint brush into icepick and box scars (for acne) or into deep rhytides or rugae anywhere in the face. An additional swipe with a cotton-tipped applicator is done in areas where additional tightening is desired (for example, on the marionette lines and buccal cheeks where wrinkles and "draping" occurs). An antiseptic, antiinflammatory powder, bismuth subgallate (Delasco or Spectrum Pharmaceuticals, Irvine, CA), is then applied to the entire face except the upper lids (where we use Aquaphor), before the patient is discharged home (Fig. 12.10). This dries into a protective mask that will stay in place for the next 7 to 8 days.

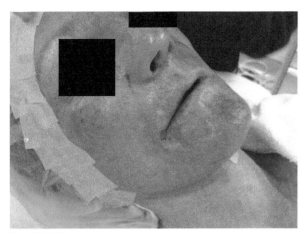

Fig. 12.6 Frosting shows when the appropriate endpoint has been reached with gray-white edema and yellow-red epidermolysis.

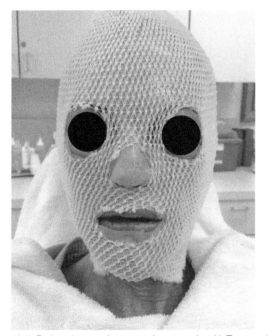

Fig. 12.7 Patient leaves the procedure wearing HyTape and a surgical net, to be removed by the physician on day 2.

Patients should be sent home with limited sleeping pills, a sedative, and analgesics (for details see Table 12.4)

Days 3 to 8

The patient is restricted to home and is not allowed to shower until the mask is ready to be removed. On approximately the eighth day, the mask spontaneously begins to separate due to skin reepithelialization (Fig. 12.11). Vaseline is then applied over the entire mask, allowed to soak in, and left on overnight. The mask is gently removed the next morning by applying more petroleum jelly under the slowly separating mask while showering. Medical barrier creams (Epionce) or Aquaphor ointment (Eucerin, Beiersdorf AG, Hamburg, Germany) is used until the skin is no longer tender or red. Most patients are 99% reepithelialized by day 9. There has been no incidence of infections following this procedure in the author's clinic.

Days 8 to 30 and Beyond

After the mask falls off, using white vinegar compresses (1 Tbsp vinegar in 1 cup of water) can be very soothing and reduces the risk of infection. Pain medication should not be needed anymore. The skin is fragile and sensitive, so using gentle cleansers, light noncomedogenic and hypoallergenic creams, and lotions is recommended. For oily patients who may still have active acne, a short course of isotretinoin (10–20 mg a day for 2–4 weeks) has significantly helped prevent acneiform eruptions, milia, and postinflammatory hyperpigmentation. This is especially effective in darker skin types. Other sebolytic measures such as spironolactone and acne medications have also been effective. Although sun and heat avoidance are required for 30 days, many patients begin a gradual return to their normal lifestyle by slowly increasing their activity in measure with how red their skin gets when hot. During this time, easily removable makeup is recommended to camouflage redness.

Touchups

Two to three months after the peel has healed, a regional or lesional (CROSS) peel can be repeated for persistent acne scars or perioral wrinkles, even in skin types IV to VI. These lighter skin types can tolerate a regional peel. The intent is to recreate an open wound inside the icepick scars or wrinkles, adding new collagen so they eventually fill in almost completely.

Postoperative Skin Care

Sweating should be avoided for 30 days to reduce redness, and tinted sunscreens or powder makeup (Oxygenetix, ColoreSCience) should be applied regularly once the skin has reepithelialized. More deeply peeled areas should be treated with Aquaphor. Previous skin conditioning can be reinitiated once the skin is no longer sensitive, red, and peeling (around day 14). Fluocinolone 0.01% cream can be used when PIH is noted or when redness persists longer than 30 days.

TABLE 12.4 Sequence of Two-day Croton Oil–Phenol Chemabrasion Peel

Day 1 (one hour)	1. Certify patient's medical qualifications for peel.
	   a. Labs (electrocardiogram, liver and kidney).
	   b. Medications explained to patient and assistant.
	   c. Provide bottles for water, food, and mouth rinse for 7 days.
	2. Perform with ACLS-certified personnel, equipment, and medications.
	3. Start IV Ringer's lactate, administer titratable sedative and analgesic, and connect all monitors.
	   d. IM triamcinolone 20 mg/2 mL
	4. Administer oral medications:
	   e. Clonidine 0.1 mg p.o.
	   f. Ondansetron 4 mg
	5. Mark five facial regions and degrease first region.
	6. Perform nerve blocks to anesthetize perioral region, nose, and glabella (first region).
	7. Apply selected croton oil–phenol formula with one cotton-tipped applicator to achieve uniform white frost.
	   g. Ensure that vital signs and pain control are normal and adequate.
	8. After waiting 15 minutes (can perform nerve blocks during this time), repeat degreasing, nerve blocks, and peel applications to second (forehead), third (right cheek to temple), fourth (left cheek and temple), and fifth (upper and lower lids) regions.
	9. Review all regions to make sure endpoints are noted, such as gray edema and epidermolysis. If not, then consider applying additional peel solution.
	   h. Perform CROSS into acne scars.
	   i. Apply solution into deep wrinkles.
	   j. Perform subcision if patient has rolling acne scars.
	10. Apply HyTape to entire face except upper and lower eyelids; secure with Surgilast netting for 24 hours.
	11. Send home with a "trained" assistant and with pain medications and antivirals for 10 days.

Day 2 (30 minutes)	1. Restart IV Ringer's and administer IV medications (as preferred by doctor).
	2. Remove HyTape and begin debridement of coagulum of necrotic epidermis.
	   a. Tongue depressor, 6 mm Fox curette.
	3. Debride individual acne scars and deeper wrinkles.
	   a. Chalazion curette 1–2 mm
	4. Apply peel solution with a fine brush into scars and/or deeper wrinkles.
	5. Apply a small amount of peel solution in regions with more severe skin laxity or acne scars.
	6. Apply bismuth subgallate powder everywhere except the upper and lower lids (use Aquaphor).

Days 2–8	1. Follow instructions for antiviral/pain medications. 2. Explain that swelling is worst on day 3 but improves quickly after that. 3. Ensure that the mask remains securely on the face and remind patient to minimize facial expressions or mastication. 4. On day 8 (assuming the mask is already spontaneously separating from the reepithelialized underlying skin), apply a petrolatum ointment all over mask and sleep with it on. 5. The next day take a long warm shower, allowing a soft water spray to melt off the mask. Do not remove any portion of the mask still adhering to skin. Instead reapply ointment for another 24 hours.
Days 8–30	1. Use Aquaphor daily and apply white vinegar compresses to sensitive areas. 2. By day 9, 99% of patients should have 99% reepithelialization of the face. a. Most patients return to work by day 12–14 and can wear makeup. 3. Slowly move away from ointments and start using barrier repair creams instead. 4. Consider low-dose isotretinoin for 2–4 weeks if the patient is very oily, breaking out, or developing postinflammatory hyperpigmentation.

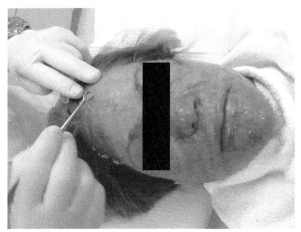

Fig. 12.8 Curettes of varying sizes are used for debriding on day 2.

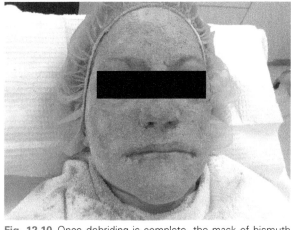

Fig. 12.10 Once debriding is complete, the mask of bismuth subgallate powder is applied and remains in place for 7 days.

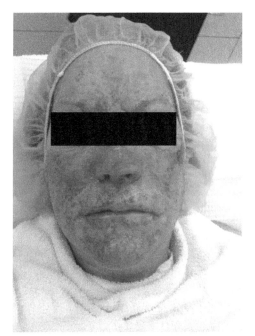

Fig. 12.9 The necrotic tissue has been removed and the epidermis can begin healing. Additional Rullan 0.35% croton oil was applied to deeper wrinkles of the perioral region.

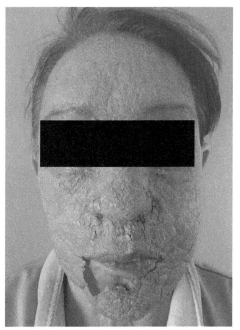

Fig. 12.11 Day 7. Once the bismuth subgallate mask begins separating, it is ready to melt off in the shower.

Full-face phenol peels are not always necessary. Segmental croton oil–phenol peels can be combined with TCA peels; regionalizing the peels by combining deeper and lighter peels can result in sufficient improvement without the risk of dyschromias or prolonged downtime. This technique for segmental croton oil–phenol peels is summarized later and has been described elsewhere in detail (Rullan et al., 2004; Rullan & Karam, 2010).

SEGMENTAL CROTON OIL–PHENOL PEELS

For many dermatologists, doing a full-face croton oil–phenol peel is not a reality. The need for cardiac monitoring, sedation, and analgesia is too restrictive.

However, for many, a combination of segmental croton oil–phenol peel and using TCA or an ablative laser on the rest of the face is a quite real option. There is no need for IV fluids (however, being hydrated is important) or for cardiac monitoring, provided that only one or two cosmetic subunits (less than 2% body surface area) are being peeled and that the peel is performed slowly over 10 to 15 minutes.

The most common cosmetic subunits that would benefit from a deeper peel are the upper lip and the periorbital region. The Hetter formulas recommended for these are 0.7% to 1.2% croton oil–phenol for the upper lip and Hetter VL 0.1% croton oil–phenol for the periorbital skin. I always tape the upper lip for 24 hours (with HyTape and Surgilast) and then debride the coagulum on day 2, before reapplying additional phenol to the deepest rhytides. The postoperative care is either bismuth powder mask for 5 days or the open technique with daily showers and Aquaphor (Fig. 12.12). For the periorbital unit, only Aquaphor is needed afterward.

For these segmental peels, the TCA peel should be applied first. The croton oil–phenol is applied next, carefully overlapping over the TCA in the smile-line cheek region or on the chin. The biggest challenge is blending skin tones in darker skin types III and IV in the chin and cheek regions. The safest option for these is to just peel the upper lip and only the lower lip's vermilion border. The ideal candidates are nonsuntanned skin types II and III. If performed in combination with laser resurfacing, the laser should be used after the peel is finished and the face is fully dry. Laser can be overlapped approximately 1 cm over peel areas to feather the results.

COMPLICATIONS

Chemical peeling complications can occur in any patient regardless of skin color. The early recognition and management of these complications is essential for a successful resolution.

Possible complications are listed below, along with suggestions for their management:

1. Herpes simplex virus (HSV) infection: Appears as erosions; can be prevented with a course of oral antivirals beginning 1 day before peel and extending until reepithelialization is completed. If there is a breakthrough of HSV despite the prophylactic dosing, the dose should be increased (valacyclovir is recommended at 1 g orally 2–3 times a day for 7–10 days).

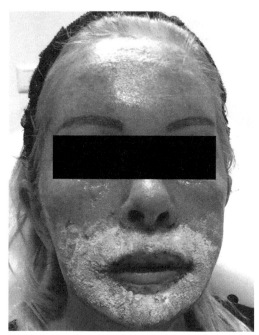

Fig. 12.12 Regional peel. Trichloroacetic acid 26% peel on the face, Hetter 0.1% on the lower eyelids, and Rullan 2-day 0.35% croton oil peel periorally.

2. Bacterial or yeast infection: Both have to be cultured and treated with white vinegar compresses. This is different from the acneiform eruption typically seen while using occlusive ointments postpeel.
3. Prolonged erythema: Treatment options include topical steroids class VI (or stronger) twice a day (fluocinolone 0.01% cream or clobetasol recommended), pulsed dye laser every 2 weeks, barrier or silicone creams, and makeup. Symptoms will subside over time if treatment is consistent.
4. Contact dermatitis: Recognize with good history; return to petrolatum and white vinegar compresses.
5. Scarring: Weekly to biweekly low dose of intralesional triamcinolone 5 mg/mL; pulsed dye laser every 2 weeks; may need to add intralesional 5-FU (monthly) to triamcinolone (equal parts); topical steroids and barrier creams.
6. PIH: Hydroquinone 4% as discussed earlier in the chapter; may add 30% salicylic peel every 2 to 4 weeks. Consider low-dose isotretinoin for 30 days when PIH starts appearing in oily skin of color.
7. Hypopigmentation: Appears insidiously and creates lines of demarcation; most obvious when peeling the chest and neck area. Repigmentation will happen gradually over a period of 2 years but can

be accelerated via targeted phototherapy with narrow-band ultravioletB (UVB).

To prevent hypopigmentation, avoid medium to deep peels in deeply tanned patients (or at the very least, get informed consent). For the neck and chest, intense pulsed light and fractional erbium may be a better option than chemical peels.

SUMMARY

The croton oil–phenol peel is the gold standard for facial rejuvenation using a resurfacing technique, even though it has been limited in usage because of inadequate training in dermatology residencies. It stands alone in its ability to correct deep wrinkles and long-term tightening of skin. It can be combined with any other resurfacing technique when doing a segmental perioral or periorbital croton oil–phenol peel.

Peels are commonly used in combination with other dermatologic procedures, or as a component of a multimodal approach, including laser ablation, electrocautery (for benign tissue growths), cosmetic surgery (blepharoplasty, rhytidectomy), dermal fillers, and neurotoxins. All peels require a preconditioning regimen and a rigorous postoperative schedule to ensure long-term satisfaction.

Patients' expectations need to be clarified. Some expect peels to control or shrink pores in a lasting manner, but this does not happen. Patients, particularly those with large pores or active acne, need to control the oiliness of their skin by using cleansers, drying agents, and acne medications such as spironolactone and especially isotretinoin. Lifestyle changes may also be required for an extended period, including avoidance of sun and the reduction of exercise-induced heat (e.g., swimming rather than running). These measures will help to ensure patients' lifelong satisfaction with their appearance after a croton oil–phenol peel.

REFERENCES

1. Rullan PP, Karam AM. Chemical peels for darker skin types. *Facial Plast Surg Cl.* 2010;18:111–131.
2. Fintsi Y. Exoderm—a novel, phenol-based peeling method resulting in improved safety. *Int J Cosmet Surg.* 2001a;1:40–44.
3. Fintsi Y. Exoderm chemoabrasion original method for the treatment of facial acne ars. *Int J Cosmet Surg.* 2001b;1: 45–52.
4. Lee JB, Chung WG, Kwahck H, et al. Focal treatment of acne scars with trichloroacetic acid: chemical reconstruction of skin scars method. *Dermatol Surg.* 2002;28:1017–1021; discussion 1021.
5. Wambier CG. Prolongation of rate-corrected QT interval during phenol-croton oil peels. *J Am Acad Derm.* 2018;78:810–811.
6. Wambier CG, Lee KC, Botini de Olivera P, et al. Comment on "surgical smoke: risk assessment and mitigation strategies" and chemical adsorption by activated carbon N95 masks. *J Amer Acad Dermatol.* 2019;80(4):e79–e80. Epub 2018 Nov 14.
7. Kass L, Kass K. The lost art of chemical peeling: my fifteen year experience with croton oil peel. *Adv Opthalmol Optomet.* 2017;2:391–407.
8. Bensimon R. Croton oil peels. *Aesthe Surg J.* 2008;28: 33–45.

FURTHER READING

Hetter GP. An examination of the phenol-croton oil peel: part I. Dissecting the formula. *Plast Reconstr Surg.* 2000;105:227–239.

Hetter GP. An examination of the phenol-croton oil peel: part II. The lay peelers and their croton oil formulas. *Plast Reconstr Surg.* 2000;105:240–248.

Hetter GP. An examination of the phenol-croton oil peel: part III. The plastic surgeons' role. *Plast Reconstr Surg.* 2000;105:752–763.

Hetter GP. An examination of the phenol-croton oil peel: part IV. Face peel results with different concentrations of phenol and croton oil. *Plast Reconstr Surg.* 2000;105:1061–1083.

Landau M. Cardiac complications in deep chemical peels. *Dermatol Surg.* 2007;33:190–193.

Obagi S, Bridenstine JB. Chemical skin resurfacing. *Oral Maxillofac Surg Clin North Am.* 2000;12:541–553.

Obagi S, Bridenstine JB. Lifetime skin care. *Oral Maxillofac Surg Clin North Am.* 2000;12:531–540.

Rullan P, Lemmon J, Rullan JM. The 2-day phenol chemabrasion technique for deep wrinkles and acne scars. *Am J Cosmet Surg.* 2004;21:199–210.

Stone PA. The use of modified phenol for chemical face peeling. *Clin Plast Surg.* 1998;25:21–44.

Stone PA, Lefer LG. Modified phenol chemical face peels: recognizing the role of application technique. *Clin Plast Surg.* 2001;28:13–36.

Truppman ES, Ellenby JD. Major electrocardiographic changes during chemical face peeling. *Plast Reconstr Surg.* 1979;63:44–48.

13

New Advances Combining the Chemical Reconstruction of Skin Scars (CROSS) and Subcision

Peter Rullan

INTRODUCTION

Minor acne scarring occurs in up to 95% of acne cases, and 22% of these patients are affected with a more significant and psychologically disturbing degree of scarring (as reported by Layton et al., 1994).[1] Various treatment modalities are used for reconstructing and improving the appearance of acne scars, including dermabrasion, punch excision, punch elevation, dermal fillers, microneedling (with/without radiofrequency), subcutaneous incision (subcision), and chemical and laser skin resurfacing (ablative and nonablative). The chemical reconstruction of skin scars (CROSS) technique significantly added to this armamentarium of options by allowing physicians to treat boxcar and icepick scars in all skin types, with little downtime required and small risk of complications (especially postinflammatory hyperpigmentation). The challenge many patients still face is that their physicians rely on resurfacing options alone instead of using combination therapies to treat their different types of scars.

REVIEW OF THE LITERATURE

The first published reference to applying an acid on the skin to treat skin scars came from Dr. G. MacKee in 1952,[2] when he used 88% phenol to produce an inflammatory action similar to that of 90% trichloroacetic acid (TCA) to treat skin alterations that affect the deeper layers of the skin. In 2002, Dr. J B Lee[3] and his colleagues published the landmark article on CROSS. They reported the use of high-concentration TCA applied focally to atrophic acne scars. The authors treated 65 patients with acne scars and Fitzpatrick skin types IV and V. The study demonstrated that 27 of 33 patients

(82%) treated with 65% TCA and 30 of 32 patients (94%) treated with 100% TCA experienced a good clinical result.

The article describes how the application of TCA to the skin causes precipitation of proteins and coagulative necrosis of cells in the epidermis and necrosis of collagen in the papillary to upper reticular dermis. Over several days the necrotic layers slough and the skin reepithelializes from the adnexal structures that are spared from chemical damage. Dermal collagen remodeling after chemical peel may continue for several months. Many investigators have observed that the clinical effects of TCA are due to both a reorganization in dermal structural elements and an increase in dermal volume as a result of an increase in collagen content, glycosaminoglycan, and elastin.

Lee's article describes their technique, where they washed the skin with soap, cleansed it with alcohol, and then applied either 65% TCA or 100% TCA focally, by pressing hard on the entire depressed area of atrophic acne scars using a sharpened wooden applicator. The skin was monitored carefully until it reached a frosted appearance after a single application within 10 seconds. CROSS was repeatedly performed every 1 to 3 months to allow dermal thickening and collagen production. There were no cases of significant complication.

Lee and his colleagues later refined their technique (2007), developing a method using a 1-mL syringe and a fine-gauge needle. They filled the 1-mL syringe with 0.1 to 0.2 mL of 100% TCA; connected a disposable fine-gauge needle, preferably a 30- or 31-gauge needle for acne scars and a 33-gauge for enlarged pores; carefully removed the piston from the syringe (being held upright); and applied the TCA onto the affected area using the needle. They felt this made it easier to control the amount and depth of TCA applied. Lee's article also states that they believe that a drug history of isotretinoin is not a relative contraindication and does not influence the clinical results, because CROSS spares the adjacent normal skin.

Complications of the CROSS method include erythema, hypopigmentation and hyperpigmentation, scarring, and development of hypertrophy and atrophy. The atrophy produced by TCA acid resembles that sometimes generated by intralesional corticosteroids. Weber et al. (2011)[4] reported a large atrophic defect caused by acid covering normal tissue beyond the bounds of the scar. This article emphasizes the care taken with this technique and that only small amounts accurately placed in the depth of the scar should be used.

Dr. Agarwal et al. (2015)[5] published a clinical study of 52 patients that provides an excellent review on CROSS. They showed that 70% TCA CROSS was more effective in treating boxcar scars than rolling or icepick scars. Their patients' sampling of scar types were 37.8% icepick scars, 39.6% rolling scars, and 22.6% boxcar scars. Patients were treated every 2 weeks for four sessions and followed monthly for 3 months.

Dr. Leheta et al. (2011)[6] compared dermarolling (manual microneedling) to 100% TCA CROSS to treat different types of scars in 30 patients and concluded that CROSS was superior in boxcar and icepick scars, whereas dermarolling was better for rolling scars. Their patients underwent four sessions (4 weeks apart) of either dermarolling or 100% TCA CROSS.

Dr. Yug et al. (2006)[7] performed a histological study of treating atrophic acne scars with 95% TCA CROSS, at 6-week intervals, for a total of six treatments. Punch biopsies approximating the diameter of representative acne scars were performed at baseline and at 1 year. At baseline, he found that depressed acne scars exhibit a loss of collagen and adnexal structures resulting in a downward pull of the epidermis. Ice pick scars also have a decrease in elastin manifested by smaller fragmented elastin fibers, an increase in type III collagen, and fibroblasts oriented parallel to the epidermis. At 1 year, during the dermal remodeling phase, type III collagen is gradually replaced by new type I collagen and elastin and presents clinically as more elevated and improved acne scars.

This author has extensive experience doing CROSS with either croton oil–phenol formulas or TCA, but the results published by Dr. Dalpizzol et al. (2016)[8] led him to change his technique to using 88% carbolic (phenol) instead of TCA. This Brazilian group compared 88% carbolic to 90%

TCA, a hemifaced paired comparison; for 15 patients with icepick and boxcar scars, they applied TCA to one cheek and carbolic to the other. This was done every 3 weeks for four sessions and assessed 1 month later. Their study confirmed the efficacy of both TCA and phenol for treating such scars but showed that CROSS phenol resulted in less severe complications such as hypopigmentation and scar enlargement (Figs. 13.1 and 13.2).

TRIPLE COMBINATION OF CARBOLIC CROSS, CANNULA SUBCISION, AND MICRONEEDLING

The successful treatment of acne scars is very challenging and requires a serial, multimodal approach (Table 13.1). Most patients are young and thus very adept at using the Internet (acne.org, etc.) to assess and find what they feel are the best options. The author's evolution into the following technique is the result of 35 years of practice and feedback from experienced patients. Many of these complain they obtained none or very little benefit from CO_2 laser resurfacing (even multiple times), yet our specialty considers this treatment the gold standard. Indeed, it is a great resurfacing technique, but by itself lacks the ability to treat acne scar types such as rolling and icepick scars. Comments such as "lasers do not treat the scars under the skin" make perfect sense once a physician experiences the rasping sounds heard while performing subcision of rolling and dermal scars. These deeper scars can be best measured with overhead shadow photography. Three sessions of the author's combined triple therapy, 6 to 8 weeks apart, are usually recommended (Fig. 13.3 and Box 13.1). Dermal fillers are essential to complete the regimen, because atrophic scars are improved but not corrected. However, the triple combination helps release scars so they become distensible, and changes icepick and boxcar scars to make their shoulders less angled and more filled in. These changes greatly improve the effectiveness of dermal fillers when used.

All three treatments are performed in one sitting, one cheek at a time, beginning with degreasing the skin aggressively with acetone, then applying 88% carbolic acid with a fine paint brush, into each icepick or boxcar scar present on the face (Figs. 13.4 and 13.5). Some spillover onto the shoulders of a scar is allowed (only with carbolic acid; this should be avoided with TCA). After the extent of the rolling scars is marked, the cheeks are tumesced; a peristaltic pump is used (as for liposuction), and one single entry point is created with a 20-gauge spinal needle. From that entry point, the skin is punctured with an 18-gauge

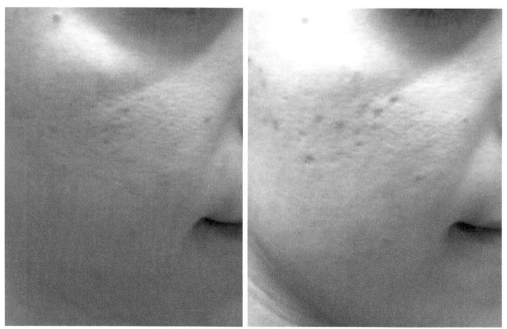

Fig. 13.1 Before (left) and after (right) trichloroacetic acid (TCA): A case of TCA CROSS causing widened acne scars.

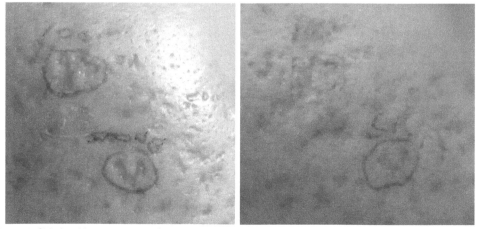

Fig. 13.2 Side-by-side comparison of 100% trichloroacetic acid (TCA) vs. Stone (0.2% croton oil/55% phenol solution) CROSS, before and after. Notice the TCA-treated scar remains deep with equal or wider edges, whereas the Stone-treated scar has filled in more and has much softer shoulders.

needle and an 18-gauge, 7-cm, fat transfer cannula (Soft-fil) is inserted, attached to an empty 3 mL syringe. A piston movement and fanning technique are used to break up the fibrotic fibers that are both vertical (tethers) and horizontal (dermal fibrosis). The face is swollen from the anesthesia, but bleeding and hematomas are very uncommon. This is in stark contrast with the author's experience using an 18-gauge Nokor for subcision, where significant bleeding and hematomas were very common. After subcision,

microneedling (Collagen PIN) is performed with a dermal infusion of a topical hyaluronic acid blend (Induction Therapies, Louisville, KY, USA) on the involved areas. The goal is to achieve punctate bleeding. The depth of the needle is around 0.5 to 1.0 mm on the temples and forehead and 1.5 to 2.5 mm on the cheeks. The hyaluronic acid gel is applied topically before and after microneedling.

Alternatively, in skin types I–III, fractional Erbium/CO_2 laser may be substituted for microneedling.

TABLE 13.1	**Various Treatments for Acne Scarring: Defect-Oriented Therapy**
Icepick scars	1 Incisional Removal, punch Excision or elevation
	2 *CROSS with 30%, 60%, or 100% trichloroacetic acid (TCA) or 88% carbolic acid (can be combined with any other resurfacing technique)*
Rolling scars	1 Subcision: 18-gauge cannula or Nokor 18-gauge needle
	2 *Surgical facelift*
Boxcar scars	1 Fractional ablative laser resurfacing: *erbium and CO2*
	2 Nonablative laser resurfacing
	3 Microneedling (skin types IV–VI)
	4 Dermabrasion
	5 2-day *phenol chemabrasion: spot or full-face scarring*
	6 TCA peels
	7 Excision
	8 Punch elevation or punch grafting
	9 Radiofrequency (microneedling)
Atrophic scars	1 Fillers (most effective in distensible scars with soft shoulders)
	2 Fillers are usually needed for atrophic scars on temples
	3 *Surgical facelift*

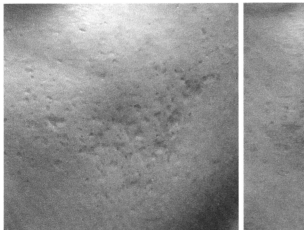 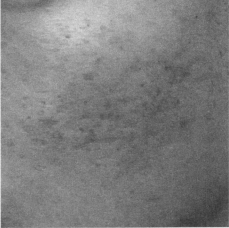

Fig. 13.3 Before (left) treatment and after (right) three rounds of CROSS combined with subcision and microneedling.

Occasionally, based on the degree of fat atrophy of the cheek, L-poly-lactic acid (10 mL) is injected subcutaneously or platelet-rich fibrin (PRF) is injected into deep dermis after the microneedling.

The downtime ranges from 5 to 6 days, with surface crusts from the CROSS falling off and leaving behind a pink mark. It takes 4 to 6 weeks for the boxcar scars and icepick scars to fill in. The following are the goals of this triple approach:

1. Make icepick and boxcar scars more shallow.
2. Round out and soften the sharp edges of these scars.
3. Make rolling scars more distensible.
4. Make all scars more responsive to dermal fillers and to resurfacing techniques.
5. Provide fastest recovery with the lowest risk of adverse effects.
6. Be financially affordable.
7. Provide a fly-in and fly-out option for out-of-towners.

REFERENCES

1. Layton AM, Henderson CA, Cunliffe WJ. A clinical evaluation of acne scarring and its incidence. *Clin Exp Dermatol.* 1994;19:303–308.
2. Mackee GM, Karp FL. The treatment of post acne scars with phenol. *Br J Dermatol.* 1952;64:456–459.
3. Lee JB, Chung WG, Kwahck H, et al. Focal treatment of acne

BOX 13.1   **Steps for the Rullan Triple Combination**

1. Take shadow photographs.
2. Degrease with acetone.
3. Apply 88% carbolic acid into all icepick and boxcar scars using a fine paint brush.
4. Mark the facial areas with rolling scars.
5. Tumesce one hemifacial region at a time.
6. From one 18-gauge needle puncture, insert an 18-gauge, 7-cm, fat transfer cannula and perform bi-level subcision until resistant fibrotic bands are broken.
7. Next perform device-assisted microneedling to achieve punctate bleeding.
8. Repeat steps 4–7 on the other side of the face.

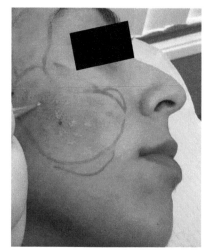

Fig. 13.5 In contrast to trichloroacetic acid (TCA), carbolic CROSS produces edema and mild epidermolysis inside the icepick and boxcar scars, effectively removing the epidermal barrier of these scars.

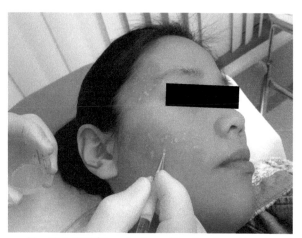

Fig. 13.4 CROSS application with a fine-tipped brush.

scars with trichloroacetic acid: chemical reconstruction of skin scars method. *Dermatol Surg.* 2002;28:1017–1021.

4. Weber MB, Machado RB, Hoefel IR, et al. Complication of CROSS-technique on boxcar acne scars: atrophy. *Dermatol Surg.* 2011;37:93–96.
5. Agarwal N, Gupta LK, Khare AK, et al. Therapeutic response of 70% trichloroacetic acid cross in atrophic acne scars. *Dermatol Surg.* 2015;41:597–604.
6. Leheta T, El Tawdy A, Abdel Hay R, et al. Percutaneous collagen induction versus full-concentration trichloroacetic acid in the treatment of atrophic acne scars. *Dermatol Surg.* 2011;37:207–216.
7. Yug A, Lane J, Howard M, et al. Histologic study of depressed acne scars treated with serial high-concentration (95%) trichloroacetic acid. *Dermatol Surg.* 2006;32:985–990.
8. Dalpizzol M, Weber MB, Mattiazzi AP, et al. Comparative study of the use of trichloroacetic acid and phenolic acid

in the treatment of atrophic-type acne scars. *Dermatol Surg.* 2016;42:377–383.

FURTHER READING

Alam M, Dover JS. Treatment of acne scarring. *Skin Ther Lett.* 2006;11:7–9.

Brodland DG, Roenigk RK, Cullimore KC, et al. Depths of chemexfoliation induced by various concentrations and application techniques of trichloroacetic acid in a porcine model. *J Dermatol Surg Oncol.* 1989;15:967–971.

Brody HJ. Variations and comparisons in medium-depth chemical peeling. *J Dermatol Surg Oncol.* 1989;15:953–963.

Butler PE, Gonzalez S, Randolph MA, et al. Quantitative and qualitative effects of chemical peeling on photo-aged skin: an experimental study. *Plast Reconstr Surg.* 2001;107:222–228.

Fabbrocini G, Cacciapuoti S, Fardella N, et al. CROSS technique: chemical reconstruction of skin scars method. *Dermatol Ther.* 2008;21(s3):S29–S32.

Goodman GJ. Post-acne scarring: a short review of its pathophysiology. *Australas J Dermatol.* 2001;42:84–90.

Rivera AE, Missouri K. Acne scarring: a review and current treatment modalities. *J Am Acad Dermatol.* 2008;59:659–676.

Stegman SJ. A comparative histologic study of the effects of three peeling agents and dermabrasion on normal and sun damaged skin. *Aesthetic Plast Surg.* 1982;6:123–135.

Whang SW, Lee KH, Lee JB, et al. Chemical reconstruction of skin scars (CROSS) method using a syringe technique. *Dermatol Surg.* 2007;33:1539–1540.

14

Chemical Peeling as an Adjunct to Facelift and Eyelid Surgery

Joe Niamtu III

In this day and age of high technology, younger patients and surgeons often think that only devices or new technology is the answer to skin rejuvenation. Although contemporary technology has in fact opened new doors, the historic chemical peel still stands as a stalwart in skin rejuvenation. Many colleagues have spent upward of $200,000 for a skin rejuvenation device that produced the same results that could have been achieved with $1.50 worth of 30% trichloroacetic acid (TCA). Just because something is new does not mean it is better. Chemical peeling has been around in some shape or form for millennia and is one of the few cosmetic procedures that has withstood the test of time in safety and results.

Chemical peeling is an appealing procedure for cosmetic practitioners for many reasons. First and foremost, it is predictable and is capable of producing significant results. Another important factor associated with the popularity of chemical peeling is the low cost of the materials. In reality, TCA chemical peeling may be the most profitable treatment in the entire cosmetic panoply. One ounce of 30% TCA can be purchased (at the time of this writing) for $28.00 from dermatologic supply companies (www.Delasco.com). Similar products can be purchased on the Internet for much less, but practitioners should only trust products purchased from a qualified and certified vendor. There are numerous ways to concoct TCA preparations, including volume/volume, weight/volume, etc. In addition, the quality of product is unpredictable when purchasing medications on the Internet. Remember, this is an acid, and it can cause permanent scarring and other health problems. There is no such

thing as a good deal on fire extinguishers, parachutes, seat belts, and TCA!

Chemical peeling is seemingly a very simple procedure, right? After all, it was performed by laypersons long before it became an accepted medical procedure. The skin is degreased with acetone, and a coat of acid solution is placed on the skin surface. There are even self-peeling videos available online. However, this sentiment is far from the truth. When I reflect on my own 25-year experience with chemical peeling, I believe I had some of my most sleepless nights related to chemical peeling and laser resurfacing. This is a simple procedure with a lot that can go wrong. It is imperative that the novice peeler has a complete understanding of the anatomy and healing of the skin, as well as the specific agents used for wounding the epidermis and dermis. As I will mention numerous times in this chapter, failure to do so can result in complications, permanent scarring, and lawsuits.

There are many articles and textbooks about chemical peeling, and Dr. Suzan Obagi is internationally recognized as an expert in this field. I recommend reading the articles and various book chapters she has written on the subject. Another excellent source is an older text by expert cosmetic dermatologist Mark Rubin, MD. The first edition (1995) of *Manual of Chemical Peels: Superficial and Medium Depth* (Lippincott Williams & Wilkins) was truly my bible. Dr. Rubin has more contemporary texts on peeling, and they are all good. The first edition, however, was especially useful because it covered skin anatomy, skin aging, skin pathology, peeling agents, peeling technique, peeling case presentations, and complications in one compact text.

PEELING AGENTS

There are more peeling agents than chapters in this book, and these are covered in depth in other chapters. It makes sense for the prudent practitioner to experiment with various agents and techniques to see what works best in his or her hands. I use the word "experiment" very cautiously, because any peeling agent can cause serious and permanent damage. A doctor new to chemical peeling should never "experiment." Before ever peeling a patient, a novice doctor should study books and videos and observe seasoned practitioners. After that, the first series of peels should be performed with a proctor to ensure safety. The golden rule of cosmetic surgery is to start conservatively, because one can always go back and do more. On the other hand, it is impossible to reverse some complications. Walk before you run, and you will rarely go wrong. After experimenting with Jessner's, TCA, glycolic acid, and phenol, I personally settled on TCA. It is not only important what agent one uses, but how it is used. The depth of penetration is subject to many variables, including but not limited to the following:

- Type of acid
- Strength of acid (%)
- Number of coats applied (volume)
- Patient's skin thickness
- Patient's skin oiliness
- The body part being peeled (thin eyelid skin versus thicker forehead skin)
- The amount of actinic damage and rhytids a patient has

All of these variables and many others can influence the depth of wounding of the skin. The effectiveness of any peel is directly related to the depth of wounding and the related healing. A very aggressive peel can equal the skin rejuvenation of a CO_2 laser, whereas a light peel may not produce any noticeable difference.

DEPTH OF PEELING

Peels can vary from very superficial to superficial, medium, and deep, and the depth of wounding is generally proportional to the length of healing and the final result. Medium-depth peels are among the safest types of chemical peeling, producing noticeable results and having low complications. Peels that do not extend into the papillary dermis provide minimal results for wrinkles and more pronounced photodamage. A medium-depth TCA peel will extend into the papillary dermis.

SKIN TYPES

With all resurfacing, lighter-skinned patients (Fitzpatrick I and II) are safer to peel, as they have less pigmentation problems. The same can be said for very dark-skinned patients. It is the midrange patients (Fitzpatrick IV and V) that can have the most pigmentation problems, and too aggressive of a peel can make them permanently lighter or darker. In my experience, any patient with brown eyes will have a higher incidence of postinflammatory hyperpigmentation (PIH). PIH will generally manifest at about 30 days and is generally responsive to hydroquinone 4%, retin A, and sunscreen within several weeks. PIH can be very disconcerting to patients, so it is imperative to educate them preoperatively about the possibility.

Technically, any skin type can be peeled with experience. I frequently peel Asians, Latinos, and African-Americans who I would not think of treating with a CO_2 laser.

PREPEEL SKIN CONDITIONING

The basis of chemical peeling requires that the peeling agent be able to penetrate the skin. Preconditioning the skin is discussed in greater detail in Chapter 3. Preconditioning the skin with retin A will thin the stratum corneum and facilitate penetration as well as afford many other positive attributes to the skin health. Starting 4% hydroquinone will also help precondition the melanocytes, which many doctors feel can lessen PIH after a peel. Sunscreen should also be added to this basic regimen. Pretreating patients also gives the doctor an idea of the patient's level of compliance. If a patient cannot maintain a simple three-step cream regimen, they may not be great candidates for proper postpeel aftercare. I start all light-skinned chemical peel patients on this triad 30 days before a peel in the ideal situation. On patients with pigmented skin, I prefer an 8- to 12-week pretreatment cycle.

ANESTHESIA

Depending on the setup of the physician's practice, one can perform the chemical peel using oral sedation, nerve

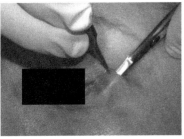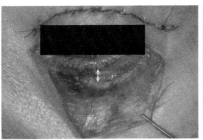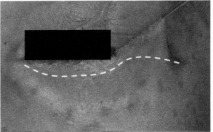

Fig. 14.1 A subciliary approach to the lower eyelids involves removing skin from the lower eyelid. This treatment will improve skin quantity but not quality and can also contribute to lower eyelid retraction.

blocks, intravenous (IV) sedation, or general anesthesia. The author performs all peels and laser resurfacing procedures with IV sedation or general anesthesia. It is crucial to have the patient as comfortable as possible to allow for the desired peel depth to be achieved.

CHEMICAL PEEL INDICATIONS

The great thing about a chemical peel is that virtually any adult (and sometimes younger) patient is a candidate. This varies from light to deep peels depending on the reason for peeling. A younger patient may benefit from a light peel to clean out pores, improve skin texture, and help acne. A middle-aged patient may benefit from a deeper peel for the same reasons and to improve fine lines. Older patients benefit from all of these plus improvement of dyschromias and deeper lines and wrinkles.

In a surgical practice the main indications for chemical peels are as follows:

- Nonsurgical patients desiring better skin health, reduction of fine lines and wrinkles, and improvement of pigmentation abnormalities
- Patients undergoing cosmetic blepharoplasty who are not candidates for or do not desire CO_2 laser skin resurfacing of the eyelids
- As an adjunct to facelifting when concomitant lift and peel are performed
- As a "hybrid" treatment with full-face CO_2 laser resurfacing to blend the lasered skin into the hairline

Chemical Peel as an Adjunct to Cosmetic Blepharoplasty

Many contemporary cosmetic surgeons feel that transconjunctival blepharoplasty is a superior approach to lower lid rejuvenation compared with subciliary skin muscle approaches.

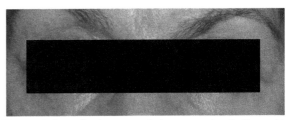

Fig. 14.2 One disadvantage of the external subciliary, skin muscle approach is the increased incidence of lower eyelid malposition.

The subciliary skin muscle approach involves making a skin incision under the lower lid lash line and dissecting the skin and muscle to access the lower lid fat pads. After the fat is reduced, a strip of skin (and sometimes muscle) is removed from the lower lid (Fig. 14.1).

Removing this excess skin causes stretching of the remaining lower lid skin, which improves the appearance of the wrinkles. There are two main problems with this method of blepharoplasty. First, this approach violates the orbital septum, which can cause septal contraction and contribute to lower eyelid malposition. Second, and most critical, is the fact that even with care, excessive skin can be removed inadvertently and also produce lower lid malposition with scleral show, canthal rounding, and dry eyes (Fig. 14.2).

Not all patients experience this by any means, but it is more common with this external approach. These are good reasons to perform the transconjunctival approach, which is retroseptal and does not carry the liability of lower lid retraction. The biggest problem with subciliary blepharoplasty is that they improve skin quantity (stretching) but do not improve inherent skin quality such as pigmentation and collagen production. So, the safety of the transconjunctival approach is desirable but

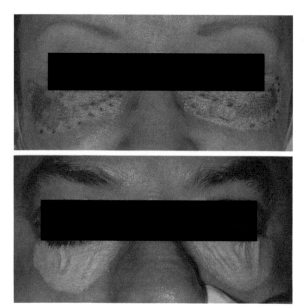

Fig. 14.3 CO_2 laser resurfacing (*top*) and TCA chemical peeling (*bottom*) are mainstay treatments for eyelid rejuvenation when performing transconjunctival blepharoplasty.

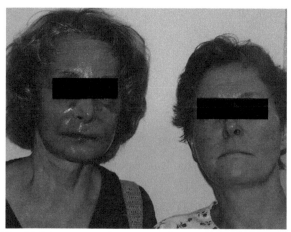

Fig. 14.4 Laser procedures generally produce more dramatic results than chemical peels but have a more unpleasant and extended recovery. The patient on the left is 1 week postmultipass, high-fluence laser skin resurfacing, and the patient on the right is 1 week post–30% trichloroacetic acid medium-depth chemical peel.

requires a separate procedure to address the excess and wrinkled skin (dermatochalasis). Simultaneous skinresurfacing procedures will improve skin quality and skin quantity at the same time with less chance of lower lid malposition. Having said this, it is possible to overtreat the lower lid skin with laser or chemical peel and produce lower lid malposition.

The author's preferred techniques for lower eyelid dermatochalasis are CO_2 laser resurfacing and chemical peel (Fig. 14.3).

There are pluses and minuses for either procedure. In general, I feel that laser treatment is more effective but has a more unpleasant recovery (Fig. 14.4).

The chemical peel is effective but is more tolerable for patients because it is a dry wound. A medium-depth TCA peel on the lower lids is not equally as dramatic as the laser but is a great alternative for those patients who do not want laser, need a faster recovery, or in darkskinned patients who may not be candidates for laser. Patients are told that if the laser is 100% effective, the peel is 80% as effective but heals much quicker with less prolonged erythema and can easily be repeated at a later date with local anesthesia. There is also less chance (but still possible) to have eyelid malposition compared with aggressive laser treatment.

LOWER EYELID CHEMICAL PEEL TECHNIQUE

After the lower transconjunctival blepharoplasty is performed, the lower lid skin is degreased with acetone. Light-skinned patients are generally treated with several coats of 30% TCA to a solid white frost (Fig. 14.5). A delay of at least 2 minutes is taken between coats of acid to allow the effect to take place and the frost (which determines the endpoint) to mature. When the desired level of frost is reached, either a white frost with a pink background or a solid white frost, the procedure is stopped and the skin coated with a suitable wound dressing.

For darker-skinned patients, a single coat of 30% TCA or several coats of 20% is applied. The endpoint frost is less dense, because darker-skinned patients tend to have less wrinkling, and this will prevent overtreatment in this patient population.

Postoperatively patients are instructed to use either Vanicream or Vaniply Ointment (Pharmaceutical Specialties, Inc, MN) (Fig. 14.6). These products are the least irritating because they do not contain preservatives, dyes, parabens, lanolin, or other potentially irritating ingredients. They are very affordable and easily found.

Postpeel care consists of 24/7 application of Vaniply until fully peeled. The patient washes the peeled area or entire face twice a day with the Vaniply cleanser and

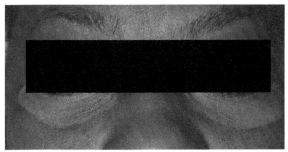

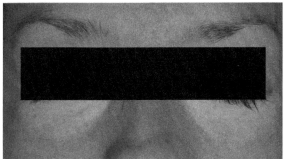

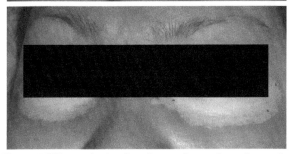

Fig. 14.5 Different depths of peeling are chosen depending on the amount of skin damage and the skin color. The top image shows two coats of 20% trichloroacetic acid (TCA) on a dark-skinned patient. The center picture shows a single coat of 30% TCA on a patient with minor to moderate wrinkling, and the bottom photo shows a denser white frost from two coats of 30% TCA for more penetration on a patient with increased dermatochalasis.

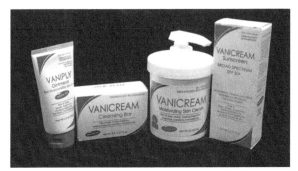

Fig. 14.6 The "Vani" line of post-resurfacing skin care products is easy to use, affordable, and nonallergenic.

reapplies the Vaniply ointment continually. After complete reepithelialization, the patient applies Vanicream moisturizer and sunscreen. I have had excellent healing and compliance with these products.

It is important for patients not to pick or peel off the dead skin, because this can cause scarring and expose the underlying skin that is not yet reepithelialized. In some cases, the dead skin can be safely removed by the doctor (Fig. 14.7).

HYBRID LASER/PEEL TECHNIQUES

Although chemical peeling is a useful treatment in and of itself, combining peeling with laser skin resurfacing has distinct advantages. My most common combination of peel and laser is using the peel to blend in the hairline when performing full-face CO_2 laser. The hair-bearing scalp will be untreated when performing laser resurfacing, because treatment would burn the hair. Failing to blend this area can produce a drastic transition of treated and untreated skin. By lasering up to the hairline, then peeling into the hair, a blending is achieved (Fig. 14.8).

Another indication for a peel/laser combo is when a specific area such as the lower lids requires more aggressive treatment than the rest of the face. I see this occasionally in younger patients with moderate full-face sun damage but accelerated lower eyelid skin aging. In these patients I may perform a multicoat 30% TCA peel on the entire face but laser the lower lids, which require a more aggressive treatment and deeper wounding (Fig. 14.9).

FACELIFT WITH SIMULTANEOUS TRICHLOROACETIC ACID CHEMICAL PEEL

Facelift with simultaneous peel or laser resurfacing is controversial, because the undermined facelift flaps are dissected from the underlying tissues and more sensitive to devitalization. I have performed more than 1200 facelifts and necklifts at the time of this writing and performed simultaneous CO_2 laser or TCA chemical peel in almost one-third of the facelifts.

This is done after the lift is completed and all suture lines are closed. The face is degreased with acetone and the central oval (nonundermined regions) is treated with multiple coats of 30% TCA to the desired endpoint. The flaps are marked to show the demarcation of

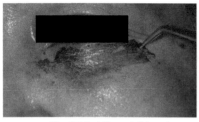
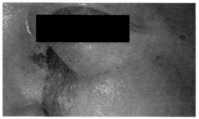
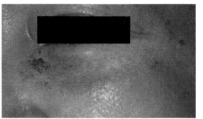

Fig. 14.7 Although it is not recommended to remove dead skin, in some cases it can be removed by the doctor if the underlying tissues are healed. This very compliant patient presented at 1 week, and the remnant skin was removed. Note the minor hypopigmentation that will improve to normal skin tone over the coming weeks.

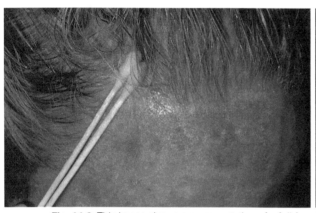
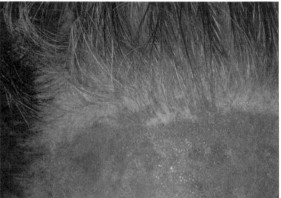

Fig. 14.8 This image shows a representation of a full-face CO_2 laser treatment with chemical peeling into the hairline to blend the treatment and avoid a frank line of demarcation.

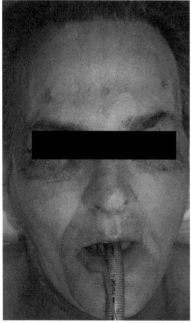

Fig. 14.9 This patient underwent blepharoplasty with full-face chemical peel. Because the lower lids had significant dermatochalasis, a CO_2 laser treatment was performed on this area.

the undermined/nonundermined area, and the undermined regions are treated with a single pass of 20% TCA (Figs. 14.10 and 14.11).

Experienced facelift/peel surgeons can treat somewhat deeper, but it is prudent to always be more conservative on the undermined skin. Identical treatment can be performed with laser as well, treating the central oval in a normal fashion with decreased fluence over the undermined flaps.

CASE PRESENTATIONS

The following patients were treated with surgical procedures and simultaneous TCA chemical peel (Figs. 14.12-14.20):

COMPLICATIONS

It is imperative to protect the eye when peeling in the periorbital region. The doctor and team must pay close attention to acid flowing into unwanted areas. A large volume of water should always be on the treatment tray to lavage the eye in the event acid comes in contact with

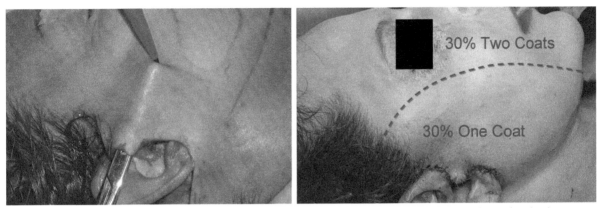

Fig. 14.10 The left image shows the undermined facelift flaps being marked to delineate the undermined region that will be treated in a more conservative manner. The right image shows the central oval (non-undermined skin) treated with two coats of 30% trichloroacetic acid and the undermined flap treated with a single coat of the same.

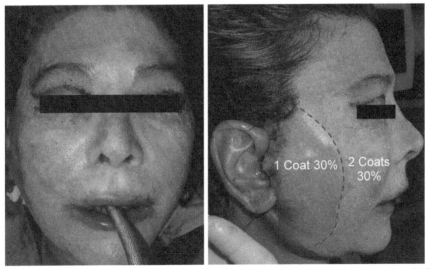

Fig. 14.11 This image shows another patient treated with multiple coats of 30% trichloroacetic acid (TCA) on the central oval of the face and a single coat of 30% TCA over the undermined flap.

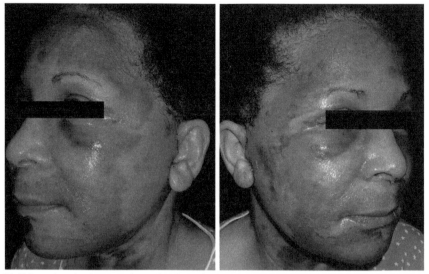

Fig. 14.12 This patient is shown 5 days after facelift with simultaneous 30% trichloroacetic acid (TCA) peel (two coats) on the central face and two coats of 20% TCA on the facelift flaps.

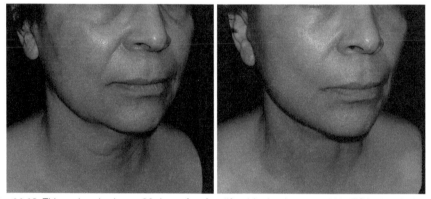

Fig. 14.13 This patient is shown 90 days after facelift with simultaneous 30% TCA chemical peel.

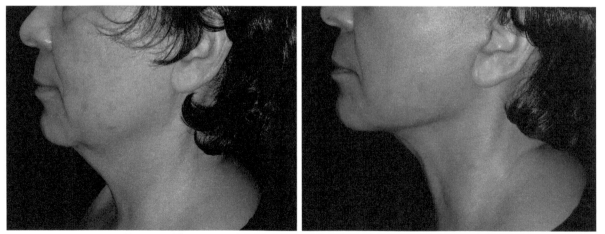

Fig. 14.14 The same patient shown in Fig. 14.13 is shown in the lateral view.

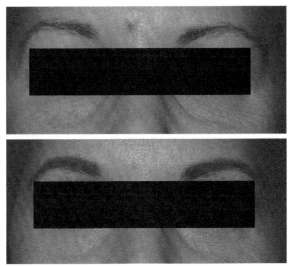

Fig. 14.15 This patient was treated with upper and lower laser-assisted blepharoplasty with lower-lid 30% TCA peel.

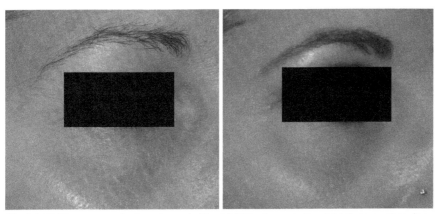

Fig. 14.16 The same patient as shown in Fig. 14.15 is shown in the right three-quarter view.

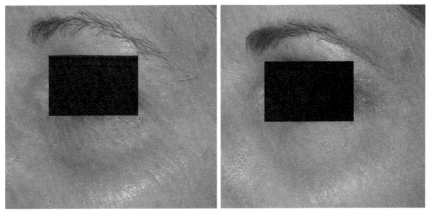

Fig. 14.17 The same patient as shown in Fig. 14.15 and 14.16 is shown in the left three-quarter view.

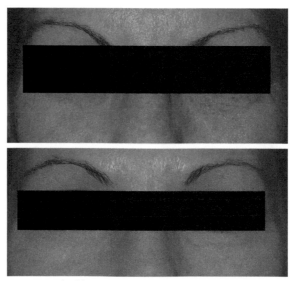

Fig. 14.18 This patient was treated with upper and lower laser-assisted blepharoplasty with lower lid 30% trichloroacetic acid peel.

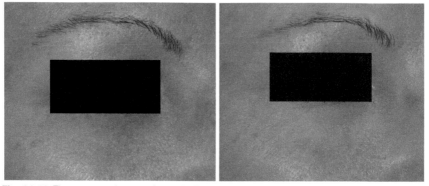

Fig. 14.19 The same patient as shown in Fig. 14.18 is shown in the right three-quarter view.

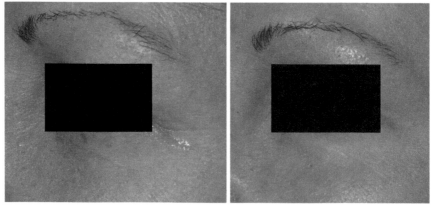

Fig. 14.20 The same patient as shown in Fig. 14.18 and 14.19 is shown in the left three-quarter view.

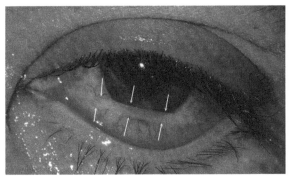

Fig. 14.21 This patient is shown immediately after a 30% trichloroacetic acid peel in which some of the acid reached the lower eyelid margin and opacified a strip of the cornea. The eye was painful and irritated but healed uneventfully.

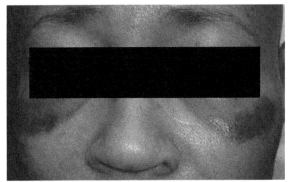

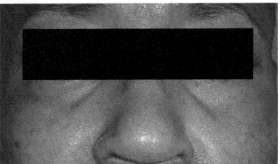

Fig. 14.22 This patient is shown in the upper picture 90 days postpeel with postinflammatory hyperpigmentation of her upper lid laser scar and periorbital regions that were peeled with several coats of 20% trichloroacetic acid. The bottom picture shows the patient 30 days after treatment with 4% hydroquinone and sunscreen.

the cornea. Minor contact is very irritating but generally heals in several days without problems. Fig. 14.21 shows such an incident.

Chemical peel sequalae such as extended erythema and PIH are common, but more serious complications are rare. Pigmentation changes are the most common considerations, especially in darker-skinned patients. It is important to discuss these potential pigmentation problems in the informed consent process. I show all patients pictures of hypopigmentation and hyperpigmentation and have them initial the pictures to indicate that they realize these changes are possible. If patients experience pigmentation problems without warning or understanding, they can become very unhappy and more difficult to manage. One key to managing these sequalae is to get these patients back to work or play as soon as possible; makeup can be the surgeons' best friend in these circumstances.

Postinflammatory hyperpigmentation is very common in darker-skinned patients and can be disconcerting to the patient and surgeon. This condition generally responds well to treatment with bleaching creams such as 4% hydroquinone and sunscreen. Fig. 14.22 shows a patient with postpeel PIH.

Hypopigmentation can also occur after a peel and generally repigments spontaneously over several weeks or months (Fig. 14.23). It is important to help these patients choose an appropriate makeup to cover these areas.

Scarring can occur but is uncommon. Textural healing changes of the lower lids can be intercepted with

a steroid cream such as Clobetasol 0.05% twice daily. Actual scars are injected with very small aliquots of triamcinolone 10 mg/mL. Fig. 14.24 shows a patient with textural changes and minor hypertrophic scarring 6 weeks post 30% TCA peel.

Although a more prevalent complication with laser treatment, lower eyelid retraction can occur with chemical peeling. This is more common in patients with previous lower lid skin excision but can occur in the unoperated patient as well (Fig. 14.25). It is not uncommon for postpeel patients to have retracted lids upon animation in the early postpeel phase, but this generally resolves spontaneously and can be improved with lower lid skin stretching.

CONCLUSION

TCA chemical peel is a very useful and safe adjunct to procedures such as blepharoplasty and facelift. The

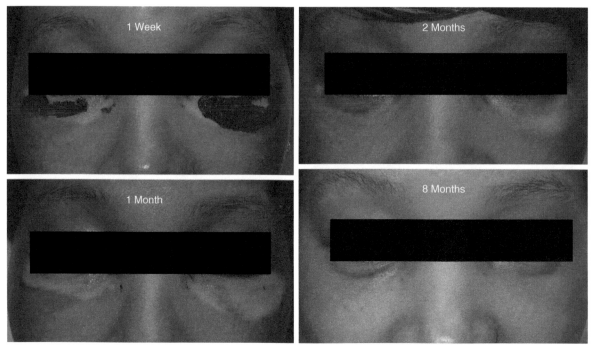

Fig. 14.23 This patient is shown at 1 week, 1 month, 2 months, and 8 months after several coats of 20% trichloroacetic acid peel of her lower eyelids.

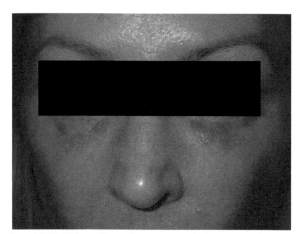

Fig. 14.24 This patient shows textural changes and minor hypertrophic scarring after chemical peel. She responded well to topical steroid and triamcinolone injection.

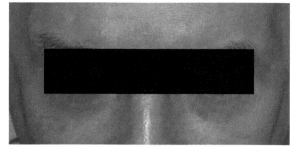

Fig. 14.25 This patient is shown 10 days after 30% trichloroacetic acid peel. The patient is opening his mouth wide, which is stretching the lower lids and causing retraction. This generally improves spontaneously and can be accelerated with stretching the lower lids. In patients who have had lower eyelid skin removed with previous blepharoplasty, this can be a permanent situation.

procedure is quick, inexpensive, and predictable. Any unpredictability is related to skin color, the peeler's experience, and the variances of skin healing. Although these factors can be unpredictable, they all generally heal without consequence with normal peeling methods. Overtreatment is the cause of more severe complications.

15

Segmental Phenol Croton Oil Peels for Brow Lifting, Eyelid Tightening, and Lip Eversion

Carlos G. Wambier

INTRODUCTION

This special topic chapter explores a still pioneering aspect of deep chemical peeling using phenol–croton oil formulas. Although the basic concepts of safety, perioperative care, formulas, and the application of deep chemical peeling were well covered by Dr. Richard Bensimon, Dr. Marina Landau, and Dr. Peter Rullan in Chapters 7, 8, and 12, some extremely important phytochemical aspects are reinforced in this chapter for adequate understanding of the mechanisms of action involved in surface retraction and dermal neocollagenesis of such procedures.

Physicians who want to focus their expertise in deep peeling should further read about the shift of paradigms that occurred with the awareness of strength gradation by titration of the *Croton tiglium* oil concentration introduced by Dr. Hetter[1-5] in an up-to-date, condensed review article recently published by the International Peeling Society (IPS) in the *Journal of the American Academy of Dermatology* continued medical education article,[6] which also has videos.

MECHANISM OF ACTION

Dr. Adolph M. Brown, the plastic surgeon who first introduced to medical applications mixtures of phenol with croton oil, brought a premature rationale that phenol was the active ingredient of his formulas, which contained vegetable oils to "retard" its action, and that phenol penetrated deeper when it was more dilute.[7]

Brown's original phenol–croton oil formula, shown as "Example 3" in his April 1959 US patent application entitled "Skin treating method and composition," was the first mixture of phorbol esters with phenol in a chemical peel formula. It consisted of 0.5% croton oil in a mixture of water, 50% phenol, and 5% cresols (methylated phenol).[7] To celebrate the 60th anniversary of Brown's invention, let's further elaborate on this formula and his efforts. Possibly because Brown apparently had no disciples to continue the application of his initial formula, and because of the patent, which would have commercial implications, his formula was never disseminated in the dermatology or plastic surgery practice. Also, Brown's actual phenol–croton oil formula was never published in a medical journal. Brown and his wife, Dr. Marthe Erdos Brown, a dermatologist who trained in Paris, published the results of their technique in the *British Journal of Plastic Surgery*[8]; however, the formula omitted croton oil for unknown reasons. Two aspects of the 1960 publication were interesting: the sequential taping technique, which is performed as soon as each small area of the face is peeled, which is appropriate for occlusion of a volatile compound, and the "thick and stout applicator," which allows better control of the surface spread of the formula.

Brownian dogmas about mechanisms of action were popularized among plastic surgeons and some dermatologists after the standard adoption of the Baker-Gordon classical formula,[9] which was published shortly before Brown's death in 1963, not leaving enough time for scientific discussions or further scientific elucidations.

Brown's rationale at that time for the mechanisms of action of deep peeling was appropriate given that the field of dermatopathology was still in its infancy. Neither the Herovici stain nor immunohistochemistry methods existed to differentiate newer type III collagen from older type I collagen. "The principal concept … is to induce a controlled fibrosis of some of the inner layers of the skin to cause shrinkage by noticeable condensations of the collagenous fibers of the dermis and by lamination and flattening of some elements of the connective tissue parallel to the skin surface."[7]

Phorbol esters were initially discovered in croton oil itself in the late 1920s,[10] and such molecules were since thought to explain the paradox of toxic and stimulative effects of croton oil for millennia in Eastern medicine and since the 1800s in Western medicine.[11] Croton oil is still recognized as the richest matrix of these complex vegetable metabolites, which were later found in other species of Euphorbiaceae.

Probably, the interaction of these tetracyclic diterpenes of croton oil with follicular and dermal stem cells and other cells of the connective tissue create the observed rejuvenation, although science still seeks data to elucidate the direct and indirect mechanisms of action of phorbol esters in the connective tissue. Phorbol 12-myristate 13-acetate (PMA) and other phorbol esters trigger numerous biochemical functions in cells; the most well understood are related to the rapid and strong membrane activation of protein kinase C (PKC) isoforms.[12] PMA, the most potent tumor-promoting agent known, is extracted from croton oil.[13] Phorbol esters are not considered carcinogens, but when applied in combination with a carcinogen, they may promote tumor growth. PMA also has anticancer properties, causing differentiation of immature cell lines.[14,15] The vast historical experience of phenol–croton oil peeling points to anticancer results by many authors, and no case of carcinogenesis was ever reported.[16-18] Baker stated in 2003 that in thousands of facial peels performed during his career, he never observed a single case of skin cancer during decades of follow-up.[16] The deep action of phorbol esters during a deep chemical peel might provide superior chemoprevention for field cancerization than any other known method; however, proper studies are still pending.[19,20]

By current dermatopathology methods, after the application of phenol–croton oil formulas, the superficial layers of the skin clearly undergo coagulative necrosis. The deeper layers remain viable and undergo severe inflammation. The epidermal cells from follicles proliferate under the necrotic eschar, whereas type III collagen is formed below the newly formed epidermis. Once the eschar is detached, epithelization completes with a new, thicker epidermis. A thick neocollagenesis band continues to form for some weeks under the new epidermis.[21] Thus skin tightening seems to occur by a deep, thick neocollagenesis band and longitudinal superficial surface shrinkage.

To better understand the effects of a deep chemical peel, one may think of the old skin as an old pillow that has a very loose, wrinkled cover over a flattened, non-elastic, old stuffing (deep dermis). The cover is completely removed, and the superficial part of the stuffing is scratched. Subsequently, in a few days, a new thicker and tightly fitted cover forms over the stuffing. After that, a new thicker and more elastic stuffing is formed between the cover and the scratched old stuffing, making the pillow more round and tight, with less cover surface area as well.

STRENGTH AND EFFECTS

The current unequivocal ways to increase the penetration of a deep chemical peel are as follows:
- Increasing the concentration of croton oil
- Increasing friction and pressure (hand weight)
- Increasing the total volume applied: in each application or sets of applications/passes
- Priming the epidermal barrier: degreasing, topical retinoids, and abrasion

The belief that there is increased action by postoperative occlusion with petrolatum jelly or tape after complete absorption of the formula is still debatable, because animal models are extremely impractical and the evidence in patients is still limited to a single split-body case report with tape performed in an extra-facial area.[22] Because postoperative occlusion for increasing the depth of wounding is still debatable, the physician should use the controlled environment in the office to apply the peel to the desired depth of penetration. The depth of penetration correlates to all the effects observed, including treatment goals: fading of deep wrinkles, superficial shrinkage, and collagen formation in the mid-dermis. However, along with deeper penetration, there is a trade-off with the risk of complications, including postoperative pain, edema, longer reepithelization time, longer periods of persistent erythema, skin dryness, postinflammatory hyperpigmentation in susceptible patients, and finally increased risks of pronounced hypopigmentation after full recovery.

SEGMENTAL (PARTIAL) PEELS

Not all patients need a full-face peel. Many patients are strictly concerned with the perioral area, periocular area, forehead,[23] or lips.[24] Some patients with acne scars or thin wrinkles may be concerned with the cheeks only. With the appropriate application technique, the surgeon may in most cases avoid demarcation lines by feathering the transition of the peeled area to an unpeeled area by some centimeters (Fig. 15.1). Some cases may be peeled without feathering, by combining a different resurfacing technique to the adjacent area, such as a medium-depth peel or a Q-switched laser peel.[21]

A major advantage of performing a segmental peel is safety.[23] If the peeled area is less than 0.5% of the body surface area (palm without fingers), the peel may be performed slowly, but without the 10-minute waiting period between each cosmetic area (safety pause) and without intravenous hydration with Ringer's lactate.

A segmental peel is also easier for the patient during the 7-day recovery period. The author refers to the recovery time as "the tunnel of metamorphosis," given the way patients feel while entering the procedure: unsafe during the downtime period and happy when leaving this tunnel.

SAFETY IS THE NUMBER ONE PRIORITY

Although arguments could be made for not monitoring patients due to the extreme safety of a short procedure, the author prefers to monitor most patients due to their age, concurrent medications, and high blood pressure. Monitoring is harmless and brings a "vital awareness" of the electrocardiogram (ECG) status and vital signs. Awareness creates a safer environment. For example, if the patient complains of their heart "beating" or "racing," one quick glance at the monitor can reassure the team and the patient, instead of reaching for a stethoscope or running for a 12-lead ECG. Most importantly, if clinically relevant changes are noted, the physician can execute a plan instantly. Furthermore, the monitor might show a preexisting arrhythmia or extremely high blood pressure before the procedure even begins.

A thorough medical history (with a focus on skin healing issues, nutrition, autoimmune status, and heart and respiratory conditions), simple laboratory tests such as a complete blood count, basic metabolic panel, and a 12-lead ECG to evaluate the rate-corrected QT interval

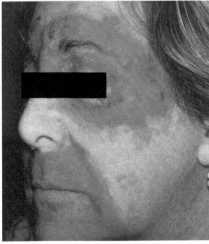 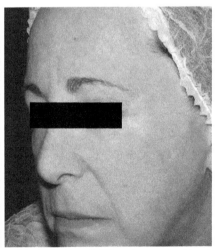

Fig. 15.1 Periocular and perioral peel with 1.2% croton oil in 35% phenol. Skin color may be blended to the untreated area by feathering. On the fourth postoperative day and after 9 months, with polarized light photographs, cautious observation reveals no demarcation lines, but the unpeeled skin presents mild melanosis that could be addressed with segmental peels using a medium-depth peel or even with 532-nm Q-switched laser peel.

(QTc) could also bring important awareness of hidden risks of undergoing a procedure that could cause an arrhythmia and severe skin inflammation. Because phenol–croton oil peels do prolong the QTc[25] even in segmental peels, the peel is contraindicated in patients with long QTc by Fridericia calculation (such as above 450 ms). QTc over 500 ms is an absolute contraindication and requires therapy by a cardiologist. Medications known to prolong QTc are antidepressants, thiazide diuretics, antiemetics, some antibiotics, antifungals, and opiates. CredibleMeds is available as an app for smartphones and may be used through the website https://crediblemeds.org; it is the most comprehensive and up-to-date list of medications known to cause QTc prolongation. The CredibleMeds list categorizes each medication by risk to cause *torsades des pointes*.

Technique Limitations

Although the skin is tightened to a certain point by deep chemical peels, a thick superficial muscular layer is certainly not tightened. To tighten and lift ptotic muscles, one must incorporate surgical procedures to shorten the supralabial area and to lift the forehead. However, in areas where the superficial musculoaponeurotic system (SMAS) is thin, such as the eyelids, cheeks, and lateral forehead, it is possible to achieve tightening effects with deep peels. Such retraction is best observed in the eyelids, where both epidermis and dermis are the thinnest.

Special attention must be given during the preoperative period to the evaluation of the lower eyelid, with particular attention for a tendency to have ectropion by the open-mouth maneuver, and also evaluating for excessive laxity by the snap-back test. A negative snap-back is a contraindication to deep peels, especially when using strong formulas or application methods.[21] Previous lower eyelid blepharoplasty may cause lower eyelid retraction, which may be accentuated by a deep peel (Fig. 15.2).

The peeled area is also an important predictor of the total volume of the neocollagenesis band created parallel to the peeled area. More collagen is built with wider areas of peeling, which creates tightening and increased volume.

THE BLEPHAROPEEL

When performing a blepharopeel, the periocular zone is peeled, and the area that would be excised during an upper blepharoplasty is peeled more deeply, either with higher concentrations of croton oil, such as 2% croton oil in the classical Baker-Gordon formula,[26] or with the same Hetter's formula that was used in the superior eyelid, but after the frosting is set, the "excision area" is peeled with more passes, more friction, and more solution.

An effective method to create this is to use the Wambier-Simão blade, which consists of a cotton-tipped, split wooden tongue depressor. The surface created by the split has a thin area, and creates more pressure and

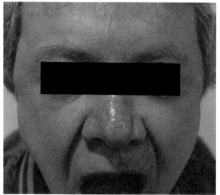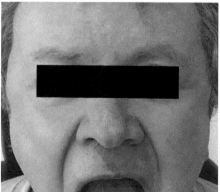

Fig. 15.2 Ectropion noticeable only with open mouth, after a lower eyelid peel with 1.2% croton oil in 35% phenol. Patient was previously submitted to blepharoplasty, facelift, and full-face peel with 1.6% croton oil in 35% phenol sparing the lower eyelids (initially contraindicated due to preexisting retraction). The photodamage in the lower eyelids became so obvious that the patient and physician decided to complete the peel in those areas. Complete spontaneous resolution occurred after 6 months. The open mouth accentuates lower eyelid retraction and cicatricial ectropion. This demonstrates how the skin contracts after the peel and how movement and time cause collagen remodeling to occur.

is not polished, so that it creates more friction. By using the "saw" surface of the Wambier-Simão blade, with repeated movements, peel depth is increased by modifying three factors: number of passes, pressure/friction, and skin abrasion. The area peeled with the "saw" takes longer to heal, which is the most objective measurement of peeling depth (Fig. 15.3).

Blepharopeelings are not able to shrink very abundant skin and do not address prolapsed fat pads. However, deep peels may substitute for minor blepharoplasties with the benefit of not leaving a scar if performed properly (Fig. 15.4).

When performing blepharopeels, various areas may be addressed: (1) upper blepharopeeling; (2) upper and lower blepharopeeling; (3) periocular peeling—"the Raccoon"; (4) periocular peeling including temples, eyebrows, and glabella—"the Robin Mask"; (5) and periocular, temples, the full forehead, glabella with feathering to the tip of the nose, with a coincident lower limit of feathering in the malar area to the cheeks—"El Zorro" (which basically spares the lower face only).

Currently, the most used formula by the author for periocular peels is Hetter's light formula, containing 0.4% croton oil in 35% phenol,[6] with the recent modification of the replacement of Septisol (banned by the Food and Drug Administration [FDA] because of triclosan) for Novisol (Young Pharmaceuticals, Inc.). Emulsions created with Novisol are more stable than those created using Septisol (Fig. 15.5 and 15.6). Some cases will require stronger formulas, such as Hetter's heavy, which contains 1.2% croton oil in 35% phenol. Regarding the stability of the emulsion, the author recommends that the vial or cup used during the peel to dip the applicator be completely transparent so the surgeon can observe whether the formula is evenly emulsified. That means that surgical steel cups are not appropriate for phenol–croton oil emulsions. Use glass shot glasses or the Novisol Emulsivial instead, which has a cap to close the vial tight to allow better agitation, and a smaller diameter, which reduces the volatilization of organic compounds.

THE BROWLIFT PEEL

Although the muscular area of the forehead is amenable to skin tightening by deep peels (see limitations sections), a mild lift is obtained if the skin is peeled deeply from the upper half of the eyebrows to about 2 cm above the eyebrow,

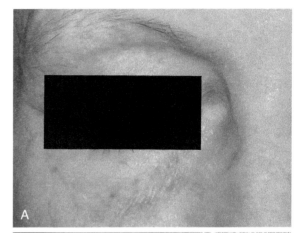
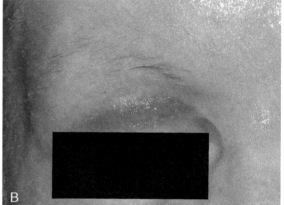
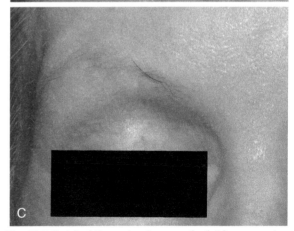

Fig. 15.3 Detail of the periocular area of a full-face procedure with 1.6% croton oil in 35% phenol. A, Before. Vigorous application in the crease of the upper eyelid causes increased retraction, with expected delayed healing. B, Tenth postoperative day (POD). C, No visible scar on the 30th POD.

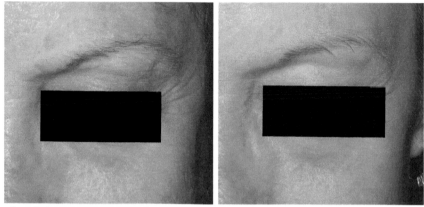

Fig. 15.4 Detail of the periocular area of a full-face procedure with 1.6% croton oil in 35% phenol. A, Before. B, Marked improvement and tightening after 1-year follow-up.

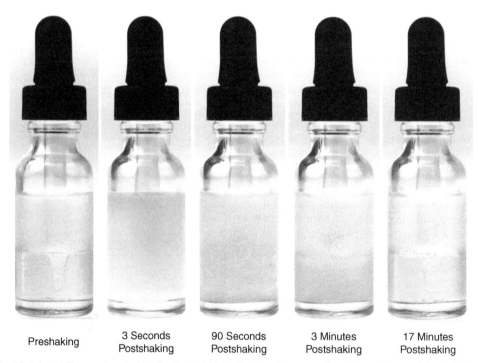

| Preshaking | 3 Seconds Postshaking | 90 Seconds Postshaking | 3 Minutes Postshaking | 17 Minutes Postshaking |

Fig. 15.5 Instability precipitated by Septisol of Hetter's phenol–croton oil peel formula containing 1.6% croton oil in 35% phenol. The upper layer is opaque and white; the lower layer has a yellowish hue. Mixing the formula creates a temporary emulsion that quickly separates back into two distinct layers. In animal studies performed at the State University of Ponta Grossa in collaboration with Dr. Beltrame and his team of researchers at the Laboratory of Phytotherapy, Phytotherapy Technology and Chemistry of Natural Products, the lower layer was observed to be active, while the upper layer was found to be inactive. Therefore agitation before placing the applicator into the emulsion was of paramount importance. (Photographs courtesy of John Kulesza, Young Pharmaceuticals, Inc.)

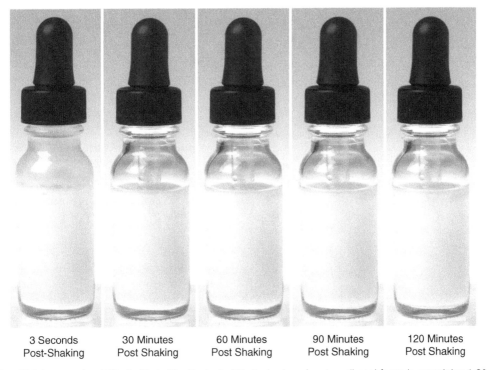

| 3 Seconds Post-Shaking | 30 Minutes Post Shaking | 60 Minutes Post Shaking | 90 Minutes Post Shaking | 120 Minutes Post Shaking |

Fig. 15.6 Improved stability facilitated by Novisol of Hetter's phenol-croton oil peel formula containing 1.6% croton oil in 35% phenol. The emulsion is stable throughout the usual procedure time. This results in improved safety by maintaining formula consistency including frost uniformity.

which is exactly the area that is not usually injected with botulinum toxin due to the risk of eyebrow ptosis.

Some patients with deep and multiple forehead wrinkles develop these lines because of brow ptosis or mild upper eyelid ptosis. Thus a correct diagnosis must be made for adequate planning. Sometimes, inspection during full frontalis relaxation will reveal a primary cause.

A surgical browlift usually has temporary effects using tread fixation to the bone, or even more temporary effects with noninvasive technology or dermal/subcutaneous threads. Surgical interventions may cause a hard-to-disguise scar over the eyebrow or in the frontal scalp. Thus a chemical peel may be indicated in cases where brow ptosis is not severe, and when the forehead skin actually requires resurfacing due to wrinkles, with a secondary gain of some millimeters of brow lift.

The peel is performed usually in combination with blepharopeeling. Rarely, a stand-alone frontal peel is indicated (Fig. 15.7), and the zones mentioned can be peeled more heavily. It is very rare to execute a stand-alone browlift peel because of the risk of color mismatch

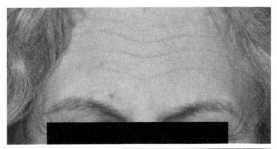
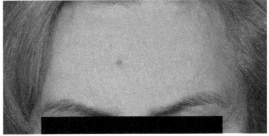

Fig. 15.7 Before and after 4 months of partial-face intervention with phenol 35% and croton oil 1.6% forehead peel (pseudo-hypopigmentation seen). The eyelids and crow's feet were peeled after 2 weeks with Jessner's solution followed by 35% trichloroacetic acid, as the patient only wanted to remove the forehead wrinkles. An expected discrete lateral browlift is achieved.

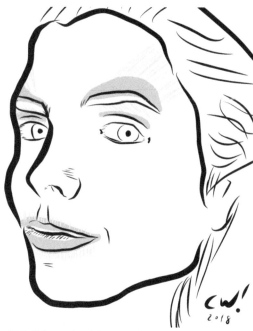

Fig. 15.8 Schematic of the most important areas to be peeled heavily to achieve skin contraction (painted in orange), and the surrounding adjuvant areas that also contribute to a better effect by a contraction at distance (surrounding yellow lines). For a mild eyebrow lift: top half of the eyebrows and supraorbital area with a wider lateral zone, with the respective fronto-temporal adjuvant area. For upper eyelid tightening/contraction: the area hidden in sulcus (wider area with the eyes closed) should be more heavily peeled for an effective blepharopeel. The adjuvant area is the remainder of the upper eyelid. For the eversion of the lips, the most important area to be peeled is the vermilion to the vermilion border. The inner part of the vermilion (near the wet-dry line) actually causes some inversion of the lip but further contributes to volume by neocollagenesis. For eversion, the outer part of the lips is peeled, leaving the inner part without peeling. The adjuvant area is about 1 cm around the lips/perioral area.

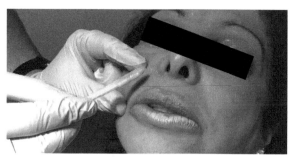

Fig. 15.9 Typical frosting of the vermilion, while the Wambier-Simão blade is soaked with 1.2% croton oil in 35% phenol for a second, more aggressive pass around the contour of the lips. The patient has petrolatum jelly over her eyelids, still shut soon after a "Robin's mask" periocular and glabellar segmental peel.

of Novisol Cleanser and 5.5 mL of distilled water. For a smaller volume, mix 2 mL of Hetter's stock with 3 mL of the following mixture: 0.25 mL of Novisol Cleanser and 2.75 mL of distilled water. This makes a total of 5 mL. To prepare 25 mL of Hetter's stock, mix 24 mL of phenol 88% with 1 mL of croton oil. The stock solution is not to be used undiluted on normal skin surfaces.

THE LIP PEEL

The application of this tightening concept for the lips,[20] the "lip peel," may be used as a stand-alone procedure or in combination with a full-face peel or segmental peel for the perioral area. In contrast to a hyaluronic acid lip injection, the peel is able to create some volume by neocollagenesis, which is limited by the surface area peeled, while addressing surface changes related to chronic solar damage (deep wrinkles and actinic keratoses). Additionally, by shrinking the vertical outer surface of the lip, the lip edge everts.

The lips are one of the few facial areas that can be peeled strongly without having to feather onto surrounding skin, because the lip color is sharply demarcated from the surrounding areas. However, by feathering onto the perilabial area or treating the entire perioral area, one can create a stronger eversion effect, because the surrounding skin tightening assists to evert the lips.

For lip peels, the author uses Hetter's heavy or very heavy formula.

The schematics of the main areas discussed in this chapter are illustrated in Fig. 15.8. A typical lip peel in

to the forehead, but with adequate feathering or combination with other modalities for color blending, a smaller area can be treated. Peeling these areas appropriately is of greatest importance to enhance results of a full-face peel or an "El Zorro" peel regarding the brow area.

For browlifts, the formulas most used by the author are the Hetter's heavy to very heavy (1.2%–1.6% croton oil in 35% phenol emulsion). For very heavy, add 4 mL of Hetter's stock into a Novisol Emulsivial that contains 6 mL of water/surfactant, for 10 mL of a peel formula. Or, mix in a glass cup 4 mL of Hetter's stock with 0.5 mL

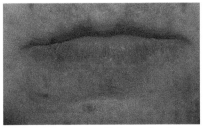
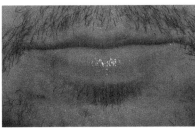
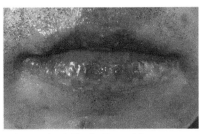

Fig. 15.10 Before, after 7 days, and the third day (middle of the "tunnel of metamorphosis") of a lip peel to improve the contour in a male patient with Hetter's heavy formula: 1 mL of phenol 88% + 3 mL of Hetter's stock + 0.5 mL of Novisol Cleanser + 5.5 mL of distilled water.

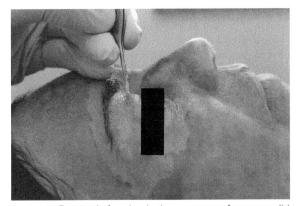

Fig. 15.11 Removal of eschar in the saw zone of upper eyelids in a combination of medium-depth peel with periocular deep peel containing 0.8% croton oil in 35% phenol (2 mL of phenol 88% + 2 mL of Hetter's stock + 0.5 mL of Novisol Cleanser + 5.5 mL of distilled water).

combination with "Robin's mask" peel is illustrated in Fig. 15.9, and a typical evolution of a lip peel is illustrated in Fig. 15.10.

STANDARD TOPICAL POSTOPERATIVE CARE

Petrolatum jelly (Vaseline) is applied as needed throughout the first week.[20] The first application is performed by the physician after the procedure. The author currently prescribes a water-based jelly containing chlorhexidine (K-Y) during the first 1 to 2 days, if the patient prefers, after testing both during the critical initial edema and exudative phase. K-Y has been used by ophthalmologists during contact lens placement for gonioscopy, without ocular side effects,[27] possibly because of a low concentration of chlorhexidine gluconate, as it is used in contact lenses antiseptic solutions[28] and eyedrops prescribed for healing corneal ulcers.[29]

Patients usually do not require debridement if the eschars are kept moist and proper hygiene is maintained with compresses and face washes. However, if needed, it is important to be very gentle when removing the eschar or fibrin without damaging the healing epidermis or fragile dermis. Soft compresses with saline or bacteriostatic water assist the in-office cleaning or debridement when needed Fig. 15.11.

FINAL WORD

The learning curve for deep chemical peels is long, but it is a procedure that gives undisputed resurfacing results if performed with the correct manual skills and peel formulas. Training in continued medical education hands-on courses/workshops or during residency or fellowships is irreplaceable for the proper technique.

REFERENCES

1. Hetter GP. An examination of the phenol-croton oil peel: part I. Dissecting the formula. *Plast Reconstr Surg.* 2000a;105:227–251.
2. Hetter GP. An examination of the phenol-croton oil peel: part II. The lay peelers and their croton oil formulas. *Plast Reconstr Surg.* 2000b;105:240–251.
3. Hetter GP. An examination of the phenol-croton oil peel: part III. The plastic surgeons' role. *Plast Reconstr Surg.* 2000c;105:752–763.
4. Hetter GP. An examination of the phenol-croton oil peel: part IV. Face peel results with different concentrations of phenol and croton oil. *Plast Reconstr Surg.* 2000d;105:1061–1083; discussion 1084–1087.

5. Larson DL, Karmo F, Hetter GP. Phenol-croton oil peel: establishing an animal model for scientific investigation. *Aesthetic Surg J*. 2009;29:47–53. https://doi.org/10.1016/j.asj.2008.11.008.

6. Wambier CG, Lee KC, Soon SL, Sterling JB, Rullan PP, Landau M, et al. Advanced chemical peels: phenol-croton oil peel. *J Am Acad Dermatol*. 2019;81(2):327 336. https://doi.org/10.1016/j.jaad.2018.11.060.

7. U.S. Patent 3,067,106 filed April 7, 1959. Issued December 4, 1962.

8. Brown AM, Kaplan LM, Brown ME. Phenol induced histological skin changes: hazards, techniques, and uses. *Br J Plast Surg*. 1960;13:158.

9. Baker TJ. Chemical face peeling and rhytidectomy: a combined approach for facial rejuvenation. *Plast Reconstr Surg Transpl Bull*. 1962;29:199–207.

10. Böhm R, Flaschenträger B. Über den giftstoff im krotonöl. *Naunyn Schmiedebergs Arch Exp Pathol Pharmakol*. 1930;157:115–116. https://doi.org/10.1007/BF01972119.

11. Hutchinson R. Croton oil. *Bost Med Surg J*. 1833;8:411–414. https://doi.org/10.1056/NEJM183308070082602.

12. Newton AC. Protein kinase c: structural and spatial regulation by phosphorylation, cofactors, and macromolecular interactions. *Chem Rev*. 2001;101:2353–2364. https://doi.org/10.1021/cr0002801.

13. Bertolini TM. Is the phenol-croton oil peel safe? *Plast Reconstr Surg*. 2002;110:715–717.

14. Polliack A. 12-0-Tetradecanoyl phorbol-13-acetate (TPA) and Its effect on leukaemic cells, in-vitro—a review. *Leuk Lymphoma*. 1990;3:173–182. https://doi.org/10.3109/10428199009050993 10.3109/10428199009050993.

15. Totterman TH, Nilsson K, Sundstrom C. Phorbol ester-induced differentiation of chronic lymphocytic leukaemia cells. *Nature*. 1980;288:176–178.

16. Baker TJ. Is the phenol-croton oil peel safe? *Plast Reconstr Surg*. 2003;112:353–354. https://doi.org/10.1097/01.PRS.0000067107.16672.04.

17. Kligman AM, Baker TJ, Gordon HL. long-term histologic follow-up of phenol face peels. *Plast Reconstr Surg*. 1985;75:652–659. https://doi.org/10.1097/00006534-198505000-00006.

18. Pyun S-H, Shim I-S, Ahn G-B. Xeroderma pigmentosum treated with advanced phenol-based peeling solution. *J Eur Acad Dermatol Venereol*. 2008;22:879–880. https://doi.org/10.1111/j.1468-3083.2007.02476.x.

19. Wambier Carlos Gustavo, Lee KC, Bertolini TM, Rullan PP, Beltrame FL. About "anti-aging effects of ingenol mebutate for patients with actinic keratosis" and phenol-croton oil peelings. *J Am Acad Dermatol*. 2019. https://doi.org/10.1016/j.jaad.2019.01.065.

20. Wambier Carlos G, Neitzke IC, Lee KC, Soon SL, Rullan PP, Landau M, et al. Augmentation and eversion of lips without injections: the lip peel. *J Am Acad Dermatol*. 2019;80:e119–120. https://doi.org/10.1016/j.jaad.2018.06.030.

21. Wambier CG, Pires F. Combining phenol-croton peeling. In: Issa MC, Tamura BM, eds. *Chemical Physical Proced. Clinical Approach Procedure Cosmetic Dermatology* (Vol 1). 1st ed., London: Springer; 2017.

22. Stegman SJ. A comparative histologic study of the effects of three peeling agents and dermabrasion on normal and sundamaged skin. *Aesthetic Plast Surg*. 1982;6:123–135. https://doi.org/10.1007/BF01570631.

23. Lee KC, Sterling JB, Wambier CG, Soon SL, Landau M, Rullan P, et al. Segmental phenol-croton oil chemical peels for treatment of periorbital or perioral rhytides. *J Am Acad Dermatol*. 2018. https://doi.org/10.1016/j.jaad.2018.11.044.

24. Wambier Carlos G, Korgavkar K, Beltrame FL, Lee KC. Response to "clinical and histologic evaluation of ingenol mebutate 0.015% gel for the cosmetic improvement of photoaged skin". *Dermatol Surg*. 2019;45(6):857–859. https://doi.org/10.1097/DSS.0000000000001948.

25. Wambier CG, Wambier SP de F, Pilatti LEP, Grabicoski JA, Wambier LF, Schmidt A. Prolongation of rate-corrected QT interval during phenol-croton oil peels. *J Am Acad Dermatol*. 2018;78(4):810–812. https://doi.org/10.1016/j.jaad.2017.09.068.

26. Parada MB, Yarak S, Gouvêa LG, Hassun KM, Talarico S, Bagatin E. "Blepharopeeling" in the upper eyelids: a nonincisional procedure in periorbital rejuvenation--a pilot study. *Dermatol Surg*. 2008;34:1435–1438. https://doi.org/10.1111/j.1524-4725.2008.34304.x.

27. Mehta HK. A new use of K-Y jelly as a gonioscopy fluid. *Br J Ophthalmol*. 1984;68:765–767.

28. Tabor E. Corneal damage due to eye contact with chlorhexidine gluconate. *JAMA J Am Med Assoc*. 1989;261:557. https://doi.org/10.1001/jama.1989.03420040091021.

29. Geffen N, Norman G, Kheradiya NS, Assia EI. Chlorhexidine gluconate 0.02% as adjunct to primary treatment for corneal bacterial ulcers. *Isr Med Assoc J*. 2009;11:664–668.

16

Skin Resurfacing Complications

Suzan Obagi

INTRODUCTION

Considering that skin resurfacing is, for the most part, an elective procedure, the tolerance for complications is very low on the part of the patient. For the physician, resurfacing the skin involves creating a controlled injury to the skin surface followed by the natural healing process of the skin. The recovery period for a medium-depth to deep peel can range from 7 to 14 days. Any adverse event during the healing process can push this time out even further and may take a large emotional toll on the patient. Unlike other cosmetic procedures where the healing process is hidden under the skin surface, during skin resurfacing, the healing process is visible to the patient, family, and the physician. Thus any complication is also highly visible and disturbing to the patient.

One must remember that the role of skin is to serve as a physiological barrier to prevent fluid loss and to protect the human body from exposure to trauma, ultraviolet radiation, infections, and toxins. Other major functions of the skin include sensory perception, immune recognition, and thermoregulation. The skin is composed of two layers, epidermis and dermis, that overlie the subcutaneous fat. The epidermis is about 50 µm in thickness and consists of three major resident cells, keratinocytes, Langerhans cells, and melanocytes. The main substance of the dermis contains collagen, elastin, and glycosaminoglycans along with vascular structures and nerve endings and provides circulation, nutrition, and structural support for the epidermis. Fibroblasts, macrophages, and dendritic cells are the main resident cells in the dermis. Fibroblasts produce the collagen, elastin, and glycosaminoglycans that constitute the

dermal matrix. Adnexal structures include eccrine glands, apocrine glands, sebaceous glands, and hair follicles. It is these adnexal structures that help to reepithelialize the skin after skin resurfacing.

COMPLICATIONS

Early recognition and management of complications is key. Regardless of the type of resurfacing modality, whether peels or lasers, many of the post-resurfacing complications are the same (Table 16.1).

Swelling

Skin-resurfacing procedures that generate a lot of heat or that penetrate to the papillary dermis or reticular dermis level will result in a variable amount of swelling that differs among patients. Typically, swelling begins the night of or the day after the procedure, peaks at 48 hours, and then begins to resolve starting at 72 hours (Fig. 16.1). Management of swelling is by having the patient apply "crushed-ice" bags or frozen peas in small plastic bags to the cheeks and periorbital areas 10 minutes an hour for the first 48 hours. Sleeping with the head elevated to at least 45 degrees helps reduce swelling. Finally, if swelling is severe and the patient's eyes are swollen almost shut, an oral steroid taper can be given as long as the patient has no contraindications to systemic steroid therapy.

Contact Dermatitis

Contact dermatitis, usually irritant in nature, is commonly seen after skin resurfacing because of an impaired epidermal barrier function. Patch testing is not generally helpful during the postoperative period, because time is of the essence in managing this issue. However, once healed, patch testing can be performed if desired. However, the dermatitis is rarely a true type IV delayed hypersensitivity reaction, because patch testing fails to reveal the allergens in most cases.

Presenting symptoms are often new-onset burning and itching of the skin along with increased redness. Healing regression and eczematous eruptions may also occur (Fig. 16.2). Patients can develop contact dermatitis at any time during the postoperative period. The denuded or deepithelialized skin allows for ingredients to easily penetrate through the skin, thus making

the skin more susceptible to topical irritants such as fragrances, propylene glycol, lanolin, and allergens in cleansers, moisturizes, and topical ointments. Patients should be instructed to adhere strictly to the postoperative products given to them to avoid self-prescribed topical "herbal" regimens or topical antibiotics (such as Neosporin [Johnson & Johnson, New Brunswick, NJ] or bacitracin) during the healing process.

If contact dermatitis is suspected, the patient should be instructed to stop all topical lotions and cleansers. Instead, the patient should wash the skin twice a day with plain water and apply a bland petrolatum ointment two to three times a day until healed. If the reaction is severe or the patient is very uncomfortable, a mid-potency topical steroid and oral antihistamines are helpful to alleviate pruritus and the cutaneous eruptions. If the patient has significant skin weeping, topical gauze dilute vinegar compresses (1 teaspoon white vinegar in 2 cups of water) can be applied for 5 to 10 minutes per hour. In severe cases, systemic steroids may be warranted to decrease the risks of postinflammatory hyperpigmentation (PIH) and scarring.

Infection

Denuded skin is a prime site for infection, because the skin barrier function is impaired. Early recognition and management of skin infections will help mitigate the risk of scarring. Postoperative infections can be yeast, viral, or bacterial. The timing of the onset of symptoms can be helpful (Table 16.2).

TABLE 16.1 Classification of Complications	
Temporary Complication	Potentially Permanent Complications
Swelling	Persistent erythema
Contact dermatitis	Scarring
Infection (viral, bacterial, fungal)	Texture change
Milia	Hypopigmentation
Acne flare/rosacea flare	Lines of demarcation
Postinflammatory hyperpigmentation	
Ocular injury	

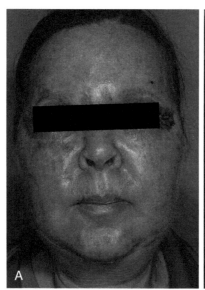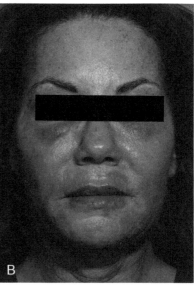

Fig. 16.1 A, Patient is postoperative day 2 following a blue peel, periorbital fractionated laser resurfacing, and an upper eyelift. B, Patient is postoperative day 3 following a blue peel, periorbital fractionated laser resurfacing, and a Hetter VL peel of the cutaneous upper lip.

Bacterial Infection

Rapid onset of discomfort, pruritic papules and pustules, focal areas of increased erythema, purulence, malodorous discharge, and crusting are signs of bacterial infection. *Staphylococcus aureus* (Fig. 16.3A) is the

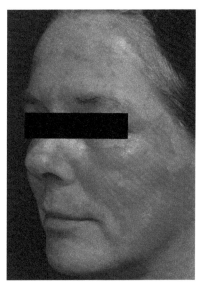

Fig. 16.2 Patient developed contact dermatitis to one of the postoperative products. Her symptoms were pruritus and healing regression manifesting on postoperative day 4 following a blue peel.

TABLE 16.2	Timeline of Skin Infection	
Infectious Agent	**Onset**	**Diagnosis**
Bacteria	Any time after 24 hours	Gram stain
		Culture and sensitivities
		Empiric coverage until culture and sensitivity results are in
		Adjust antibiotic if needed
Virus	Usually after 48 hours but can occur at any time until skin is fully reepithelialized up to postoperative days 7–14	Tzank prep PCR, DIF, or DFA Viral culture
Yeast	Usually after day 5	KOH prep

DFA, Direct fluorescent antibody assay; *DIF,* direct immunofluorescence; *KOH,* potassium hydroxide; *PCR,* polymerase chain reaction.

most commonly isolated species, but even *Pseudomonas aeruginosa* and *Serratia marcescens* (Fig. 16.3B) can occur. *S. marcescens* is a gram-negative anaerobic bacillus belonging to the Enterobacteriaceae family. However, if the wound is occluded for more than 48 hours or if prophylactic antibiotics are used, the incidence of a gram-negative infection, including *P. aeruginosa,* is significantly increased.

Any patient suspected to have an infection should have skin swabs sent for Gram stain as well as culture and sensitivity. An antibiotic can be prescribed to treat the suspected infection and then modified once the sensitivities are available. In the author's practice, bacterial skin infection post-resurfacing is almost nonexistent once patients were instructed to apply mupirocin ointment to the nares of the nose three times a day starting 1 week before their procedure and for 1 to 2 weeks afterward (until fully healed).

Minimizing the risk of infection is key. Therefore meticulous wound care with decreased duration of occlusion, frequent dressing changes, and thorough cleaning of the wound with 0.25% acetic acid solution are effective in reducing the bacterial colonization. The routine use of prophylactic antibiotics is controversial, although it is recommended in patients with increased risks of infections.

Viral Infection

A flare of herpes simplex virus (HSV) or an eruption of varicella zoster virus (VZV) during the recovery period can be disastrous. It is critical to recognize and treat the infection to prevent delayed wound healing, disseminated viral infection, secondary bacterial infection with *S. aureus,* and, most importantly, scarring. The nature of the infection with VZV and HSV viruses results in deep erosions that can heal with extensive scarring. Because the skin is deepithelialized, viral infection may only present as superficial erosions that spread and enlarge, as opposed to the classic vesiculopustules that appear on normal skin (Fig. 16.4A–B). Typically, the patient presents with new-onset healing regression and rapidly spreading erosions that do not necessarily start on the lips. These erosions are accompanied by pain and discomfort. Touching them and then touching other areas of open skin can transmit the virus to that region. Prior HSV infections can be subclinical; therefore all patients who plan to undergo full-face or perioral resurfacing should receive oral antiviral prophylaxis such as acyclovir, famciclovir,

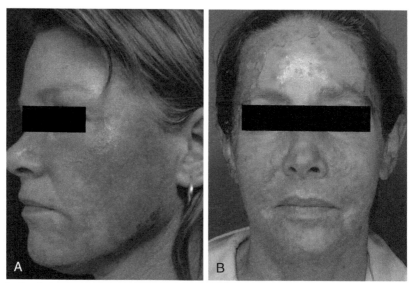

Fig. 16.3 A, *Staphylococcus aureus* infection manifesting as crusting, tenderness, and healing regression on postoperative day 4. B, *Serratia marcescens* manifesting as pruritic papules, tenderness, and healing regression on postoperative day 6.

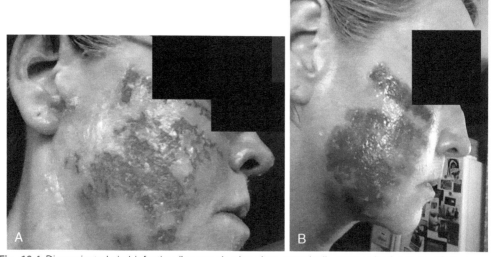

Fig. 16.4 Disseminated viral infection (herpes simplex virus or varicella zoster virus) can manifest aggressively as quickly spreading erosions and ulcerations with a high likelihood to scar if early intervention is missed. A, Patient at postoperative day 5 from a trichloroacetic acid blue peel of the face and a Hetter VL peel of the eyes. B, Same patient several weeks later still with erosions. In between, she developed a secondary *S. aureus* infection requiring oral antibiotics.

or valacyclovir. The prophylaxis should be initiated 1 to 2 days before the resurfacing and continued for 7 days (medium-depth peels or light laser resurfacing) to 15 days (dermabrasion, laser resurfacing, and deep peels) until reepithelialization of the skin is complete.

However, despite appropriate prophylactic antiviral therapy, some patients can still experience an outbreak while on a suppressive regimen. If an HSV or VZV infection is suspected, a viral culture or a swab for polymerase chain reaction (PCR) for VZV and HSV should be sent as soon as possible, and the dosing of antiviral therapy should be increased to the dose used to treat a zoster infection (i.e., valacyclovir 1000 mg three times a day for 10 days). Viral infections can sometimes yield a false negative if the lesion that is cultured is older than 48 hours. Therefore, even if the viral culture or PCR are negative, the course of antiviral therapy should be continued. I believe strongly that many viral infections are reactivated VZV rather than disseminated HSV. Both can then spread quickly to denuded areas; thus they may not appear as a typical viral infection would.

Yeast Infection

Candida albicans is the most common fungal/yeast species causing wound infections after skin resurfacing. Typically, around postoperative day 5 patients begin to develop regression of wound healing along with pruritic papules and pustules. An in-office potassium hydroxide (KOH) slide preparation should be performed if *Candida* infection is suspected. If an occlusive dressing was used, switching to an open wound care protocol will help. Furthermore, cleaning the wound with diluted acetic acid, topical antiyeast cream, and oral fluconazole can be used.

Other Infections

One must keep in mind that other unusual infections may also occur after skin resurfacing. Atypical mycobacterial infection with *Mycobacterium fortuitum* after full-face skin resurfacing with CO_2 laser has been reported. The patient developed nontender erythematous nodules that resolved after multiple incisions and drainage and a 4-week course of oral ciprofloxacin. Another case series cites two cases of mycobacterial infection following fractionated laser resurfacing. If a mycobacterial infection is suspected, one must specify this on the culture request so that the culture can be held long enough to grow these slow-growing organisms. Although atypical mycobacterial infection is a rare complication of skin resurfacing, it is important to keep it in the differential diagnosis when a patient does not respond to traditional wound care, antibiotics, or antifungal or antiviral therapies.

Milia

The development of multiple small keratin-retention cysts, milia, usually occurs between 3 and 8 weeks after ablative skin resurfacing and is often related to the depth of wounding. In most cases, milia resolve spontaneously as the skin continues to reepithelialize. Topical application of retinoic acid, alpha- or poly-hydroxy acid

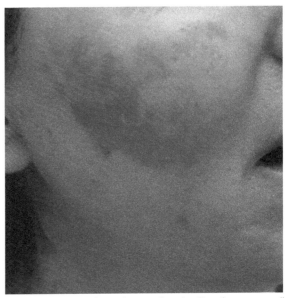

Fig. 16.5 Prolonged erythema after healing from a medium-depth trichloroacetic acid peel. Healing was complicated by overly icing the skin (frostbite).

creams, and manual extraction are also helpful modalities to facilitate the resolution of milia.

Acne and Rosacea Flare

Postoperative acne and rosacea flares are relatively common after skin resurfacing. Patients whose acne and rosacea are not well controlled before skin resurfacing are more prone to flares after the procedure. Proper topical regimens in combination with oral antibiotics such as tetracycline and doxycycline should be used to curtail the flare before any scarring occurs. Rarely, a more aggressive systemic agent, such as isotretinoin, is required to control a significant flare-up.

Prolonged Erythema

Postoperative erythema is an expected consequence of skin resurfacing. However, prolonged erythema (more than 3 weeks postoperatively) can be a challenging complication (Fig. 16.5) because it may be a harbinger of an impending scar or it may just be the natural course of a deep skin resurfacing (with laser resurfacing or phenol peels). When it lasts for more than 3 months, it can be very frustrating to both patients and physicians. Although prolonged erythema can occur with any skin resurfacing modality, it appears to occur more often with ablative laser resurfacing and deep chemical peels. It is more likely to occur in areas that had delayed wound healing or in areas resurfaced to the level of the reticular dermis. The exact mechanism of prolonged erythema is uncertain but may be associated with resurfacing-induced inflammatory response, reduced absorption of light by melanin, and decreased optical scattering in the dermis.

Treatment of prolonged erythema should not be started until the skin has healed fully. Topical therapy consists of conservative use of retinoic acid or retinaldehyde to normalize cell turnover and collagen production, ascorbic acid to mitigate erythema, a mineral sunscreen for daily protection, and judicious use of a mid-potency topical steroid 2 days a week (i.e., 0.1% triamcinolone cream). The role of topical corticosteroids in the treatment of postoperative erythema is controversial. Some studies indicate that postoperative use of topical corticosteroids appeared to be a cause of prolonged erythema and telangiectasias because of the effects of vasoconstriction and vasodilation through a nonintact barrier.

However, if the area of erythema is very "angry" or is showing textural changes (fibrosis, thickening), it could be a sign of impending scarring. In this instance, the topical application of ultrapotent class I steroids (i.e., 0.05% clobetasol cream or ointment) to the area 2 days a week for several weeks can be used to prevent scar formation. These patients require close monitoring to ensure improvement or to intervene with laser treatment or intralesional steroid injections if no improvement is seen. Pulsed dye lasers (PDL) are indispensable tools in the treatment of postresurfacing erythema by targeting the redness, aberrant telangiectasias, and to help with collagen remodeling. Treatment with PDL can be performed using nonpurpuric energy settings at 2 to 4 week intervals until the erythema subsides (Fig. 16.6).

Scarring

To achieve "tightening" of the skin, skin resurfacing must reach the level of the papillary dermis. At this level, it will strengthen the anchoring fibrils that span the epidermis to dermis, thus tightening the skin. On the other hand, to level the skin, as one would for deep wrinkles or deep scars, the wound depth must approach the upper to midreticular dermis. Thus skin laxity is addressed with "tightening" levels of skin resurfacing, whereas certain acne scars and deeper rhytides require a "leveling" depth of wounding.

The trade-off with leveling types of procedures is the significant risk of permanent pigmentary change, textural change, and scarring that goes with it. Therefore it is essential to control the depth of the wounding to obtain the maximal desired clinical effects with minimal complications. One of the most devastating and serious complications of skin resurfacing is scarring.

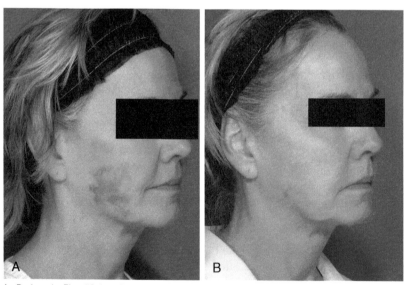

Fig. 16.6 A, Patient in Fig. 16.4 at 1 year postoperatively with overall healing but still with persistent erythema. During this time she was seen weekly for pulsed dye laser, when indicated, intralesional steroids, and proper skincare. B, Patient is shown 4 years later fully healed with only one small area (8 mm) of hypertrophic scarring at the jawline.

Scarring can take the form of reticulate atrophy or can be hypertrophic or keloidal in appearance (Fig. 16.7). Scars often develop in areas of pruritus, infection (especially viral), prolonged erythema, or delayed wound healing. Patients at increased risk for scarring are those with a tendency to develop keloids, a history of radiation therapy to the treated area, and perioperative isotretinoin use within 3 months of a reticular dermis–level peel. Furthermore, certain anatomic areas such as the thin skin of the neck, perioral, and periorbital regions, or areas over bony projections such as the chin, mandibular border, and malar areas are more prone to scar formation.

Mitigation of the scarring hinges on early detection and intervention (Fig. 16.8). Areas of delayed wound healing should be treated with low-level lasers (low-fluence Nd:YAG laser, low-fluence alexandrite laser, low-fluence broadband light) or sub-purpuric PDL weekly to encourage wound healing. Areas that are healed but have become indurated/thickened or are very red should be treated with low-level laser or PDL in addition to the topical application of ultrapotent class I corticosteroids (two times a week) and silicone gel sheeting daily.

Alternatively, the hypertrophic or keloidal scars can be treated with intralesional steroids with or without intralesional 5% 5-fluorouracil. The combination of intralesional triamcinolone acetonide and 5-fluorouracil has shown favorable results in the treatment of hypertrophic scars and keloids with less risk of atrophy and telangiectasias. The concentration of triamcinolone acetonide used (ranging from 1–10 mg/mL) and the injection interval

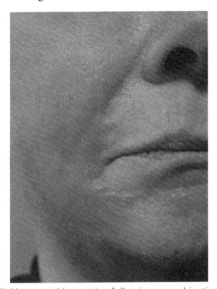

Fig. 16.7 Hypertrophic scarring following a combination trichloroacetic acid peel (face) and dermabrasion (perioral). No operative report was available to determine the order of procedures, but either the dermabrasion was too deep or the peel got onto the dermabraded skin and penetrated deeply.

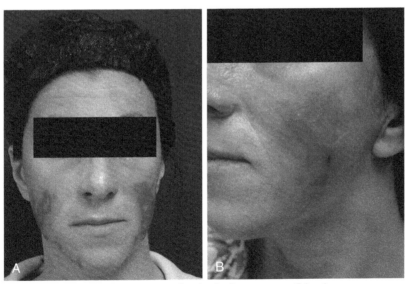

Fig. 16.8 A, Healing regression seen at postoperative day 9 after an uneventful early recovery process. B, Same patient at postoperative day 13 showing improvement with low-level laser, bland topical emollient, and conservative topical steroid use. This patient went on to a full recovery but required weekly visits until the skin had fully healed.

(every 2–4 weeks) are based on the scar thickness. Thicker scars require more frequent injections at a higher concentration, whereas thinner scars require lower concentrations. Rarely should the concentration of triamcinolone acetonide exceed 10 mg/mL.

Delayed Wound Healing

Rarely, cases of wound healing regression have been reported with no underlying identifiable causes. Several case reports and one case series describe patients with actinic damage who underwent uneventful laser or chemical peel skin resurfacing that developed healing regression, erosions, or pustules with no identifiable viral, bacterial, or fungal/yeast etiology. Skin biopsies were nonspecific. Lacking any other identifiable etiology, patients were given a diagnosis of facial erosive pustular dermatosis, a very recalcitrant and hard to-treat condition. Treatment included long-term minocycline, isotretinoin, systemic steroids, or dapsone.

Pigmentary Alteration

Hyperpigmentation

PIH can occur as the skin heals following medium-depth and deep skin resurfacing in susceptible patients. PIH can even occur with light peels if a patient with darker skin does not start a proper preconditioning regimen (see Chapter 3) before starting the light peels. Although typically not permanent, PIH can be distressing to the patient and can take away from the overall success of the procedure. The severity and longevity of PIH usually correlates with wound depth. It can occur in about one-third of patients postoperatively regardless of their skin type. In Caucasian patients, those with darker skin tones (brunettes) are more at risk for PIH compared with more fair-complexion patients. However in Asian skin or Black skin, patients with lighter skin tones are more prone to PIH. A red flag is a darker-skinned individual who presents with freckling, melasma, or other dyschromia at baseline. This shows that their pigment cells are more unstable or reactive. Darker-skinned patients with uniform skin color or a lack of freckling are less likely to develop PIH. Tanned skin also puts the patient at increased risk for PIH, because their melanocytes are already stimulated. Although most PIH is transient, it is usually noticeable, and the majority of patients would like to speed up its resolution (Fig. 16.9).

The regular use of broad-spectrum sunscreens for at least 6 to 8 weeks before the resurfacing procedure

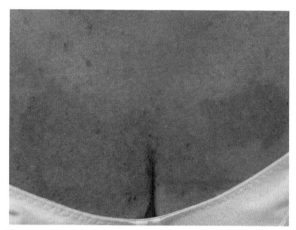

Fig. 16.9 Postinflammatory hyperpigmentation following a trichloroacetic acid peel of the chest. This resolved with topical retinoic acid, 4% hydroquinone, sunscreen, and several 30% salicylic acid peels.

and postoperatively are critical to prevent ultraviolet light–induced melanin synthesis and thus to achieve and maintain the optimal result of resurfacing. Topical bleaching agents such as hydroquinone (gold standard), Kojic acid, retinoic acid, azelaic acid, ascorbic acid, glycolic acid, and physical sunblock are first-line treatments for PIH. A typical regimen would include twice daily 4% hydroquinone to the whole face and extra to the browner areas, 6% glycolic acid lotion or 8% polyhydroxy acid lotion in the morning, 50 SPF mineral sunscreen daily, and 0.5% retinoic acid or 0.1% retinaldehyde in the evenings.

In recalcitrant cases, superficial light chemical peels with 30% salicylic acid biweekly can hasten the resolution of hyperpigmentation. Before tackling PIH, once must ensure that the skin has fully healed. Starting a topical treatment regimen before reepithelialization of the skin can further aggregate the severity of PIH.

Reducing the risk of PIH is crucial before performing a skin resurfacing procedure. The proper use of a skin-conditioning program both before and after resurfacing greatly reduces the risk of PIH (see Chapters 2 and 3). The duration of the preconditioning program is adjusted to the patient's skin type and their risk of PIH. Therefore patients deemed to be at risk for PIH should be preconditioned for 3 months rather than the standard 6 weeks. Likewise, the duration of the postconditioning program should be prolonged in patients prone to PIH.

Hypopigmentation

Hypopigmentation is an uncommon late complication of deep skin resurfacing that usually becomes apparent 6 to 12 months after the procedure once the initial erythema and PIH subside. Once the depth of resurfacing reaches the reticular dermis, permanent hypopigmentation can occur. However, true hypopigmentation is rare with most medium-depth procedures. Skin lightening in post–medium-depth peels is most likely pseudo-hypopigmentation. Pseudo-hypopigmentation appears as a lighter skin color in the newly resurfaced skin compared with the surrounding skin because of its healthier state (lack of photodamaged) compared with the adjacent photodamaged skin (Fig. 16.10). The newly resurfaced skin is simply skin color that is back to the patient's baseline skin color. It can also be seen temporarily in darker-skinned patients until their pigment fully returns. To minimize this contrast and minimize lines of demarcation, one should consider using topical agents or lighter peels to blend in the skin adjacent to the treated area.

When multiple facial areas need to be resurfaced, treating the entire face instead of individual areas might be a better option to avoid lines of demarcation. Alternatively, one can choose variable-level resurfacing procedures to address areas with the most prominent scars or rhytides more deeply while areas that are not quite as damaged can be resurfaced in a lighter manner so that all the areas blend together nicely after healing is complete.

Ocular Injury

Getting the peeling solution into the eye can cause corneal damage and be very uncomfortable for the patient, may require an ophthalmology consultation, and will add to the discomfort during the postoperative days. Sedated patients sometimes will manifest with lag ophthalmos and be at risk of solution getting into their eyes. Because they are sedated, they will not be able to vocalize that the peel solution has gotten into their eyes (Fig. 16.11). Therefore extreme caution and constant vigilance is needed while performing a peel on a sedated patient. All physicians should adhere to the following measure to reduce the risk of ocular injury (Table 16.3): Acid should never be passed over the patient's eyes to avoid accidental dripping into the eyes. Furthermore, if peeling the eyelids, a slightly moist cotton-tipped

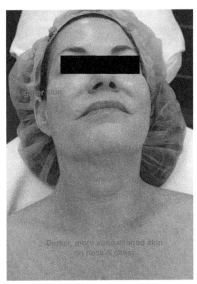

Fig. 16.10 Pseudo-hypopigmentation. This patient has had many medium-depth peels and laser resurfacing over 15 years for her facial skin. She protects her face extremely well from the sun, but comparing her face to the neck and chest (which is tan on examination) makes the skin on the face look even lighter.

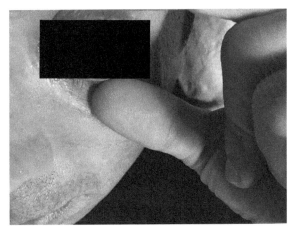

Fig. 16.11 Ocular injury following trichloroacetic acid peel of the face and eyes. A linear band of coagulated protein (frosting) is seen across the globe where the acid trickled into the eye during the procedure. (Photo courtesy Dr. Joe Niamtu.)

applicator should be used and the physician should control the position of the eyelid during the application of the peel (Fig. 16.12). During the course of applying the peel to the eyes, do not allow the cooling units or fans to blow the acid toward the lid margins.

TABLE 16.3 Reducing the Risk of Ocular Injury During Peels	
Measures for Prevention	**Management of Acid into the Eye**
Keep a tissue in your nondominant hand to constantly blot excess acid from the skin	Nonphenol solutions—flush the eye with copious amounts of saline or water
	Phenol solutions—flush the eye with mineral oil
Make sure fans and cooling devices are turned down or off while the eyelid skin is being peeled to reduce the risk of the acid being "blown" into the eye	Ophthalmology consultation if phenol or a strong TCA solution was used
Never pass the acid-soaked gauze or sponge across or over the eyes	Ophthalmology lubricants two to three times a day until healed
Keep the gauze or sponge on the drier side, and make sure there is no acid on your fingertips that might accidentally drip onto the eyelids	
Remove all contact lenses or corneal eye shields before performing a peel	

TCA, Trichloroacetic acid.

A delayed ocular risk is scleral show and exposure keratitis if the lower eyelid overly retracts during the healing process. Patients at risk for this are those with lower lid laxity or preexisting scleral show or prior upper and lower eyelid surgery. Preoperatively, this can be assessed by retracting the lower lid inferiorly and holding it down for 5 seconds; if it takes more than 2 seconds for the lid margin to pull back up to the globe, tightening the lateral canthus is indicated before deep skin resurfacing periorbitally. If, during the healing process, the physician begins to notice lower eyelid retraction, ectropion, or scleral show, the patient should be instructed to perform firm eyelid massage and pull the skin in an upward and cephalic-lateral direction to slowly stretch the skin as it is healing. This may need to be continued for 4 to 6 weeks while the healing process is ongoing.

Last, a disturbing permanent complication with lower eyelid resurfacing is the folding of the lower eyelid upon itself during the healing process and creating a permanent fold along the lower eyelid. Keeping an eye on the healing skin and gently pulling it apart with two cotton-tipped applicators can help spread apart a fold as it is forming.

Uneven Peel Penetration

Early on as one learns to perform peels, they may find that they are getting variable depths of penetration with the peel solutions. The main reason could be "hot spots" (Fig. 16.13) where there is a collection of acid sitting on the skin. The acid will keep penetrating into the skin in these spots. The key to even acid penetration is to prepare the skin so that the stratum corneum is smooth and compact; the acid should be applied in firm even strokes without leaving "hot spots," and care should be taken to wait long enough between passes to see the extent of frosting and to see where more solution is needed. If laser resurfacing is being performed the same day, the peel should be performed first and the skin cleansed of residual acid. Otherwise, if the laser is performed first, the peel can trickle into the open wound and penetrate very deeply.

Complications From Deep Phenol Peels
Cardiac Arrhythmias

Phenol is absorbed through skin, subsequently metabolized by the liver, and excreted by the kidneys. Patients who have impaired liver or kidney functions are more susceptible to the toxicity of phenol. In addition, the extent of cutaneous absorption of phenol is associated with the total area of exposed skin rather than the concentration of the phenol used. Cardiac arrhythmias including tachycardia, premature ventricular contractions, bigeminy, paroxysmal atrial tachycardia, ventricular tachycardia, and atrial fibrillation can be seen in phenol-based peels with rapid application in the full-face treatment. Therefore it is important to use cardiac monitoring during the resurfacing procedure and in the recovery period, allowing for immediate detection of potential cardiac complications. Hydrating the patient with intravenous fluids just before and during the peel further reduces the cardiac risk. Probably the most

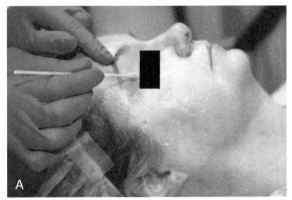
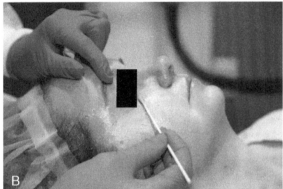

Fig. 16.12 Proper technique for peeling eyelids. A, Upper eyelid: Hold the brow up and approach the eye either from the side or from the cephalad region to avoid having to cross the opening of the eye. The cotton-tipped applicator should be moist but not dripping. The physician should have tissue in his/her non-dominant hand to blot any drips. B, Lower eyelid: Similar technique with holding the brow taut enough to pull the upper eyelid up a little to help expose the entire lower eyelid region. Approach the eye from the side or from the caudal direction to avoid crossing the opening of the eye.

important manner in which to reduce cardiac risk is by treating the face in small cosmetic units with a 15 to 20 minute pause before moving on to the next area. This allows a total of 90 to 120 minutes for the whole face procedure, thus allowing for ongoing metabolism of the phenol when treating the entire face. Other important points made by authors in this textbook (see Chapters 7 and 8) is keeping the patient comfortable to reduce any adrenergic surge and to avoid the use of epinephrine in any local anesthetics or nerve blocks.

Laryngeal Edema

Laryngeal edema is an uncommon complication in patients undergoing phenol peels. There is one case

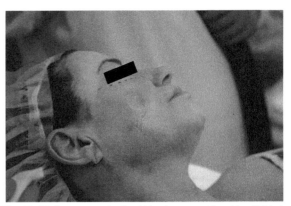

Fig. 16.13 A wet streak of acid is shown on the skin. If this is not quickly blotted, it will penetrate more deeply in this area and create a "hot spot."

series of three patients (all heavy smokers) developing laryngeal edema along with stridor, hoarseness, and tachypnea within 24 hours after phenol peeling that resolved within another 24 hours after heated mist inhalation therapy. The hypothesis is that this was an additive effect of irritation to the larynx by ether fumes and cigarette smoke or a hypersensitivity reaction to phenol.

CONCLUSION

Chemical skin resurfacing is a very gratifying procedure that yields amazing rejuvenative results. However, as beautiful as the ultimate outcome may be, any scarring or prolonged erythema or dyschromia can detract from the end result and require a lot of hand holding on the part of the physician. The best way to reduce the likelihood of long-term sequelae from resurfacing procedures is to correctly identify and manage these issues as they arise. Having the patient come in frequently during the first 1 to 2 weeks and having them call to notify the physician of any changes during the recovery period is essential.

FURTHER READING

Alam M, Pantanowitz L, Harton AM, Arndt KA, Dover JS. A prospective trial of fungal colonization after laser resurfacing of the face: correlation between culture positivity and symptoms of pruritus. *Dermatol Surg.* 2003;29(3):255–260.

Alster TS, Lupton JR. Prevention and treatment of side effects and complications of cutaneous laser resurfacing. *Plast Reconstr Surg.* 2002;109(1):308–316; discussion 317-8.

Alster TS, Nanni CA. Famciclovir prophylaxis of herpes simplex virus reactivation after laser skin resurfacing. *Dermatol Surg.* 1999;25(3):242–246.

Alster TS, Williams CM. Treatment of keloid sternotomy scars with 585 nm flashlamp-pumped pulsed-dye laser. *Lancet.* 1995;345:1198–1200.

Beeson WH, Rachel JD. Valacyclovir prophylaxis for herpes simplex virus infection or infection recurrence following laser skin resurfacing. *Dermatol Surg.* 2002;28(4):331–336.

Beeson WH. The importance of cardiac monitoring in superficial and deep chemical peeling. *J Dermatol Surg Oncol.* 1987;13(9):949–950.

Bernstein LJ, Kauvar AN, Grossman MC, Geronemus RG. The short- and long-term side effects of carbon dioxide laser resurfacing. *Dermatol Surg.* 1997;23(7):519–525.

Botta SA, Straith RE, Goodwin HH. Cardiac arrhythmias in phenol face peeling: a suggested protocol for prevention. *Aesthetic Plast Surg.* 1988;12(2):115–117.

Brody HJ. Complications of chemical resurfacing. *Dermatol Clin.* 2001;19(3):427–438, vii–viii.

Costa IMC, Damasceno PS, Costa MC, Gomes KGP. Review in peeling complications. *J Cosmet Dermatol.* 2017;16(3):319–326.

Culton DA, Lachiewicz AM, Miller BA, et al. Nontuberculous mycobacterial infection after fractionated CO_2 laser resurfacing. *Emerg Infect Dis.* 2013;19(3):365–370.

Dan Li, Lin Shi-Bin, Cheng Biao. Complications and posttreatment care following invasive laser skin resurfacing: a review. *J Cosmet Laser Ther.* 2018;20(3):168–178. https://doi.org/10.1080/14764172.2017.1400166. Epub 2017 Dec 13.

Demas PN, Bridenstine JB. Diagnosis and treatment of postoperative complications after skin resurfacing. *J Oral Maxillofac Surg.* 1999;57(7):837–841.

Gross BG. Cardiac arrhythmias during phenol face peeling. *Plast Reconstr Surg.* 1984;73(4):590–594.

Khetarpal S, Kaw U, Dover JS, Arndt KA. Laser advances in the treatment of burn and traumatic scars. *Semin Cutan Med Surg.* 2017;36(4):185–191. https://doi.org/10.12788/j.sder.2017.030.

Klein DR, Little JH. Laryngeal edema as a complication of chemical peel. *Plast Reconstr Surg.* 1983;71(3):419–420.

Landau M. Cardiac complications in deep chemical peels. *Dermatol Surg.* 2007;33(2):190–193; discussion 193.

Lowe NJ, Lask G, Griffin ME. Laser skin resurfacing. Pre- and posttreatment guidelines. *Dermatol Surg.* 1995;21:1017–1019.

Mervak JE, Gan SD, Smith EH, Wang F. Facial erosive pustular dermatosis after cosmetic resurfacing. *JAMA Dermatol.* 2017;153(10):1021–1025.

Nanni CA, Alster TS. Complications of carbon dioxide laser resurfacing. An evaluation of 500 patients. *Dermatol Surg.* 1998;24:315–320.

Nikalji N, Godse K, Sakhiya J, Patil S, Nadkarni N. Complications of medium depth and deep chemical peels. *J Cutan Aesthet Surg.* 2012;5:254–260.

Ozturk MB, Ozkaya O, Karahangil M, Cekic O, Oreroğlu AR, Akan IM. Ocular complication after trichloroacetic acid peeling: a case report. *Aesthetic Plast Surg.* 2013;37(1):56–59.

Rao J, Golden TA, Fitzpatrick RE. Atypical mycobacterial infection following blepharoplasty and full-face skin resurfacing with CO_2 laser. *Dermatol Surg.* 2002;28(8):768–771; discussion 771.

Rapaport MJ, Rapaport V. Prolonged erythema after facial laser resurfacing or phenol peel secondary to corticosteroid addiction. *Dermatol Surg.* 1999;25(10):781–784; discussion 785.

Sriprachya-Anunt S, Fitzpatrick RE, Goldman MP, Smith SR. Infections complicating pulsed carbon dioxide laser resurfacing for photoaged facial skin. *Dermatol Surg.* 1997;23:527–535; discussion 535-526.

Truppman ES, Ellenby JD. Major electrocardiographic changes during chemical face peeling. *Plast Reconstr Surg.* 1979;63:44–48.

van Gemert MJ, Bloemen PR, Wang W, et al. Periocular CO_2 laser resurfacing: severe ocular complications from multiple unintentional laser impacts on the protective metal eye shields. *Lasers Surg. Med.* 2018;50:980–986. https://doi.org/10.1002/lsm.22951.

Walia S, Alster TS. Cutaneous CO_2 laser resurfacing infection rate with and without prophylactic antibiotics. *Dermatologic Surgery.* 1999;25(11):857–861. https://doi.org/10.1046/j.1524-4725.1999.99114.x.

Zhang AY, Obagi S. Diagnosis and management of skin resurfacing–related complications. *Oral Maxillofac Surg Clin North Am.* 2009;21(1):1–12. https://doi.org/10.1016/j.coms.2008.11.002.

Note: Page numbers followed by "f" indicate figures; "t" indicate tables, and "b" indicate boxes.